CLINICAL
WOUND
Management

CLINICAL WOUND Management

Prem P. Gogia, PhD, PT

Clinical Director
Rehabilitation Services
Park Plaza Hospital
Houston, TX

Adjunct Assistant Professor
Department of Physical Therapy
University of Texas Medical Branch
Galveston, TX

SLACK Incorporated, 6900 Grove Road, Thorofare, NJ 08086-9447

Note to the Reader

As new scientific information becomes available through basic and clinical research, recommended treatments and drug therapies undergo changes. The editor and publisher have done everything possible to make this book accurate, up-to-date, and in accord with accepted standards at the time of publication. The authors, editor, and publisher cannot accept responsibility for errors or exclusions or for the outcome of the application of material presented herein. There is no expressed or implied warranty of this book or information imparted by it. Any practice described in this book should be applied by the reader to the unique circumstances that may apply in each situation. The reader is advised to always review the provided product literature and use caution when using new or infrequently ordered drugs.

Any review or mention of specific companies or products is not intended as an endorsement by the author or by the publisher.

Acquisitions Editor: Amy E. Drummond
Publisher: John H. Bond
Production Editor: Debra L. Clarke
Associate Editor: Jennifer J. Dyer

Clinical wound management/[edited by] Prem P. Gogia.
p. cm.
Includes bibliographical references and index.
ISBN 1-55642-234-2
1. Wounds and injuries—Treatment. 2. Wound healing. I. Gogia, Prem P.
[DNLM: 1. Wounds and Injuries—therapy. 2. Physical Therapy. 3. Wound Healing. WB 460 C6417 1995]
RD93.C57 1995
617.1'406—dc20
DNLM/DLC
for Library of Congress

94-48426

Printed in the United States of America

Published by: SLACK Incorporated
                     6900 Grove Road
                     Thorofare, NJ 08086-9447

Last digit is print number: 10   9   8   7   6   5   4   3   2

Dedication

To my wife Suman and daughters Reena and Ruchi for love and support, and for their patience during the preparation of this manuscript.

Contents

Acknowledgments

I would like to thank each of the contributors for sharing their experience, knowledge, and judgment with the readers. Thanks to Fred Steinberg for the editorial assistance. Thanks to the staff at SLACK Inc. for their patience and support.

Prem P. Gogia, PhD, PT
Editor

Contributors

Saroj M. Bahl, PhD, RD, LD
Associate Professor, Program in Nutrition and Dietetics, School of Allied Health Sciences,
    University of Texas Health Science Center, Houston, Texas

Laura L. Bolton, PhD
Director, Scientific Affairs, ConvaTec Wound and Skin Care, Skillman, New Jersey

Marybeth Brown, PhD, PT
Assistant Professor, Department of Physical Therapy, Washington University School of
    Medicine, St. Louis, Missouri

Jan Cuzzell, MA, RN
Charles R. Baxter Wound Center, Dallas, Texas

Mary Dyson, PhD, CBiol, MIBiol
Director, Tissue Repair Lab, Guy's Hospital, London, England

Ann-Jeanette Fattu
Pre-Medical Student, State University of New Jersey
    New Jersey ConvaTec Research Intern, ConvaTec, a Division of Bristol-Myers Squibb,
    Princeton, New Jersey

Prem P. Gogia, PhD, PT
Clinical Director, Rehabilitation Services, Park Plaza Hospital, Houston, Texas
    Adjunct Assistant Professor, University of Texas Medical Branch, Galveston, Texas

Carole L. Johnson, PhD, PT
Assistant Director of Outpatient Rehabilitation, Providence Hospital, Seattle, Washington

Diane Krasner, MS, RN, CETN
ET Nurse Consultant, Doctoral Student, University of Maryland School of Nursing,
    Baltimore, Maryland

Robin Ryan Marquez, MS, PT
Clinical Education Associate, Texas Woman's University and Hermann Hospital,
    Houston, Texas

Mary Matwhich, RN, CCRN
Burn Unit Research Nurse, The New York Hospital and Cornell Medical Center, New
    York, New York

Gil Micheletti, MD
Dermatologist, Park Plaza Hospital, Houston, Texas

Michael J. Mueller, PhD, PT
Assistant Professor, Department of Physical Therapy, Washington University School of
    Medicine, St. Louis, Missouri

David R. Sinacore, PhD, PT
Assistant Professor, Department of Physical Therapy, Washington University School of
    Medicine, St. Louis, Missouri

Lia van Rijswijk, RN, ET
Nurse Consultant, Newtown, Pennsylvania
    RN-MSN Student, LaSalle University School of Nursing, Philadelphia, Pennsylvania

David J. Wainwright, MD, FRCS(C), FACS
Assistant Professor of Plastic Surgery, University of Texas Health Science Center,
    Houston, Texas

Foreword

Evaluating and treating patients with open wounds is a challenging part of health care. These clients typically have associated medical conditions, such as diabetes or peripheral vascular disease, that affect the process of wound healing. Sensory and/or motor function may be impaired as in patients with spinal or brain injuries. Clients often are elderly or have poor nutritional status. In addition, clients may not have the financial or social resources to follow through with home care for their wounds. The diverse nature of this group of clients requires the services of a multidisciplinary team of health care professionals. The contributing authors of this text are varied in professional education and clinical experience and provide expert information in each of their fields.

Evaluation is an integral part of the management of open wounds. Clinical measurements that are reliable and provide meaningful information are essential to accurately evaluate response to treatment. The evaluation should include not only the local area of involvement, but also characteristics that reflect the health and well-being of the individual. The desired treatment outcome for the patient is to return to the highest possible functional level. By sharing expertise in each of the disciplines, health care professionals can guide patients toward this goal. As with many medical conditions, there are multiple treatment options. This text reviews the many treatment modalities that are used to facilitate wound healing and provides current references on treatment effectiveness. The information can be used by clinicians to evaluate their current treatment programs and to guide changes that may improve patient outcomes. The literature will continue to grow in this area as research is published to support or refute the efficacy of each of the modalities. Treatment approaches then may need to be modified based on research findings.

This text provides a comprehensive review of the management of patients with open wounds, including pathophysiology, evaluation methods, and treatment options. Directions for clinical research, which is an essential area because of the need to establish both efficacy and cost-effectiveness of the various treatment modalities, are addressed. The text will serve as a resource for clinicians who strive to provide effective and efficient services.

Claire Peel, PhD, PT
Associate Professor and Chair
Department of Physical Therapy
University of Texas Medical Branch
Galveston, Texas

Preface

Management of wounds presents a great challenge to clinicians. A multitude of problems associated with wounds cause the clinician considerable frustration. Effective management of wounds requires a multidisciplinary team approach including physicians, nurses, dieticians, social workers, and physical therapists.

This book is written for students and health care practitioners practicing in a variety of specialties. Every effort is made to write this book as a clinical reference guide based on scientific research. This book provides a systemic approach to carry out wound assessment as well as appropriate treatment. This includes pressure and leg ulcers, nutrition, pharmacology, dressings, total contact casting, and a variety of modalities including electrical stimulation, ultrasound, oxygen therapy, and low-energy laser. An overview of surgical procedures is also presented.

The contributing authors share their knowledge in their field of expertise. Each chapter includes general introduction, literature review, and treatment procedures followed by excellent up-to-date references. Illustrations and tables are included as needed to enhance the clarity of the text. It is hoped that this book will assist students and practicing clinicians in improving treatment outcomes in wound management.

Prem P. Gogia, PhD, PT
Editor

Physiology of Wound Healing

Prem P. Gogia, PhD, PT

A clear, fundamental understanding of wound healing and the factors that adversely affect healing is important for effective evaluation and appropriate management of wounds. The purpose of this chapter is to describe anatomy and physiology of the skin, normal epidermal and dermal wound healing, and the factors affecting the healing process.

ANATOMY AND PHYSIOLOGY OF THE SKIN

The skin is the largest organ of the body. Being the major interphase between the body and its environment, the skin is adapted to serve many different functions. It is constantly engaged in biological and biochemical activities. The skin is composed of two distinct primary layers (Figure 1-1). The outer layer, the epidermis, is an epithelial layer. The inner layer, the dermis, is a connective tissue layer. The epidermis is attached to the dermis by a basement membrane. The area between the epidermis and the dermis has a ridge and groove interdigitation which prevents the shearing of epidermis from dermis with external stresses.

The epidermis is composed of several layers. The thin, outermost, horny layer of the epidermis, the stratum corneum, is composed of dead, keratinized cells. It is dry, waterproof, and rich in the protective protein keratin. The next layers of the epidermis (the stratum lucidum, stratum basale, stratum granulosum, and stratum germinativum) contain living cells. The epidermis is a protective covering that provides a barrier to injury, contaminants, and light. It also prevents dehydration of the underlying tissues, retains fluid and nutrients within the skin, and produces melanin, which is responsible for the color of the skin.

The dermis is composed primarily of collagen and elastin fibrous connective tissues. These fibers are interspersed within mucopolysaccharide matrix and provide strength and elasticity to the skin. The hair follicles, sebaceous glands, and sweat glands are contained in the dermis. A network of lymphatics, blood vessels, and cutaneous nerve endings serve the skin appendages. The dermis produces hair, regulates body temperature, houses sensory receptors, supplies nutrients and oxygen, and synthesizes various chemical substances.

Underneath the dermis are loose connective and fat tissues called the subcutaneous layer. It provides insulation, support, and cushion for the skin and other tissues to withstand stresses and pressures. It also stores energy for the skin. Beneath this layer, fascia and muscles lie to provide additional cushion over the bony structures.

EPIDERMAL WOUND HEALING

Epidermal wounds involve the epidermal layer and may also involve the superficial layer of the

Figure 1-1. Cross-section of the skin showing epidermis and dermis.

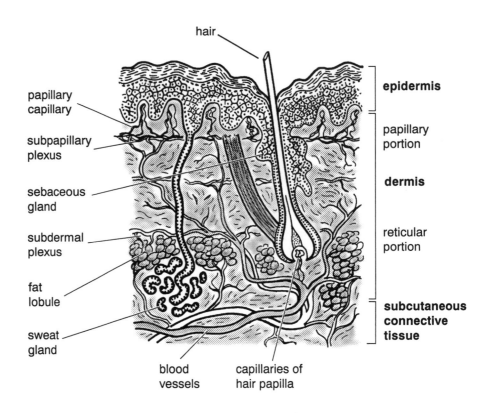

dermis. These wounds are called partial-thickness wounds. The wounds are initially covered by a crust which is formed by blood and debris particles. Epidermal wounds heal by regeneration. The process of regeneration is called re-epithelialization. The epithelial cells respond to injury within 24 to 48 hours. These cells detach from the basal layer, migrate toward the defect, and proliferate by mitosis. The new cells gradually thicken the epithelial layer. Once the healing is complete under the crust, the crust sloughs off. The proliferated cells then differentiate into mature epidermal cells and begin to keratinize. The epidermal wounds heal without any scar tissue and the duration of healing is relatively much shorter than the dermal wound healing.

DERMAL WOUND HEALING

Dermal wounds involve the complete epidermis, dermis, and subcutaneous tissues. They may also involve muscles and bone. These wounds are called full-thickness wounds. They heal by scar formation. The healing of dermal wounds is highly complex as compared to the epidermal wound healing.

The dermal wound healing process goes through three phases before complete healing occurs:
(1) inflammatory phase
(2) fibroplastic phase
(3) remodeling phase

The number of phases as well as the terms used to identify each phase varies with the author. The inflammatory phase prepares the wound for healing and cleans up the debris. The fibroplastic phase rebuilds the damaged structures and provides strength to the wound. Finally, the remodeling phase modifies the immature scar to a mature scar to fit the wound and provides the final form to the wound. These phases of normal wound healing are complex and highly organized. The phases of wound healing overlap each other and the end of one phase stimulates the beginning of the next phase. Figure 1-2 is a flow diagram of the phases of normal wound healing.

INFLAMMATORY PHASE

The inflammatory response is a natural reaction to any acute injury. The inflammation is prerequisite to the healing process. If there is no inflammation, the wound healing will not take place.[1] The acute inflammation phase usually lasts for 24 to 48 hours and is completed in 2 weeks followed by a subacute phase of approximately 2 weeks.[2]

The inflammation is a vascular and cellular response to dispose of bacteria, foreign material, and dead tissue. The initial stages of inflammation are characterized by vascular changes. Following the injury, the damaged blood and lymphatic vessels undergo vasoconstriction to slow or stop blood loss in the affected area. Norepinephrine secreted by blood vessels and serotonin secreted by platelets and mast cells are responsible for the vasoconstriction of the vessels. The vasoconstriction lasts for about 5 to 10 minutes.[3] Platelets play a key role. Besides secreting vasoconstrictive substances, the platelets also aggregate along the endothelium of the injured blood vessels and form platelet plugs to slow or stop blood loss.

Concurrent with the transient vasoconstriction, leukocytes begin to cluster together. The endothelial wall of the vessels becomes sticky and the leukocytes begin to adhere to the vessel wall. This process is called neutrophilic margination. Immediately following the vasoconstriction, the non-injured vessels dilate and the capillary permeability increases in response to chemicals released from the injured tissues. These chemical changes are due to the histamine released by the mast cells and the prostaglandin released by the injured cell membrane.[3] Vasodilation lasts for less than an hour. The histamine reaction is very short-lived, while the prostaglandin causes long-term permeability. Increased vessel permeability allows the plasma to leak into the wound area. Fibrin plugs arising from the escaped plasma block the lymphatic flow, seal off the wound, localize the inflammatory reaction, and prevent the spread of infection. At this stage, the area around the wound is red, hot, swollen, and painful.

Leukocytes, erythrocytes, and platelets adhere to the dilated endothelial walls of the blood vessels.

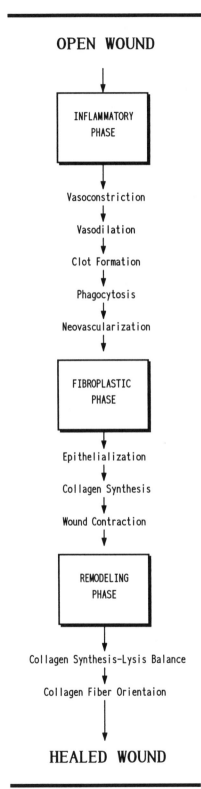

Figure 1-2. Flow diagram of normal wound healing.

Chemical changes in the wound induce and attract these cells to leak through the enlarged capillary pores and enter the wound area. The polymorphonuclear leukocytes are the first to migrate to the wound and engage in phagocytosis of debris and foreign substances. The main purpose of the phagocytosis is to prevent or rid infection. The leukocytes form pseudopods around debris particles, encircle them, and then enzymatically dissolve and digest the debris particles. As the polymorphonuclear leukocytes die, their intracellular enzymes and debris are released into the wound area and become part of the wound exudate or pus.

Next, monocytes, mononuclear leukocytes, emigrate from the capillary into the wound and are transformed into macrophages. The macrophages are the most important cells of the inflammatory stage that aid in phagocytosis. The macrophages ingest the material that has not been solubilized by the polymorphonuclear leukocytes. They also engulf leftover polymorphonuclear leukocytes. As the macrophages ingest microorganisms, they also excrete products of digestion, i.e., ascorbic acid, hydrogen peroxide, and lactic acid.[4] Hydrogen peroxide aids in controlling anaerobic microbial growth. Ascorbic acid and lactic acid signal the extent of damage.[5] As these acids accumulate at the wound site as by-products, more macrophages are produced for further phagocytosis. The accumulation of pus in the wound can impair wound healing. Clinically, wound cleansing results in a clean wound bed that helps to further the healing process.

As this phase comes to an end, fibrinolysin from blood vessels is produced to assist in dissolving the blood clots. The lymphatic channels then open to assist in reducing the wound edema. As mentioned earlier, inflammation is a vital part of wound repair. If too little inflammation occurs, the healing is slowed. If too much inflammation occurs, excessive scar is produced.[4] Therefore, it is important to control the factors which contribute to inflammation.

FIBROPLASTIC PHASE

This phase is also called proliferative phase. Once the wound is cleaned by the leukocytes through phagocytosis, the rebuilding of the damaged tissues continues. This phase continues until the wound is healed. The re-establishment of epidermis is initiated within hours after the injury occurs.[6] Epithelial repair goes through a sequence of mobilization, migration, proliferation, and differentiation. Mobilization begins when the epidermal cells flatten and develop actin filaments at the cytoplasmic edges of the cell. The epithelial cells migrate from the periphery into the wound area. The epithelial cells continue to proliferate and lay down the multiple layers of epithelium beneath the clot, and later, beneath the crust. The epithelial cells finally differentiate into their original cuboidal or rectangular shapes. Initially there is a thin, silvery, epithelial layer around the periphery of the wound. Gradually epithelialization covers the surface of the wound to close the epithelial defect. Epithelialization provides a protective barrier to prevent fluid and electrolyte loss from the wound and to reduce the chances of infection.

As the epithelium gradually undermines, the crust loosens and detaches from the wound leaving a thin, transparent covering over the skin. The crust is believed to be a temporary barrier for the wound and should not be disturbed until the epithelialization is completed. However, the crust impedes the rapid re-epithelialization; therefore, the wound should be kept moist.[7] Application of occlusive moist dressing helps minimize the crust formation. If the dressing is allowed to dry out, it will function as debridement when removed.

While the re-epithelialization is occurring, the wound contraction process is initiated. Wound contraction has been defined as the remodeling of the area of the wound by mobilization of the surrounding tissues. This decreases the size of the defect by a centripetal movement of the normal full-thickness skin.[8] It is believed that it is the forces exerted by the retraction of the granulation tissue which provoke the contraction of the wound. Contraction of wound margins begins 5 days after the wounding and peaks at 2 weeks.[7] If the wound is not closed by 2 to 3 weeks post-injury, the contraction stops. Wound contraction pulls the entire wound together resulting in a smaller wound to be repaired by scar formation.

Myofibroblast cells are the primary cells responsible for wound contraction. Fibroblast cells transform into myofibroblasts. These cells have the ability to extend and retract. The rate of contraction is proportional to the cell population at and under the wound margins, and inversely proportional to the lattice collagen contraction.[9]

Contraction proceeds at a fairly uniform rate of about 0.6 to 0.75 mm per day.[10] The size of the wound does not affect the rate of contraction,[10] whereas the shape of the wound has been reported to affect the contraction process.[11] Linear wounds contract rapidly, square or rectangular wounds contract at a moderate pace, and circular wounds contract slowly.

The myofibroblasts attach to the skin margins and pull the entire epidermal layer inward. Clinically, range of motion exercises control contraction.[12] Application of pressure and tension ameliorate contraction.[13] The ability of the wound to contract is limited if the surrounding skin is not mobile. If the contraction progresses, it may result in a debilitating deformity known as contractures. Smooth muscle relaxants have been suggested to prevent contractures.[14,15]

The healing of the surface wound by epithelial cells is not adequate for the integrity of the wound. The healing wound also needs to have strength to withstand mechanical stresses. The fibroplastic phase provides this strength. The primary cells responsible for the fibroplastic phase are the fibroblasts. Fibroblasts are produced from the undifferentiated mesenchymal cells that migrate into the wound. Lactic acid, ascorbic acid, and other cofactors present in the wound are responsible for stimulation of the fibroblasts to synthesize collagen tissue.

The integrity of the wound depends upon the collagen tissue which provides strength and stiffness to the wound. Fibroblasts synthesize three polypeptide chains which aggregate into a triple helix called procollagen. The procollagens are then secreted from the fibroblasts into the extracellular space where they undergo cleavage. They are then called tropocollagens, and they coil together with other tropocollagens to form collagen fibrils. Collagen fibrils are composed of bundles of collagen filaments, which further combine to form collagen fibers (Figure 1-3). The collagen molecules cross-link intramolecularly and intermolecularly to provide strength to the wound (Figure 1-4).

It is not the quantity of collagen tissue but the collagen cross-linking that provides the tensile strength to the wound.[16,17] However, only 80% of the original tensile strength of the skin is ever regained.[18] The fibroblasts also synthesize a viscous, gel-like ground substance called glycosaminoglycans (GAG) which occupies the spaces between the connective tissue fibers.[19] The GAG provides lubrication and density to the connective tissue. The number of fibroblasts in the wound diminishes as a sufficient quantity of collagen is produced. The disappearance of fibroblasts marks the end of the fibroplastic phase and the beginning of the maturation phase of wound healing.

Additional oxygen supply and nutrition to the injured tissues are essential for cell proliferation. This oxygen and nutritional requirement is provided by newly formed blood capillaries. Endothelial cells form buds at the end of the intact capillaries and grow into the wound area to join other buds to form a capillary network. This new capillary network fills the entire wound bed, and along with collagen tissue forms granulation tissue. It is the capillary network that gives healthy granulation tissue a bright red and granular appearance. This process is called angiogenesis or neovascularization. The granulation tissue at this stage is very delicate and therefore should be protected from any repetitive microtrauma or chemical irritation.

REMODELING PHASE

This phase is also called the maturation phase. After approximately 2 to 4 weeks, depending on the site and size of the wound, the remodeling phase begins. The scar formed during fibroplasia is an enlarged, dense structure of collagen fibers which are highly disorganized. During the remodeling phase, changes in the form, bulk, and strength of the scar occur.

Throughout the healing process, new collagen is produced while the old collagen breaks down. For

Figure 1-3. Collagen synthesis.

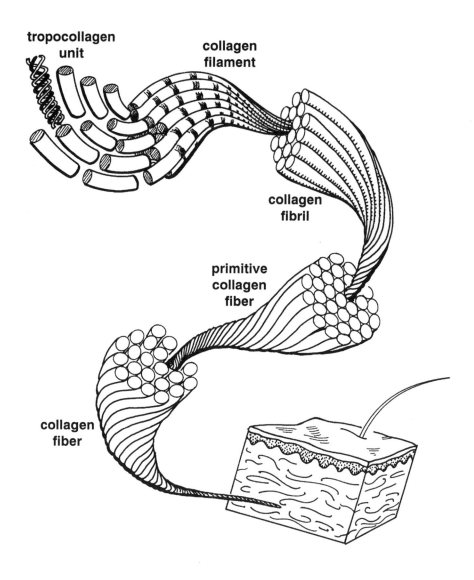

tropocollagen
unit

collagen
filament

collagen
fibril

primitive
collagen
fiber

collagen
fiber

normal scar formation, this synthesis and lysis occurs in a balanced fashion. However, if the rate of breakdown exceeds the rate of production, this results in a softer and less bulky scar; if the rate of production exceeds breakdown, this results in a hypertrophic scar or keloid.

Hypertrophic scar and keloid are due to overabundant collagen deposition. Keloid extends beyond the boundaries of the original wound and invades surrounding tissue, whereas hypertrophic scar, although raised, remains within the normal boundaries of the original wound and tends to abate gradually.[20] Clinically, the hypertrophic scar can be controlled by the application of prolonged pressure. This renders an ischemic condition and lowered oxygen tension, resulting in decreased synthesis of collagen tissue while lysis continues.[21]

The physical weave of the collagen fiber is largely responsible for the final function of the wound. The arrangement of collagen fibers in scar tissue is

Figure 1-4. Intramolecular and intermolecular cross-linking of the collagen filaments.

Intramolecular cross-links

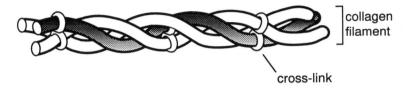

collagen filament

cross-link

Intermolecular cross-links

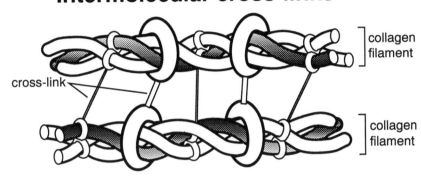

collagen filament

cross-link

collagen filament

Figure 1-4. Intramolecular and intermolecular cross-linking of the collagen filaments.

disorganized and distinctly different from that in the surrounding tissue. Collagen turnover allows the randomly deposited scar tissue to be arranged in both linear and lateral orientation. As the scar ages, fibers and fiber bundles become more closely packed.

There are two theories which explain the realignment of the collagen tissues: the induction theory and the tension theory. According to the induction theory, the scar attempts to mimic the characteristics of the tissue it is healing.[22] The tissue structure induces the collagen weave. Thus, dense tissues induce dense scarring whereas pliable tissues induce loose scarring. The tension theory refers to internal and external stresses that affect the wound area during the remodeling phase.[23] Physical change of scar length could be achieved through the application of stress during the appropriate healing phase.

Clinically, range of motion helps in remodeling the collagen tissue.[13] Range of motion exercises ignore myofibroblast pull and concentrate on remodeling the collagen as it is laid down. As the remodeling process goes forward, the bright pink scar of an immature wound of 6 to 12 weeks begins to give way to a softer lavender, and finally faintly pink scar.[24] As the scar softens and flattens, the raised hypertrophic appearance of many scars gives way to the soft, white, flat, mature scar tissue characteristic of the mature wound. This process takes 12 to 15 months in most cases. The capillary loops slowly close, resulting in a visible spectrum of color loss as the wound flattens and matures.

TYPES OF HEALING WOUNDS

PRIMARY CLOSURE

Primary closure, or healing by first intention, occurs when full-thickness surgical incisions or other acute wound edges with minimal skin loss are approximated and sutured together. Further healing takes place by re-epithelialization only. This type of wound healing is least complicated.

SECONDARY CLOSURE

Secondary closure or healing by secondary intention, occurs in open, large, full-thickness wounds with soft tissue loss. These wounds take longer to heal and the process is much more extensive. They undergo collagen deposition, wound contraction, and granulation followed by epithelialization. Wound contraction is the most important phenomenon in secondary closure. The wounds heal with scar.

DELAYED PRIMARY CLOSURE

Delayed primary closure, or healing by third intention, occurs in more extensive wounds which are either heavily contaminated or at risk of developing an infection during an acute phase of healing. By delaying the closure, the healing progress can be monitored and, if the wound is infected, therapeutic intervention can be initiated. Delayed primary closure does not delay the development of tensile strength. The wounds are finally sutured and further healing takes place by re-epithelialization.

FACTORS AFFECTING WOUND HEALING

There are numerous factors that affect the normal healing of the wounds. Both systemic and local factors have an adverse impact on wound healing. These factors may cause inflammatory arrest, failure of contraction, failure of epithelialization, failure to produce and cross-link collagen, and failure to neovascularize. These factors are numerous; however, the most common and important clinical factors will be described here.

SYSTEMIC FACTORS

Normal wound healing primarily depends upon the individual's general condition. The major systemic factors adversely affecting wound healing include nutrition, vascularity, systemic medications, systemic diseases, and age.

Nutrition

Nutrition has a profound effect on wound healing. Balanced nutrition is crucial for normal wound healing. Deficiency of any nutrient during the healing process may result in impaired or delayed wound healing. Patients with chronic or non-healing wounds often require special nutrients. Some nutrients are more important than others, and the deficiencies of these nutrients have specific effects on the healing process (see Chapter 5 for more detailed information).

Protein is one of the most important nutrients. A deficiency of protein impairs new capillaries formation, fibroblastic proliferation, proteoglycans and collagen synthesis, and wound remodeling.[25] Deficiency of protein also affects phagocytosis, leading to a higher risk for infection. Deficiency of vitamin A results in retardation of epithelialization, closure of wounds, rate of collagen synthesis, and cross-linking of collagen fibers.[26] Deficiency of vitamin A also causes diminished macrophage production resulting in decreased resistance to infection. Deficiency of vitamin E in the body adversely affects wound healing by affecting collagen production and intermolecular collagen cross-linking.[25,27] Deficiency of vitamin C results in the failure of fibroblasts to produce collagen, increases the sensitivity of capillaries to rupture, and also makes the wound susceptible to infection.[28] Similarly, deficiency of vitamin K results in excessive bleeding and hematoma formation.[25]

Minerals and other elements also play an important role in wound healing. Deficiency of zinc causes decreased rate of epithelialization and collagen synthesis, and results in decreased tensile strength.[29] Deficiency of magnesium may cause decreased collagen synthesis. Deficiency of copper may lead to altered cross-linking, thereby affecting the tensile strength.[25] Although iron is necessary for collagen synthesis, research has not confirmed whether iron deficiency further compromises wound healing by virtue of anemia.[28] Severe anemia has been reported to interfere with wound repair.[29] Furthermore, obese people with high contents of body fat and poor dietary habits are at high risk of delayed healing, wound dehiscence, and infection.

Vascularity

Both arterial and venous insufficiency play major roles in the development of lower extremity ulcers. Cardiovascular insufficiency may also affect healing of wounds.

Arterial insufficiency due to arteriosclerosis and diabetes mellitus causes tissue hypoxia and results in chronic, nonhealing wounds. These wounds are also highly susceptible to infection due to inadequate oxygen tension in the tissues.

Venous insufficiency, due to venous valve dysfunction, impedes blood flow towards the heart resulting in edema. Sustained venous pressure due to edema causes leakage of fibrinogen around the capillaries into the dermis. This pressure results in the formation of a fibrin layer which blocks tissue oxygenation, nutrient exchange, and waste removal.[30] Venous stasis ulcers are difficult to heal and are at high risk for developing infections.

Systemic Medications

Patients with open wounds frequently take systemic medications. Although medications such as antibiotics do prevent and/or eliminate infection, some of the systemic medications have adverse effects on wound healing. Steroids are known to decrease tensile strength of closed healed wounds,[31] rate of epithelialization,[32] and neovascularization,[33] and also severely inhibit wound contraction.[34] Steroids suppress the immune system which makes the wounds susceptible to sepsis. Similarly, nonsteroidal anti-inflammatory drugs (NSAIDs) cause vasoconstriction and suppress the inflammatory response.[10] NSAIDs also decrease collagen synthesis and reduce tensile strength and wound contraction.[35] These drugs also interfere with leukocyte migration into the wound, thus causing increased susceptibility to infection.

Chemotherapeutic agents interfere with cell proliferation,[10] prolong inflammation, inhibit protein synthesis, and decrease collagen synthesis.[1] Anti-neoplastic and immunosuppressive medications impair fibroblast production resulting in decreased tensile strength. These drugs significantly impair the healing process. Anticoagulant medications affect hematoma formation and decrease tensile strength.[25] Certain antibiotics also have a toxic effect and inhibit wound healing.

Systemic Diseases

Numerous systemic diseases affect wound healing, either directly or indirectly. Diabetes mellitus is one major systemic disease that adversely affects wound healing. Uncontrolled diabetes decreases collagen synthesis, decreases phagocytosis, and increases the risk of infection.[1,36] Decreased sensations due to diabetic neuropathy make the feet vulnerable to injuries. Diabetes also commonly causes atherosclerosis resulting in circulatory insufficiency.

Atherosclerosis and other vascular diseases reduce the blood supply to the wound and have adverse effects on wound healing. Acquired immune deficiency syndrome (AIDS) makes the wound susceptible to infection, and also affects phagocytosis, fibroblast function, and collagen synthesis.[37] Renal dysfunction is reported to interfere with granulation formation and fibroblast proliferation.[35] Cardiovascular problems and chronic renal and liver failure significantly impair wound healing.[38]

Age

The physiologic changes that occur with age cause the elderly to heal slower than younger persons. Decreased inflammatory response, as well as delayed granulation, is common in older people. The cross-linking of collagen fibers and their organization is superior in younger people.[39] Older people have low tensile strength and rate of epithelialization, as well as poorly organized, cutaneous small vessels.[40,41] The overall effect of aging is slow rate of healing and high risk of multiple breakdown of wounds.

LOCAL FACTORS

Common local factors that adversely affect wound healing include local infection, blood supply, local medications, dressings, necrotic tissue and eschar, and desiccation.

Local Infection

All wounds are contaminated, but all are not necessarily infected. Wound infection has been defined as a bacterial concentration greater than 10^5 organisms per gram of tissue. Infection within the wound is the most problematic local factor that affects wound healing. Among wound complications, 50% are due to local wound infection.[42] Infection has its greatest negative effect on collagen metabolism. The infection is reported to reduce the amount of collagen produced[38] while collagen lysis is increased.[43] The presence of bacterial infection also decreases the availability of the nutrients necessary for wound healing.[35] Finally, the bacterial toxicity kills the important wound cells needed for the healing process.

Blood Supply

The healing of wounds is largely dependent upon the availability of blood and oxygen to the wound cells. The nutritional status, the inflammatory response, and the oxygen tension of the wound all depend on the delivery of their components to the local area by microcirculation.[1] Decreased oxygen tension to the wound area due to decreased blood supply inhibits fibroblast migration as well as collagen synthesis. The result is decreased tensile strength of the wound.[1,10] Further, the wounds with reduced blood supply are susceptible to infection. Therefore, wound healing can be markedly impaired by decreased blood supply to the wound area, and if the wound heals, the risk of breakdown is markedly increased.

Local Medications

Topical agents are commonly used in all types of wounds. They are used to irrigate wounds, to prevent or rid infection, and to promote healing. Although these agents are known to have profound effects on wound healing, reports of adverse effects also appear in the literature. The toxicities of topical antimicrobials (povidone-iodine, acetic acid, hydrogen peroxide, and sodium hypochlorite) at certain concentrations have been reported to adversely affect fibroblast function.[44] Povidone-iodine, which has been commonly used for many years for wound management, retards epithelialization and decreases wound tensile strength.[44] Topically applied fluorinated steroids retard epidermal resurfacing and reduce collagen synthesis.[45] Certain topical antibiotics, e.g., Furacin,™ significantly retard the rate of re-epithelialization.[46] Therefore, appropriate concentrations of the various antimicrobials is the most important factor to be considered in order to avoid the adverse effects of these agents on wound healing.

Dressings

The mechanics of wound dressing is also one of the important factors that can facilitate, as well as inhibit, wound healing. The choices of dressing may range from a totally occlusive impermeable to semi-occlusive semi-permeable to non-occlusive permeable. Conventional gauze permeable wet-to-dry dressings function as debridement and help with wounds having a large amount of necrotic tissue. However, when this type of dressing is applied to a newly formed granulation tissue, it may damage the granulation tissue when the dressing is removed.[47] Further, the dry gauze dressing may cause dehydration of the wound resulting in prolonged inflammation.[48] All dressings have some advantages and some disadvantages. Choosing the right type of dressing for a given wound type is an important clinical decision during the different stages of healing. The wrong choice may have a detrimental effect on the healing process.

Necrotic Tissue and Eschar

The presence of necrotic tissue in the wound significantly impairs healing. Necrotic tissue or foreign material increases the likelihood of infection resulting in a chronic nonhealing wound. Similarly, eschar also impedes the healing process. It interferes with wound contraction resulting in a prolonged healing process.[49]

Desiccation

It is now well established that moist wounds heal much faster than dry wounds. A moist wound environment facilitates epithelialization and minimizes crust formation.[7] The rate of epithelialization is 50% faster in a moist environment.[50] Angiogenesis is also believed to be stimulated in a moist environment.[51]

CONCLUSION

Wound healing is a complex physiological process. A thorough knowledge of normal wound healing is of utmost importance for the clinicians involved in the care of patients with open wounds. It is imperative for every clinician involved in wound care to know the process which prevents, minimizes, and eliminates those factors which adversely affect wound healing.

REFERENCES

1. Carrico TJ, Mehrhof AI, Cohen IK. Biology of wound healing. *Surg Clin North Am.* 1984;64:721-733.
2. Zarro VJ. Mechanisms of inflammation and repair. In: Michlovitz S. *Thermal Agents in Rehabilitation.* Philadelphia, PA: FA Davis; 1986:3-17.
3. Bryant WM. Wound Healing. *Clin Symp.* 1977;29:1-36.
4. Hardy MA. The biology of scar formation. *Phys Ther.* 1989;69:1014-1024.
5. Rutherford RB, Ross R. Platelet factors stimulate fibroblasts and smooth muscle cells quiescent in plasma serum to proliferate. *J Cell Biol.* 1976;69:196-203.
6. Werb A, Gordon S. Elastase secretion by stimulated macrophages. *J Exp Med.* 1975;142:361-377.
7. Daly TJ. The repair phase of wound healing: re-epithelialization and contraction. In: Kloth LC, McCulloch JM, Feedar JA. *Wound Healing: Alternatives in Management.* Philadelphia, PA: FA Davis; 1990:14-30.
8. Van Winkle W. Wound contraction. *Surg Gynecol Obstet.* 1967;125:131-142.
9. Bell E, Ivarsson B, Merrill C. Production of a tissue-like structure by contraction of collagen lattices by human fibroblasts of different proliferative potential in vitro. *Proc Natl Acad Sci, USA.* 1979;76:1274-1278.
10. Peacock EE. *Wound Repair.* Philadelphia, PA: WB Saunders Co; 1984.
11. McGrath MH, Simon RH. Wound geometry and the kinetics of wound contraction. *Plast Reconstr Surg.* 1983;72:66-73.
12. Baur PS, Larson DL, Stacey TR, Barratt GF, Dobrkovsky M. Ultrastructural analysis of pressure-treated human hypertrophic scars. *J Trauma.* 1976;16:958-967.
13. Baur PS, Barratt G, Linares HA, Dobrkovsky M, de la Houssaye AJ, Larson DL. Wound contractions, scar contractures, and myofibroblasts: a classical case study. *J Trauma.* 1978;18:8-22.
14. Morton D, Steinbronn K, Lat M, Chvapil M, Peacock EE. Effects of colchicine on wound healing in rats. *Surg Forum.* 1974;25:47-51.
15. Peacock EE, Madden JW. Administration of betaamino propionitrile to human beings with urethral strictures: a preliminary report. *Am J Surg.* 1978;136:600-605.
16. Enquist IF, Adamson RJ. Collagen synthesis and lysis in healing wounds. *Minn Med.* 1965;48:1695-1698.
17. Peacock EE, Madden JW. Some studies on the effects of *B-aminopropionitrile* on collagen in healing wounds. *Surgery.* 1969;60:7-12.
18. Schumann D. The nature of wound healing. *AORN J.* 1982;35:1068-1077.
19. Dingman RO. Factors of clinical significance affecting wound healing. *Laryngoscope.* 1973;83:1540-1544.
20. Peacock EE, Madden JW, Trier WC. Biologic basis for the treatment of keloids and hypertrophic scars. *South Med J.* 1970;63:755-760.
21. Hunt TK, Van Winkle W. *Wound Healing—Normal Repair: Fundamentals of Wound Management in Surgery.* South Plainfield, NJ: Chirurgecom Inc; 1976.
22. Madden JW. Wound healing: the biological basis of hand surgery. *Clin Plast Surg.* 1976;3:3-11.
23. Arem AJ, Madden JW. Effects of stress on healing wounds. I. Intermittent noncyclical tension. *J Surg Res.* 1976;20:93-102.
24. Cocke WM, White RR, Lynch DJ, Verheyden CN. *Wound Care.* New York, NY: Churchill Livingstone; 1986.
25. Pollack SV. Wound healing: a review. III. Nutritional factors affecting wound healing. *J Dermatol Surg Oncol.* 1979;5:615-619.
26. Freiman M, Seifter E, Connerton C, Levenson SM. Vitamin A deficiency and surgical stress. *Surg Forum.* 1970;21:81-82.
27. Brown RG, Burton GW, Smith JF. Effect of vitamin E deficiency on collagen metabolism in rats' skin. *J Nutr.* 1967;91:99-106.
28. Pollack SV. Systemic drugs and nutritional aspects on wound healing. *Clin Dermatol.* 1984;2:68-80.
29. Sandblom P. The tensile strength of healing wounds. *Acta Chir Scand.* 1944;89(suppl):71-85.
30. Silane MF, Oot-Giromini B. Systemic and other factors that affect wound healing. In: Eaglestein WH. *New Directions in Wound Healing: Wound Care Manual.* Princeton, NJ: ER Squibb & Sons Inc; 1990:39-53.
31. Ehlrich HP, Hunt TK. The effect of cortisone and anabolic steroids on the tensile strength of healing wounds. *Ann Surg.* 1969;170:203-206.

32. Baker BL, Whitaker WL. Interference with wound healing by the local action of adrenocortical steroids. *Endocrinology.* 1950;46:544-551.

33. Howes EL, Plotz CM, Blunt JW, Ragan C. Retardation of wound healing by cortisone. *Surgery.* 1950;28:177-181.

34. Stephens FU, Dunphy JE, Hunt TK. The effect of delayed administration of corticosteroids on wound contraction. *Ann Surg.* 1971;173:214-218.

35. Hunt TK. Disorders of wound healing. *World J Surg.* 1980;4:271-277.

36. Goodson WH, Hunt TK. Studies of wound healing in experimental diabetes mellitus. *J Surg Res.* 1977;22:221-227.

37. Peterson MJ, Barbul A, Breslin RJ, Wasserkrug HL, Efron G. Significance of T-lymphocytes in wound healing. *Surgery.* 1987;2:300-305.

38. Irvin TT. *Wound Healing: Principle and Practice.* London: Chapman and Hall; 1981.

39. Holm-Pedersen P, Viidik A. Tensile properties and morphology of healing wounds in young and old rats. *Scand J Plast Reconstr Surg.* 1972;6:24-35.

40. Goodson WH, Hunt TK. Wound healing and aging. *J Invest Dermatol.* 1979;73:88-91.

41. Carter DM, Balin AK. Dermatological aspects of aging. *Med Clin North Am.* 1983;67:531-543.

42. Schilling J. Wound healing. *Surg Round.* 1983;6:46-62.

43. Irvin TT. Collagen metabolism in infected colonic anastomoses. *Surg Gynecol Obstet.* 1976;143:220-204.

44. Lineaweaver W, Howard R, Souey D, et al. Topical antimicrobial toxicity. *Arch Surg.* 1985;120:267-279.

45. Zitelli J. Wound healing for the clinician. In: Callen JP, Dahl MV, Golitz LE, Rasmussen JE, Stegman SJ. *Advances in Dermatology.* Vol 2. Chicago, IL: Year Book Medical Publishers Inc; 1987:243-266.

46. Geronemus RG, Mertz PM, Eaglstein WH. The effects of topical antimicrobial agents. *Arch Dermatol.* 1979;115:1311-1314.

47. Cohen IK, McCoy BJ, Diegelmann RF. An update on wound healing. *Ann Plast Surg.* 1979;3:264-272.

48. Feedar JA, Kloth LC. Conservative management of chronic wounds. In: Kloth LC, McCulloch JM, Feedar JA. *Wound Healing: Alternatives in Management.* Philadelphia, PA: FA Davis; 1990:135-172.

49. Rudolph R, Noe JM. *Chronic Problem Wounds.* Boston, MA: Little, Brown & Co; 1983.

50. Winter GD. Formation of the scab and the rate of epithelialization of superficial wounds in the skin of the young domestic pig. *Nature.* 1962;193:293-294.

51. Falanga V. Occlusive wound dressings: why, when, which? *Arch Dermatol.* 1988;124:872-877.

Chapter 2

Wound Evaluation

Robin Ryan Marquez, MS, PT

When evaluating patients with dermal wounds one must perfect the ability to retrieve and process patient information, to interpret laboratory tests results, and to maximize observational skills. A complete wound evaluation includes three components:

(1) history and subjective examination
(2) review of laboratory tests and procedures
(3) objective examination

The purpose of this chapter is to describe an organized approach for evaluating patients with dermal wounds. The information gained from the evaluation helps to clarify the primary problem and allows the clinician to better understand how the condition affects the normal phases of wound healing and the patient's ability to heal.

HISTORY AND SUBJECTIVE EXAMINATION

Prior to the objective examination it is essential that the clinician interview the patient, and in some cases the primary caretaker. This information is needed to establish a baseline history and cause of events leading to the development of the wound. Subjective information and findings can provide the examiner with a more complete picture of the patient. Knowledge gained from the patient interview process can help to clarify the primary problem and allow the examiner to make necessary decisions regarding the course of therapy.

Early in the history gathering process, information should be obtained concerning the patient's past medical history, age, sex, and occupation. Review of past medical history should include significant traumas, illnesses or diseases, and previous treatment intervention. Pre-existing medical conditions such as diabetes, hypertension, and peripheral vascular disease often complicate and delay the normal process of wound healing. The age of the patient is also an important factor in wound healing as discussed in Chapter 1. Certain disease processes may be more prevalent in one sex versus the other. The individual's occupation, as well as the type of lifestyle, can provide valuable information suggesting a possible cause for the wound. The history may also indicate the amount of activity or exercise the individual performs on a daily basis.

Once preliminary information has been obtained the examiner must inquire about the events leading to the development of the wound. This process should include onset of wound, mechanism of injury, and wound symptoms. The examiner must determine how the patient's symptoms respond to varying situations. For this reason, it is important to first localize the symptoms to determine whether the patient is having problems related to the wound or to another area. Is the pain located within or around the lesion or in other parts of the body? Does the patient complain of associated paranesthesia which could be indicative of initial nerve pathogenesis? An ulcerative lesion with true anesthesia could indicate a condition such as diabetes or a peripheral neuropathic process. Further investigation should be made to determine how the pain is affected by different body positions. For example, lower extremity ulcerations due to venous insufficiency will generally be aggravated by exercise and the gravity-dependent position.[1]

In addition to the general history, the clinician should ask certain specific details which the patient may not offer voluntarily. To identify systemic disease processes the following questions should be routinely asked:

- Is the patient a diabetic? If yes, it is important to establish the patient's age at onset of diabetes as well as the method and quantity of insulin required. This will help to determine the extent and severity of secondary neuropathic and vascular changes.
- Does the patient use any tobacco products? If so, how much and for how long? Nicotine causes immediate vasoconstriction and vasospasm of the arteries. Long-term use of tobacco can lead to arteriosclerotic plaque formation in the walls of the blood vessels.[2]
- Does the patient have a history of circulatory disturbances including peripheral vascular disease, hypertension, or congestive heart failure? Demonstration of symptoms such as cold, cyanotic hands or feet; dry, flaky skin; or lack of hair growth on the lower extremity may suggest the existence of a pathologic condition that causes arterial insufficiency and tissue hypoxia.
- Is the patient currently taking any medications? Certain prescription as well as non-prescription medications such as steroids, aspirin, antihistamines, and birth control pills may delay wound healing.
- Does the patient have any allergies to medications or topical agents? This information will help to rule out contact dermatitis versus an allergic reaction to certain agents that may be used during treatment, i.e., whirlpool additives or topical medications.
- Has the patient received previous treatment for this condition? If so, what treatments have and have not

proven to be successful? This will enable the clinician to avoid using the same treatments that may have been used in the past without success.

REVIEW OF LABORATORY TESTS

The patient's general health and the condition of all body systems has an important impact on wound healing. Results from laboratory tests can provide valuable information about the functioning of an individual's metabolic and autoimmune systems, as well as their nutritional and vascular status (Table 2-1). Impairment or compromise to any of these systems may result in delayed or nonhealing wounds. Additional tests may include:

- Wound cultures, both aerobic and anaerobic, to identify the etiogenic agents of an infectious process. It is important to remember that all dermal wounds are contaminated but not necessarily infected. Clinical infection is determined by the colony count. A bacterial load of greater than 100,000 per gram of tissue is indicative of an infection (Table 2-2).
- Tissue biopsies to rule out malignancy or tumors.
- MRI and radiographs to rule out the presence of osteomyelitis or any abscess formation.

OBJECTIVE EXAMINATION

The clinician has a multitude of objective tests available to determine the patient's wound status. Obviously, all objective tests are not appropriate for all patients. The clinician must determine which tests are pertinent for a particular patient based on the history, subjective information, and basic observations of the wound.

RISK ASSESSMENT TOOLS

Clinicians are encouraged to select and use a method of risk assessment that ensures systemic evaluation of individual risk factors. Many risk assessment tools exist, but the Norton Scale and the Braden Scale have been tested extensively for their

Table 2-1. Laboratory Tests for Routine System Functioning

	Test	Use	Normative Value/ Referred Range
Nutritional	Plasma protein Serum albumin Serum transferrin	Test for protein malnutrition (Kwashior kor)	Adult 2.8-4.3 g/dL, 200-400 mg/dL
	Hemoglobin	Measures ability of red blood cells to transport oxygen to cells; anemia	M: 42-52% F: 37-47%
	Hematocrit		M: 14-18 g/dL F: 12-16 g/dL
	Nitrogen balance (urinary nitrogen excretion)	Measures metabolic expenditure, a guide to caloric needs during illness	BUN-adult 10-20 mg/dL
	Cholesterol, Total	Used to determine patients with increased risk of coronary heart disease	Desirable 150-200 mg/dL Marginal risk for CHD 200-240 Substantial risk for CHD>240 mg/ dL
	Total lymphocyte count	Checks protein malnutrition	25-33%
Vascular	Palpation of pedal pulse	Measures arterial blood flow to the extremity	2 + = normal 1 + = diminished 0 = absent
	Doppler Arteriogram Venogram	Measures efficiency of blood flow when palpation is ineffective due to obstruction, edema, or soft tissue restriction	Normal flow No obstructions
	Prothrombin time	Measures time it takes for blood to clot	<2 sec. deviation from control
Immune system	Hematology profile	Test for body's response and ability to fight foreign bodies and infection	WBC: 4.8-10.8 x 10 RBC: M: 4.7-6.1 x 10 F: 4.2-5.4 x 10
	HIV-I/HIV-2 antibody		Negative
Metabolic	Urinalysis	Test to determine kidney, pancreas, liver functioning; also used to rule out trauma or bacterial growth	Protein—negative Glucose—negative Bilirubin—negative Blood—negative pH—4.5-8.0 Bacteria—negative

reliability. Risk assessment tools include the following risk factors: mobility/activity impairment, moisture/incontinence, and impaired nutrition. Altered level of consciousness and altered sensory perception are also identified as risk factors in most assessment tools. The greater the patient's risk assessment score the more likely he or she is at risk of developing skin breakdown or experiencing delayed wound healing. These scores are designed to identify potential at-risk patients and to allow early implementation of preventative measures.

WOUND CLASSIFICATION

Wounds develop on many parts of the body in different shapes, sizes, and depths for a variety of reasons. Despite their similarities, all wounds should

---

Table 2-2. Indications for Wound Culture and Sensitivity Testing

A. **Signs of local infection**
Edema
Erythema
Purulent or foul-smelling drainage
Increased pain
Induration
Heat around the wound

B. **Signs of systemic infection**
Fever
Leukocytosis

C. **Bone involvement**
Full-thickness wound at increased risk for osteomyelitis

D. **Nonhealing wounds**
Silent infection

---

not be classified the same way. There are several classification systems that can be used to help the clinician identify wounds seen in the clinics.

Wounds are commonly classified into two categories: partial-thickness and full-thickness. The partial-thickness wounds involve the epidermal layer and may also involve the superficial layer of the dermis, while full-thickness wounds involve the complete epidermis, dermis, subcutaneous tissue, and may also involve muscles and bone (see Chapter 1). This classification includes those wounds in which the etiology or primary cause is something other than pressure. Examples include skin tears, lacerations, surgical wounds, and venous stasis ulcers. When using this method to classify wounds, the clinician should include length, width, and depth of the wound.

Another commonly used classification for all types of wounds is by color, i.e., the red-yellow-black system. Red wounds are healthy wounds that are in the healing phase. Yellow wounds are infected wounds or wounds filled with slough. Black wounds are those wounds covered with eschar.

Wounds that develop secondary to pressure are usually classified using a four-staging system developed by the National Pressure Ulcer Advisory Panel (NPUAP). For details on staging of the wounds see

Chapter 6. The staging of pressure ulcers is only one anatomical parameter which measures the extent and depth of tissue destruction. It is therefore only necessary to measure length and width in Stage I ulcers since the epidermis remains intact. When documenting Stages II, III, and IV ulcers, length, width, and depth measurements are included.

Regardless of which classification system is used to classify the wounds, it is important to describe the wound by using consistent terminology.

PHYSICAL EXAMINATION AND OBSERVATION

Performing an accurate wound assessment is an important part of good wound care. The wound assessment should include objective measurements which will allow for serial monitoring of progress towards healing. It is preferred that wounds are assessed at least weekly and the assessment reflect changes in the depth and surface area of the wound. Factors such as wound location, shape, and depth of tissue injury need to be considered carefully when choosing a measuring technique. For example, an acetate tracing is usually more reliable than surface dimensions particularly when measuring a large, irregular wound such as a leg ulcer. Consistency in measurement is also important in maintaining accuracy. Having the same person measure the wound each time and using the same technique for each measurement will enhance precision.

CLINICAL MEASUREMENTS

Location

The examiner should begin by noting the location of the wound. The location of an ulcer can be one of the first indicators of its cause. For example, venous stasis ulcers are most commonly found over the area of the medial malleoli and only rarely appear on the anterior or lateral aspect of the shin. The opposite is true of ulcers resulting from chronic arterial disease which typically exhibit symptoms above the lateral malleoli or in small infarcted areas of the toes.[3] When documenting the location of a wound, anatomical landmarks should be used for clarity, i.e., natural creases/skin folds, joints, or bony landmarks. The involved surface area should also be documented, i.e., plantar versus volar. This is particularly important in diabetic patients who classically demonstrate ulcers on the weight-bearing surfaces on the plantar aspect of the foot due to decreased sensitivity and increased pressure. The location of the wound should be charted on a body diagram and/or photograph taken to illustrate the physical characteristics of the wound.

Size and Depth

Length and width are used to describe and document the size of the wounds. They are measured as the longest and the shortest distance from the wound edge and are documented using consistent units of measure, preferably centimeters. Using a piece of sterile acetate and a permanent marking pen is a more reliable means of objectively documenting wound size. A clear film with a calibrated grid is superimposed on the wound and the borders are traced (Figure 2-1). Depth can be determined by inserting a sterile cotton tip applicator into the deepest part of the wound bed and grasping the applicator where it meets the wound's edge (Figure 2-2). For wounds with a base of varying depth, a range should be stated from the shallowest to the deepest. An alternative technique can be utilized to measure depth if the wound can be positioned perpendicular to the line of gravity. This technique uses a syringe filled with a predetermined amount of water and then injected into the wound cavity until the cavity is filled. The water left in the syringe is subtracted from the initial amount to indicate the volume in cubic centimeters required to fill the wound.

Tunneling, also known as rimming or undermining, is a term used to describe tissue destruction underlying intact skin along the wound margins. It is imperative that the clinician assess the wound for tunneling with each dressing change. When describing tunneling, one may describe it in centimeters and o'clock numbers in relationship to the hands of a clock, with the patient's head being at 12 o'clock.

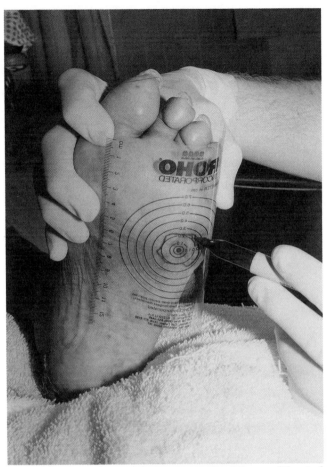

Figure 2-1. Tracing technique used with a calibrated grid to determine wound size.

Drainage

In addition to the size and depth of an ulcer, note any drainage that might be present. It is important to identify whether the drainage is active or inactive. An inactive drainage may be evident on a dressing, but at the time of examination no drainage is observed in the wound or periphery. An active drainage includes fluid that is free flowing or able to be expressed from the wound with pressure or "milking" of the peripheral borders. To assess the drainage from a wound, the following characteristics should be noted:

- *Type*: serous, purulent, sanguineous
- *Amount*: none, minimal, moderate, or copious amounts
- *Color*: clear, red, yellow, white

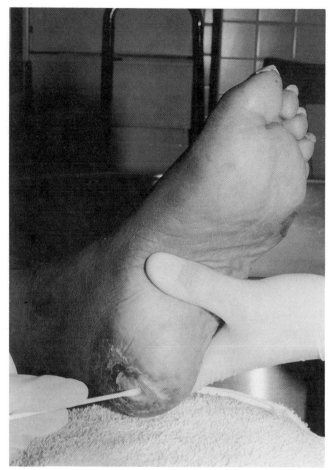

Figure 2-2. The use of a sterile cotton-tipped applicator in the measurement of depth in a tracking lesion.

- *Odor*: absent, mild, moderate, or foul smelling
- *Consistency*: thin/watery, thick/opaque

The type of drainage should be identified based on the specific make-up of the fluid:

- *Serous*: thin, watery-like serum.
- *Purulent*: containing, consisting of, or forming pus. Pus is a protein-rich, liquid inflammatory product made up of leukocytes and cellular debris.
- *Sanguineous*: bloody fluid consisting primarily of red blood cells and water.

The color, as well as the odor of the drainage, provides useful information about infection. Certain bacteria will produce distinctive colors and characteristic aromas, e.g., pseudomonas has a greenish-blue color with a sweet smell. The consistency of wound drainage can provide information relative to the source of the drainage. A sudden increase in the amount of drainage may be a sign of a worsening condition, or may indicate an abscess that has spontaneously begun to drain. When an increase in wound drainage is seen in conjunction with localized signs of infection such as foul odor, increased temperature and cellulitis, a quantitative culture should be taken.

Temperature

Variations in temperature measurements taken over the wound or around the periphery indicate the severity and limits of the inflammation. Often the clinician is not able to detect and differentiate slight temperature changes by touch alone. Several commercial instruments are available for measuring temperature. A thermistor is the least expensive and most frequently used device. This instrument consists of a temperature probe that measures temperature by surface contact. A radiometer is an alternative device which measures surface temperature by infrared radiations from the body, and does not require any surface contact with the wound. The advantage of using this device is that adjacent areas can be scanned to detect differences with the intact periphery. Thermographs are also available but rarely used in the clinic due to cost and preparation time. These thermographic devices produce a multicolor picture of the involved area, each color representing a gradient change in temperature (Figure 2-3).

Girth

To measure the extent of limb atrophy or edema, circumferential girth measurements are taken with a calibrated tape measure on both the involved and non-involved limbs (Figure 2-4). A disposable paper tape measure is recommended for areas with drainage. It is important to measure the girth with reference to bony landmarks to ensure reproducible measurements. Volumetric tests have been found to be more accurate in assessing the size of irregular shaped areas. These tests use water displacement as a means of objectifying extremity volume. The body part is lowered into a filled volumeter with water and the water overflow is collected and measured in a graduated cylinder.

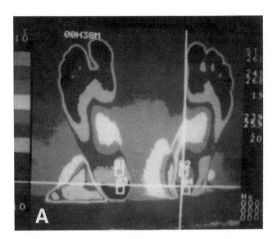
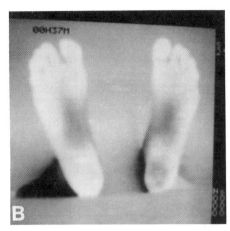

Figure 2-3. Liquid crystal thermography used in surface temperature measurement.

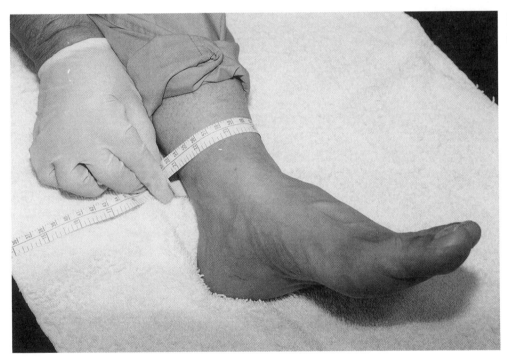

Figure 2-4. Measurement of leg girth.

Identification of Tissue/Structures

The wound evaluation should include a description and identification of tissue structures. Stating the color of the tissue is necessary because this indicates the vascularity and viability of the structure. Tissue within the wound or around the periphery will exhibit associated color changes with maceration, dehydration or hypoxia. The color of the wound bed may be described as red, yellow, or black. Red wounds usually indicate clean, healthy, granulating wounds. Yellow wounds may be filled with fibrous tissue or hydrated necrotic or dead tissue referred to as slough. Black wounds usually are covered with dried eschar. The following tissue structures are most commonly found in wounds: eschar, granulation tissue, adipose tissue, fascia, muscle, tendons, and bones. Foreign debris and necrotic tissue should be identified and removed from the wound as quickly as possible to prevent bacterial colonization and infection.

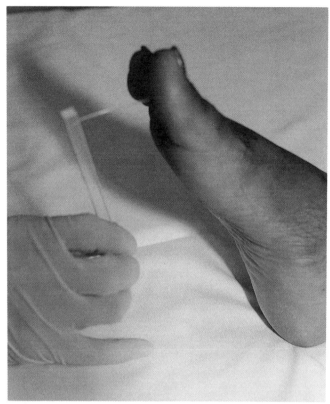

Figure 2-5. Semmes-Weinstein nylon sensory filament used to determine cutaneous sensibility.

Describing the skin around the wound, also known as peri-wound skin, is important. For example, a ring of redness or halo of erythema around the wound may be indicative of an infection. Trophic changes (e.g., dry skin, brittle nails, hair loss) are indications of poor arterial nutrition to the area. Changes in skin color will provide information relative to the functional status of the circulatory system. Areas with arterial insufficiency will demonstrate a cyanotic appearance as compared to areas of venous insufficiency where the peri-wound skin discolors due to the pigment hemosiderin being deposited.

CUTANEOUS SENSIBILITY ASSESSMENT

Patients' inability to perceive changes in sensation, temperature, or joint proprioception in the feet increases their risk for undetected trauma and/or pressure resulting in skin breakdown. For

this reason, an assessment of the patient's sensory status must be made. A sensory evaluation should always be performed on the involved side and compared to the contralateral side. A simple method to test the patient's perception of touch is to use a light object such as the tip of a cotton applicator and gently swipe over the involved area. For a more objective assessment, the Semmes-Weinstein monofilaments are preferred (Figure 2-5). The graded nylon filaments vary in thickness and are designed to bow after a specific force has been applied thus indicating the cutaneous sensibility of the area tested.[4]

ASSESSMENT OF THE PERIPHERAL ARTERIAL SYSTEM

BLOOD PRESSURE

Blood pressure should be routinely checked on all patients. This test is quick and simple, and it provides the clinician with information about the present status of the cardiovascular system. This enables the clinician to screen out patients who are at high risk for developing hypertensive ulcers. Patients with hypertensive ulcers or those at risk may be placed on antihypertensive therapy as a preventive measure.

PULSES

Peripheral pulses should be routinely taken on all patients. The quality and presence of pulses will be indicative of blood flow through the arteries. Patients with lower extremity ulcers should have pulses tested at various levels (common iliac, femoral, popliteal, dorsalis pedis, posterior tibial) to determine the location of compromise or occlusion. A significant decrease or absence of an arterial pulse is most frequently related to arteriosclerosis. Additional causes for decreased arterial pulses include trauma to the blood vessel, soft tissue restriction due to excessive swelling, and increased compartment pressures.

To properly examine lower extremity pulses, the patient should be positioned in supine with the

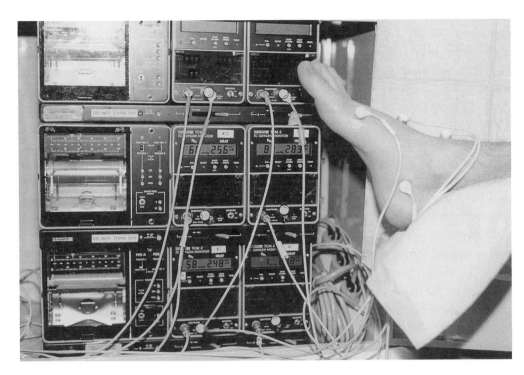

Figure 2-6. Measurement of transcutaneous oxygen concentration in the foot.

entire leg exposed. The majority of lower extremity arteries are superficial and reasonably easy to palpate. The depth of the popliteal artery often makes it more difficult to palpate. The popliteal pulse may be more easily obtained if the patient is positioned in prone with the knee extended. Pulses can be graded as 2+, 1+, and 0 indicating normal, diminished, and absent, respectively.

TISSUE OXYGEN TENSION TEST

This is a noninvasive method to measure arterial tissue oxygen tension by heating the skin through a tissue surface. This procedure utilizes a Clark polarographic electrode containing a heating element and a thermistor. The electrode must be heated to 43° to 44° C in order to produce measurable PO_2 values, and these values should closely approximate the blood values of the dilated, underlying microvessels in the involved area (Figure 2-6).

RUBOR OF DEPENDENCY TEST

This is a simple test used to determine the adequacy of blood flow in the arterial system by assessing changes in the skin color in response to elevation and dependency of the limb. In order to perform this test, the patient must be positioned in supine with the lower limb elevated to 60 degrees for approximately 1 minute. The skin color on the plantar aspect of the foot is examined once it is in the elevated position. Individuals with normal arterial circulation will exhibit no significant change in skin color. However, individuals with arterial compromise will show a pallor of the skin in the elevated position due to inadequate pressure and compromised blood flow. The second part of this test checks for skin color changes associated with the limb placed in a dependent position. Again, individuals with normal arterial circulation will show no significant skin color change, but those with arterial insufficiency will develop a reactive hyperemia or rubor with dependency as the arterial system attempts to compensate for tissue hypoxia.[5]

DOPPLER ULTRASOUND

Doppler ultrasound assessment is an effective, noninvasive diagnostic technique for determining vascular status.[6] This test is frequently used in the clinic due to the relatively low cost and ease of use. Doppler ultrasound can be used as an evaluation tool to detect abnormalities in the peripheral vascular system and to screen for venous obstructions and incompetent valves. This procedure determines the relative velocity of blood flow in the major arteries and veins in the arms and legs. A hand-held ultrasound probe contains an oscillator which vibrates at a frequency of 5 to 10 MHz which, in turn, causes the piezoelectrical crystals in the probe to emit an ultrasound beam. In order for the ultrasound wave to be transmitted transcutaneously across an artery or vein, an ultrasound coupling medium must be used (i.e., gel). The normal movement of cells in the blood vessels will cause a shift in the frequency of the ultrasound beam. This shift is known as the Doppler effect. The second crystal in the Doppler probe receives the reflected sound waves. When no movement exists within the blood vessel, the reflected sound waves will have the same frequency as the transmitted waves and there is transmission silence.[7] Any shift in frequency that occurs between the time the ultrasound beam is emitted and the time the reflected sound waves are received produces an audible signal.[7] This signal may then be analyzed in its auditory form by a skilled clinician to determine the presence of arterial disease, arterial or venous obstruction, and valvular competency.

The procedures for Doppler ultrasound will vary for arterial and venous systems. Subjective information and wound symptoms should guide the clinician in determining which system to examine. In some cases patients will exhibit compromise in both systems (Table 2-3). When the Doppler ultrasound is used to assess the peripheral arterial system, two measurements are performed. The first measurement is the Ankle-Arm Index Ratio, which is used to detect and quantify arterial vascular disease. The second measurement is the Segmental Blood Pressures, which are used to locate obstructions.

Ankle-Arm Index Ratio

Prior to initiating the test, the patient should be in a comfortable position with the knees slightly bent and hips externally rotated. The posterior tibial artery is located by manual palpation. A sphygmomanometer cuff is placed around the leg at the malleoli level. The ultrasound probe (with coupling medium) is held over the artery at a 45 degree angle and moved until the audible signal is at its strongest (Figure 2-7). Excessive pressure of the probe on the surface area should be avoided as this will decrease the auditory signal. The sphygmomanometer cuff is inflated until the sound is no longer heard; at this point it is slowly deflated and the systolic blood pressure is recorded when the sound first appears. The posterior tibial systolic blood pressure is then divided by the brachial systolic blood pressure to determine the ratio. A ratio of 1.0 or greater is considered normal.

Segmental Blood Pressures

Segmental blood pressure readings are taken at the ankle, below the knee, above the knee, and high up on the thigh. The Doppler probe is held constant on the posterior tibial artery while the sphygmomanometer cuff is moved to the specific level of testing and measurements are recorded.[8] Any artery (i.e., pedis dorsalis) can be used below the sphygmomanometer cuff to measure blood pressure at the level of the cuff placement (Figure 2-8). Segmental blood pressure readings from adjacent levels should not vary by more than 30 mmHg. If variation in adjacent segmental pressures is greater than 30 mmHg, it indicates an obstruction between those two segments.

ASSESSMENT OF THE PERIPHERAL VENOUS SYSTEM

DOPPLER ULTRASOUND

A Doppler ultrasound evaluation of the peripheral venous system is a more subjective test compared to the peripheral arterial system because the examiner must interpret the auditory signal rather than quantifying it into a systolic blood pressure reading.[9] The audible signal should be tested with the Doppler probe over the posterior tibial, common femoral, superficial femoral, and the popliteal veins. When performing a venous evaluation, the patient should be long sitting or lying down with the hips in

Table 2-3. **Doppler Ultrasound Assessment of Peripheral Systems**

	Symptoms	Indications for Use	Measurements	Procedure	Normative Values
Arterial	Intermittent claudication or resting pain in limb Tissue necrosis Decreased or absent peripheral pulse with palpation Cyanosis of digits or limb	Arterial disease or arterial obstruction	Ankle-arm index ratio	Systolic brachial pressure and systolic posterior tibial artery pressure recorded. Divide posterior tibial systolic BP by brachial systolic BP to determine ratio.	1.0 or greater = normal; no indication of arterial vascular disease. 0.8-0.9 = correlates with symptoms of intermittent claudication. 0.5-0.7 = correlates with rest pain. 0.4 or less = indicates tissue necrosis.
			Segmental pressure readings	Segmental pressure taken at ankle, below knee, above knee and upper thigh. BP cuff moves to specific level of testing. Doppler probe remains constant over artery.	Adjoining segmental readings should not vary by more than 30 mmHg. >30 mmHg between adjoining segments indicative of obstruction
Venous	Localized limb pain (especially on deep pressure or palpation) Limb is warm to touch Severe edema	Deep vein thrombosis, venous obstruction, and valvular competency	Augmentation	Pressure in the form of a quick, manual squeeze applied distally to probe to enhance auditory signal.	All vein locations tested should be augmentable.
			Spontaneous vs. non-spontaneous auditory signal	Doppler probe placed over the posterior tibial vein and checked for auditory signal.	Audible signal present.
			Compression	Manual compression applied to the limb proximal to the location of Doppler probe.	Sound should cease with compression and resume with release of compression.

slight external rotation, the knees slightly flexed, and the medial border of the foot exposed. It should be noted that the popliteal vein is more accurately tested with the patient in prone and the knee extended.

The auditory response over each of the four veins in the lower extremity should be recorded as either spontaneous (present) or not spontaneous (absent). All signals, spontaneous or not, are tested

Figure 2-7. Doppler ultrasound assessment of the posterial tibial artery.

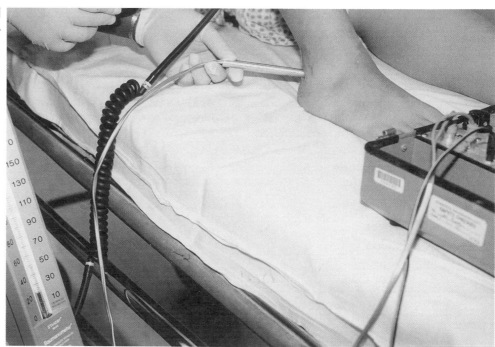

Figure 2-8. Pedis dorsalis systolic blood pressure below the knee.

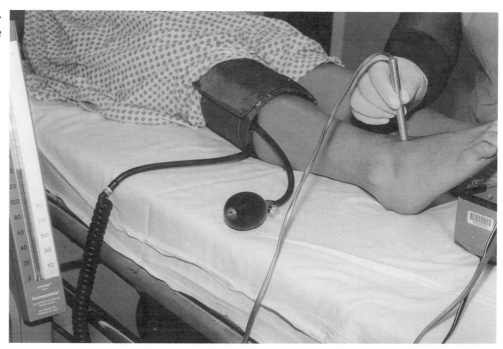

for augmentation.[10] To test for augmentation, a quick manual squeeze is applied distal to the probe to enhance the auditory signal. All locations should be augmentable. If a signal does not augment, an occlusion can be suspected between the area where the clinician is providing the augmentation and the location of the Doppler probe. Compression is a technique used to assess valvular competency. The examiner manually compresses the limb proximal to the location of the Doppler probe. If the venous valves are competent, compression will cause termination of auditory signal and release of compression will resume auditory signal. If the examiner detects a signal while providing compression, this indicates a malfunctioning of the valves allowing a back flow of blood to the area.

PERCUSSION TEST

This test is used to evaluate the potency of the venous valves. The patient should be in a standing position to allow varicosities to fill with blood. The examiner places one hand on the dilated vein and the other hand approximately 20 cm proximally on the leg. The upper hand administers percussions to the proximal segment of the vein while the lower hand checks for impulse transmission. Competent valves will not allow the transmission of the impulse. If the impulse is transmitted to the lower hand, this is indicative of incompetent valves.

TRENDELENBURG TEST

The Trendelenburg test assesses valvular competency in the communicating veins and saphenous system by measuring the retrograde filling time in the lower extremities. To empty the venous blood from the limb, the patient should be positioned in supine with the leg elevated to 90 degrees. Venous blood flow is further occluded by applying a tourniquet around the proximal thigh. The patient is then asked to stand while the examiner observes the manner in which the veins refill. The normal refilling of veins should take approximately 30 seconds.[11] Rapid filling of the superficial veins with the tourniquet still in place would indicate incompetent valves in the communicating veins. The examiner should then observe the response following the release of the tourniquet. If superficial veins continue to show rapid filling, the values of the saphenous veins are incompetent.

TEST FOR DEEP VEIN THROMBOPHLEBITIS (HOMAN'S SIGN)

This test is performed to rule out the possibility of a deep vein thrombophlebitis. When perform-

ing this test, the examiner squeezes the patient's gastrocnemius while forcefully dorsiflexing the patient's ankle with the knee held in extended position. Increased firmness and tenderness elicited upon deep palpation of the gastrocnemius suggests a deep vein thrombophlebitis. This test can be rather subjective depending on the amount of force exerted by the examiner. To make this a more objective test, a blood pressure cuff may be placed around the calf and inflated to the point at which the patient experiences discomfort. Normally, individuals with deep vein thrombophlebitis cannot tolerate pressure greater than 40 mmHg.[11]

ASSESSMENT

In the assessment, the examiner compiles all subjective and objective data and uses this information to formulate short- and long-term goals of treatment. All goals should be specific and measurable. Once the goals have been established, the clinician can determine the appropriate treatment techniques to achieve these goals and ensure optimal wound management. It is in the assessment part of the evaluation that the clinician may make recommendations regarding positioning programs, pressure relief devices, edema control, method of wound cleansing/debridement, and dressing regimen.

CONCLUSION

The basic components of the wound examination have been provided. The subjective examination stresses the importance of gathering subjective information through the patient interview process. The objective examination emphasizes the importance of reviewing laboratory test results, utilizing observational skills, taking concise clinical measurements, and administering specific objective tests to determine the cause of various lesions. It is also important to look at the patient as a whole, remembering to evaluate the individual's neurological status, range of motion, strength, and mobility. The clinician has numerous objective tests available as presented in this chapter, but careful consideration should be given to select the tests that can provide the most valuable information. The assessment is the last part of the examination in which the clinician draws all information together to make realistic measurable goals and recommendations. The assessment is the basis from which a formulated treatment plan is developed.

REFERENCES

1. McCulloch J. Peripheral vascular disease. In: O'Sullivan SB, Schmitz TJ. *Physical Rehabilitation: Assessment and Treatment.* 2nd ed. Philadelphia, PA: FA Davis; 1988:371-383.
2. Correlli F. Buerger's disease: cigarette smoker disease may always be cured by medical therapy. *J Cardiovasc Surg.* 1973;14:28-36.
3. Lazarus GS, Goldsmith ZA. *Diagnosis of Skin Disease.* Philadelphia, PA: FA Davis; 1987.
4. Bell JA. *Semmes-Weinstein Monofilament Testing for Determining Cutaneous Light Touch/Deep Pressure Sensation. The Star.* Carville, LA: National Hansen's Disease Center; Nov/Dec 1984.
5. Spittell JA. *Clinical Vascular Disease.* Philadelphia, PA: FA Davis; 1983.
6. MacKinnon JL. A study of Doppler ultrasonic peripheral vascular evaluations performed by physical therapists. *Phys Ther.* 1983;63:30-34.
7. MacKinnon JL. Doppler ultrasound assessment in peripheral vascular disease. In: Kloth LC, McCulloch JM, Feedar JA. *Wound Healing: Alternatives In Management.* Philadelphia, PA: FA Davis; 1990:119-131.
8. Barker WF. Diagnostic methods in peripheral arterial disease. *Am J Surg.* 1973;39:543-548.
9. Barnes RW, Russell HE, Wilson MR. *Doppler Ultrasonic Evaluation of Venous Disease/Doppler Ultrasonic Evaluation of Peripheral Vascular Disease.* Iowa City, IA: University of Iowa; 1975.
10. Sigelk B, Popky GL, Wagner DK, Boland JP, Mapp EM, Feigl P. A doppler ultrasound method for diagnosing lower extremity venous disease. *Surg Gynecol Obstet.* 1968;127:339-350.
11. McCulloch JM, Kloth LC: Evaluation of patients with open wounds. In: Kloth LC, McCulloch JM, Feedar JA. *Wound Healing: Alternatives in Management.* Philadelphia, PA: FA Davis; 1990:99-118.

Chapter 3

General Principles of Wound Management

Lia van Rijswijk, RN, ET

During the past 50 years our knowledge of wound healing and the effect of wound treatments on this process has increased substantially. We now know that certain treatments can hinder as well as foster repair. The need to assess the outcome of treatment modalities and to use data of controlled clinical studies has gained increased attention during the past several years.[1-3] This is even more important with respect to wound care. Devices are the most commonly used wound treatment modalities. Before marketing these devices, regulatory agencies (including the United States Food and Drug Administration) do not evaluate their safety and efficacy in the same manner as they evaluate pharmaceutical agents.[4] This chapter describes specific requirements of different types of wounds, a summary of the results of wound healing research as it relates to commonly used dressings, and a review of the general principles of wound management. The effect of topical agents on wound repair are reviewed in Chapter 4. Although usually well defined and precise, the results of in vitro and in vivo research do not always accurately predict what happens in the clinic. Therefore, this chapter will focus on the results of controlled clinical studies as a basis for the recommendations in order to help apply current research findings to clinical practice.

HOW TO HELP WOUNDS HEAL

Before discussing the general principles of wound management, we should emphasize that wounds are attached to patients. Providing optimal local care should be one part of the total care plan. The cause of the wound has to be ameliorated and systemic factors that delay healing should be addressed.[3] Also, most wounds will heal without any major problems if we let the body do what it is supposed to do. In general, topical agents, dressings, and treatment modalities do not make wounds heal faster, rather, some do not hinder the repair process as much as others and are better at fostering the natural healing process.

Wound treatments are generally used to treat infection, cleanse the wound, debride the wound, provide an optimal environment for healing, relieve pain and discomfort, and prevent complications.

TREAT INFECTION

An infected wound cannot heal and should be treated appropriately. Infection can be defined as "invasion and multiplication of microorganisms in body tissues, which may be clinically inapparent or result in local cellular injury because of competitive metabolism, toxins, intracellular replication, or anti-

Figure 3-1. Assessment of risk of infection.

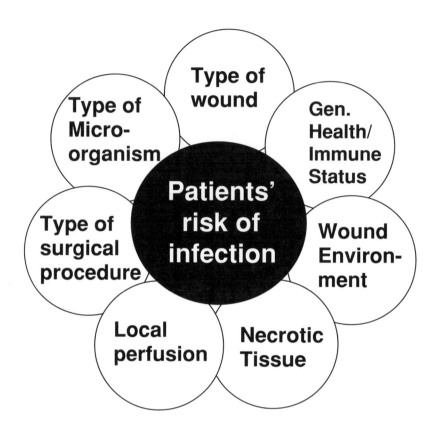

gen-antibody response."[5] Signs of microorganisms invading the surrounding tissue include: local erythema, edema, pain, impaired mobility/movement, unexplained fever, or purulent and odorous exudate.[6]

All wounds are contaminated with a variety of microorganisms, yet the majority will not get infected in part because, as Pasteur observed more than 10 decades ago, "The germ is nothing, it is the terrain in which it is found that is everything."[7] Obviously, the virulence of the microorganism is important. However, host-specific factors have been found to be very reliable predictors of the risk of infection including: the type of wound (acute or chronic) and type of surgical procedure performed, local perfusion, the presence or absence of necrotic tissue, the patient's general health and immunological status, and the wound

environment (Figure 3-1).[8-10] If a wound infection is suspected and results of a culture reviewed, it is important to remember all these risk factors and to carefully examine the wound before prescribing an antibiotic treatment regimen. Resistance to antimicrobial drugs is rapidly becoming a very serious worldwide problem.[11]

Although the best way to culture wounds remains controversial, the most accepted method is by means of a quantitative or qualitative swab. Some researchers have reported good correlation between biopsies and quantitative swab cultures.[12,13] Swab cultures sample most bacteria from the wound sur- face, whereas biopsies do not. However, if the wound is not cleansed properly prior to swabbing, the results may reflect surface colonization only.[14] An alternate method, wound fluid aspiration or swabbing the wound following careful debridement, has been shown to work quite well for diabetic ulcers, and may be helpful for other types of wounds.[15]

Once the presence of an infection has been confirmed and the infection-causing organism identified, appropriate systemic antibiotic treatment should be initiated. Penicillamines and cephalosporins are two commonly used systemic antimicrobials with a broad spectrum of activity. However, it should be noted that *Pseudomonas sp* and *enteroscoccus faecalis* are resistant to some cephalosporins.[16] Gentamicin is often used to treat infections caused by Methicillin Resistant *Staphylococcus Aureus* (MRSA). Topical agents will destroy the bacteria on the surface of the wound but most cannot penetrate into the tissue.[17]

Local wound treatment modalities can remain the same when systemic antibiotics are administered, providing the product is approved for use on infected wounds as indicated by the product package insert. If no mention is made of infected wounds, either as "indicated" or "contraindicated," it is best to discontinue use of the product. Regardless of the type of dressing or treatment used, the wound and the patient should be assessed regularly.

CLEANSE THE WOUND

Wound debris should be removed prior to dressing application, to facilitate both repair and assessment. In the clinic, wound cleansing has often been translated into "wound decontamination," even though it has been known since the late 1960s that disinfectants can damage tissue and blood vessels, and interfere with tissue function.[18,19] Refer to Chapter 4 for further detail. The use of sterile saline (under pressure if indicated) is often sufficient to achieve the goal of removing debris. Saline is also cost-effective. Evidence suggests that fluids other than saline are effective cleansers, however, at this time there are no controlled clinical studies with results that translate into indication of more expedient healing.

The recommended maximum amount of pressure to cleanse wounds is 8 to 14 psi. This can be achieved by using a 19 gauge needle (or catheter) and a 35 mL syringe, even though higher pressure may be indicated in severely contaminated or soiled wounds such as those encountered in the emergency department.[20] Whenever high-pressure irrigation is required, one should be aware of the possibility of fluid dispersion into the tissue.[21]

DEBRIDE THE WOUND

The presence of necrotic tissue or foreign matter in a wound predisposes it to infection.[22] Presence of necrotic tissue has been found to be associated with the presence of *Pseudomonas aeruginosa* and *Proteus mirabilis* in pressure ulcers.[23] These pressure ulcers were also found to heal slower. It has been postulated that once bacteria have colonized dead or foreign materials, including sutures, they are less susceptible to host defense mechanisms and antibiotic therapy.[24] Necrotic tissue also delays healing by actually splinting the wound and holding it open.[25] The necessity to debride wounds can probably be best appreciated by reviewing burn wound healing times and mortality rates of burn patients prior to and after it was feasible to excise all necrotic tissue shortly after injury.[26-28] Following debridement, the number of bacteria in the wound is decreased and the host's defense mechanism can be more effective.

There are four basic methods of debriding wounds: mechanical debridement, sharp/surgical debridement, enzymatic debridement, and autolytic debridement. For debridement techniques, also refer to Chapter 8.

Mechanical Debridement

In the past, mechanical removal of necrotic tissue by means of wet-to-dry dressings was common practice. While easy to perform, this practice may inadvertently remove healthy tissue, as well as cause trauma and pain.[3]

Sharp/Surgical Debridement

Sharp/surgical debridement is quick. Therefore, it is often recommended for wounds with a thick, leathery eschar or a compromised immune or general health status. Pain control is often required, and a skilled health care professional should perform the procedure.[29] There is some evidence that suggests that after surgical debridement, patients should be monitored for bacteremia, and coverage with a systemic antibiotic may be indicated for immunocompromised patients.[30]

Enzymatic Debridement

Enzymatic debridement is accomplished by the use of an agent to lyse fibrin, collagen, and elastin. It can be relatively quick and effective if used correctly.[31] Its use should be discontinued, however, as soon as the wound is clean and free of necrotic tissue. It should also be noted that enzymatic debriding agents do not work well on thick, leathery eschar, and that most enzymes need moisture to do their job expediently. In a controlled in vivo study, all sutilains and hydrocolloid covered necrotic wounds were debrided after 24 hours, whereas none of the sutilains and wet-to-dry gauze covered wounds were debrided.[32]

Autolytic Debridement

Autolytic debridement is nature's way of cleansing the wound by using the body's own enzymes. It is painless and selective, i.e., does not harm healthy tissues. However, it may not be very effective if the necrotic tissue is thick, leathery, and/or attached to the wound margins, and it should not be the treatment of choice in patients who are immunosuppressed.[33] Proteinase has been found in the fluid of wounds dressed with a hydrocolloid dressing (DuoDERM®, ConvaTec, a division of Bristol-Meyers Squibb, Skillman, New Jersey) as well as those dressed with a polyurethane film dressing (OpSite®, Smith & Nephew United, Key Largo, Florida).[34,35] Some of the dressings have been found to lyse fibrin, a large component of necrotic debris. All dressings that keep the wound moist will encourage autolytic debridement. However, preclinical and clinical studies have shown that the rate of fibrinolysis does differ significantly among occlusive dressings.[36,37] However, at this time it is not known whether these findings translate into more expedi-

ent autolytic debridement in the clinic. The "best" debridement method depends on the status and needs of the patient, the wound, and whether or not the patient is hospitalized. Unfortunately, there are no controlled clinical studies comparing the efficacy of the four different debridement methods described.

PROVIDE OPTIMAL ENVIRONMENT FOR HEALING

The discovery that a moisture-retentive dressing may be more beneficial for wound healing than the dressings used for centuries is one of the most important turning points in wound care, and followed a scenario that is common in medicine. Gilje treated a patient with a leg ulcer. He covered one half of the ulcer with an occlusive tape and the other half with a gauze type dressing and found that the tape-covered side healed faster.[38] Similar findings were observed by Winter in subsequent preclinical studies, and clinically it was confirmed that neither the body's own scab nor the gauze type dressings commonly used were very conducive to healing.[39-41] Many years later it was discovered that use of moisture retentive dressings not only facilitated re-epithelialization, but also influenced inflammation, as well as granulation tissue and collagen formation.[42-45] The clinical implications of these findings will be discussed later since they depend on the type of wound.

RELIEVE PAIN AND DISCOMFORT

Dressings can have a profound effect on pain. First, if the dressing adheres to the tissues, removal can be very painful. This often happens when wound exudate is absorbed into a gauze-type dressing and left to dry out. For instance, calcium alginate dressings will not dry out provided the wound is moderately or highly exudative, and, as a result, pain upon removal can be significantly reduced.[46,47] Second, dressings can also cause pain when in place, particularly when patients are ambulating. In a controlled clinical study, investigators compared Fine Mesh Gauze to DuoDERM dressings in the management of skin graft donor sites and found differences in the amount of pain as soon as patients became mobile

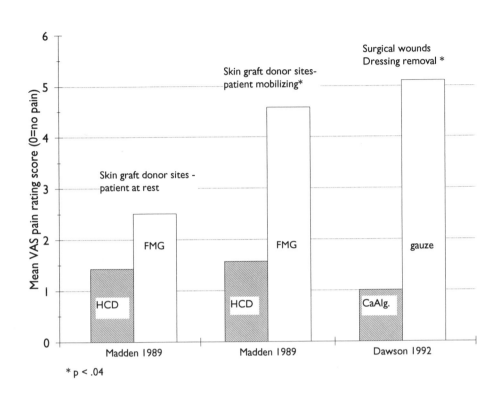

Figure 3-2. Effects of various dressings on pain level. HCD = hydrocolloid; FMG = fine mesh gauze; CaAlg = calcium alginate.

(Figure 3-2).[48] Similarly, patients with second-degree burns have consistently been found to experience less pain and be more comfortable when a moisture-retentive dressing was used, as compared to gauze with a topical antimicrobial ointment.[48-52]

Other controlled clinical studies of acute and chronic wounds have also shown that the use of moisture-retentive dressings results in less pain and discomfort than traditional gauze type dressings.[53-57] The reason for the reported reduction in pain is not clear, although it seems likely that protection of exposed nerve endings, as well as reduced inflammation, may play a role. To date, only three studies have compared skin graft donor site pain following treatment with two different moisture-retentive dressings (hydrocolloid versus polyurethane film dressing). In one study, no differences were reported, whereas in the other two studies, the hydrocolloid dressing was found to be more comfortable.[48,58,59]

Pain may affect rehabilitation, time away from work, and possibly healing since stress may also play an important role in the healing process.[48,60-63] Finally, no matter what kind of additional benefits can be achieved by increasing patient comfort, it is important to remember that "patients have a right to treatment that includes prevention or adequate relief of pain."[64]

PREVENT COMPLICATIONS

Loss of skin integrity can cause complications. One way in which treatment modalities can reduce the chance of complications is by enabling a wound to close as expediently as possible. However, studies have shown that wound care practices can reduce the incidence of complications in more ways than one.

Prevention of Dehydration and Infection

First, treatments can prevent wound dehydration. If a wound dries out, cells die, become necrotic, and the wound becomes deeper. This phenomenon has been aptly demonstrated by Zawacki, who found that superficial, second-degree burn wounds will convert to deep second-degree burns if they dry out.[65,66] Second, wound treatments can play a very important role in the prevention of infections. In addition to preventing necrotic tissue formation, which acts as a foreign body predisposing the wound to infection, moisture-retentive dressings allow the cells designed to protect against microbial invasion to be kept alive. Viable polymorphonuclear leukocytes, macrophages, lymphocytes, and monocytes have been found in the fluid that accumulates underneath these dressings.[67] Control of wound pH may also be important for this reason. A low pH of 5.8 to 6.6 may correlate to a reduced bacterial proliferation, and dressings have been found to influence the pH of wounds.[68]

Even though research in this area is limited, there are a number of clinical reports that corroborate these findings. Analysis of published infection rates showed that the rate of wound infections can range from 7.1% for wounds dressed with conventional, non-occlusive dressings, to 2.4% for foam and 1.3% for hydrocolloid dressed wounds.[69] Similarly, in prospective, controlled clinical studies, the infection rate of hydrocolloid dressed wounds was lower as compared to gauze dressed wounds.[48,70]

In addition to the effect of dressings on the wound environment, there may be other reasons for this phenomenon. Preclinical studies have shown that some dressings provide a barrier against microbial invasion.[71] Depending on the physical characteristics of the dressing, i.e., adhesion and permeability, bacteria and other external contaminants such as urine or feces will not come in contact with the wound. A few studies exploring the effect of dressings on cross-contamination have also been conducted. In a noncontrolled study, it was found that MRSA present in a wound did not penetrate the hydrocolloid dressing used, thus eliminating the need for patient isolation.[72] In another study, dressing type significantly influenced the number of organisms released into the air following removal.[73] With the increasing incidence of MRSA, particularly in chronic wounds, these discoveries merit further investigation.[74] Similarly, the findings by Bowler and associates, which showed that neither the human immunodeficiency virus (HIV) nor the hepatitis B virus (HBV) penetrated the DuoDERM dressings tested, could

have significant implications for patients and health care professionals alike.[75]

Prevention of Allergic Reactions

Patients with chronic wounds, particularly leg ulcers, often become sensitized to topical agents and adhesives. Approximately half of all leg ulcer patients have been reported to be allergic to routine topical medications.[76] Common allergens include: wool alcohols (lanolins), Parabens (preservatives), Cetylstearyl alcohol base, neomycin sulphate, Framycetin, and bandage additives such as Ester gum resin, colophony, and MBT thiuram (rubber). As a result, the use of hypoallergenic and non-sensitizing products is very important, specifically in patients with chronic wounds.

Allergic reactions are not always related to treatment modalities. Increasing numbers of patients have been found to be allergic to rubber-based products, and contact with the Latex gloves of the health care practitioner can provoke a reaction. Latex is found in a wide range of products. Patients with congenital defects (e.g., spina bifida) are most at risk for developing serious reactions as a result of frequent exposure to Latex products at an early age. Health care professionals are another "high-risk" group for developing allergies to Latex.[77]

Prevention of Skin Breakdown

When the surrounding skin of wounds breaks down, there is more tissue to repair and wound healing is delayed. Skin breakdown in patients with chronic wounds is most often a direct result of an underlying pathology such as shear, friction, or pressure in patients with pressure ulcers, and inadequate compression in patients with venous ulcers. Even the best topical treatment modality cannot compensate for inadequately addressing the underlying etiology of these wounds. However, sometimes wound treatment modalities do cause skin irritation and subsequent breakdown.

First, if a treatment modality is used inappropriately, the newly formed epithelium may break down again. Examples include application of enzymatic debriding agents onto the surrounding skin, or leaving an occlusive dressing in place when it has been completely saturated causing wound exudate to pool onto the surrounding skin for a number of days. Second, when caring for patients with surgical wounds, the use of tapes and adhesives can cause irritation and papular eruption.[78]

General Complications Related to Product Usage

While complications secondary to the use of a device (including dressings) are often considered "patient or caregiver related," that may not always be the case. If it is suspected that it may be related to the product itself and/or the way it interacts with the patient, it is important to report it to the manufacturer or the appropriate regulatory agency, particularly when a product has just been released for marketing. This type of feedback could prove very valuable and may have the potential to save unnecessary pain and suffering.[79] Most countries have regulatory reporting systems designed to encourage health care professionals to report adverse events and product problems. In the United States call the FDA at 800-FDA-1088.

Finally, unless a product package insert indicates otherwise, it is usually not recommended to "combine" different wound care products. First, the efficacy of the "combination" may be unknown, and second, if a complication develops, it will be difficult to ascertain which product caused the problem.

DIFFERENT WOUNDS HAVE DIFFERENT NEEDS

Acute wounds are different from chronic wounds, and superficial wounds cannot be compared to deep wounds. When trying to ascertain treatment efficacy, it is particularly important to distinguish one type of wound from another. While an overview of the literature by wound type is provided, it must be remembered that systemic as well as other local factors (including size and location) also influence a

Table 3-1. **Wound Types and Depth**		
Type of Wound	Skin Structures Involved	Wound Depth
Abrasion Blister Tape damage	Epidermis	Superficial
Abrasion Skin graft donor site Shave biopsy Second-degree burn Partial-thickness leg or pressure ulcer*	Epidermis and dermis	Partial-thickness
Surgical incision Punch biopsy Third-degree burn Penetrating wound Full-thickness leg or pressure ulcer**	Epidermis, dermis, adipose tissue (muscle)	Full-thickness

*Usually referred to as a Stage II pressure ulcer.
**Usually referred to as a Stage III pressure ulcer (National Pressure Ulcer Advisory Panel, 1989).

wound's response to treatment. The effect of these factors is discussed in Chapter 1.

ACUTE WOUNDS

Acute wounds are either sutured or left to heal by secondary intention and can be superficial involving the dermis, or involving the dermis as well as underlying structures (Table 3-1).

Surgical and Traumatic Sutured Wounds

To close a wound with sutures, the tissues should be clean and handled with care. Inappropriate wound-closure materials and/or poor technique can interfere with wound healing.[80] Wounds closed with sutures usually heal rapidly and re-epithelialization may occur as soon as 24 hours after surgery.[81] Traditionally, these wounds have been covered to protect the incision, and sometimes more importantly, to hide the wound from the patient's view. However, preclinical data suggest that the type of dressing used can influence the repair process of sutured wounds, and specifically, reduce inflammation.[42] In the clinic, this may result in a finer, less pigmented and flatter scar, at least up until 1 month after healing has occurred.[53,82,83] The exact mechanisms involved are, as of yet, not completely understood. However, there is evidence to suggest that a reduced inflammatory and cytokine response will result in less scarring without compromising wound strength.[84] In a series of case studies involving 3637 patients, Rubio found that the use of three different types of polyurethane film dressings, following clean surgical procedures, was convenient, safe, and facilitated patient mobility and hygiene.[85] In his comparison of three different methods of wound closure (polyurethane film versus nylon sutures versus clips) Eaton found that OpSite dressed incisions healed well, and the cosmetic results were better as compared to the control treatments.[86] Recent studies of the use of a thin hydrocolloid dressing (DuoDERM Extra Thin CGF) have focused on patient convenience issues such as ease of use and the ability to bathe or shower.[87] In a controlled clinical study of 88 children who underwent outpatient surgical procedures, the thin hydrocolloid dressing was found to be significantly less painful than conventional gauze and tape dressings. Parents especially appreciated not having to change the dressings and being able to bathe children who were still in diapers.[88] Thus, even though research into the area of surgical wound dressings is very limited at this time, there is evidence to suggest that they can influence the repair process as well as the patient's quality of life.

In summary, a dressing for sutured wounds should be safe and protect the wound from physical or chemical damage and microbial contamination. It should not interfere with the healing process and should be comfortable, flexible, easy to use and facilitate personal hygiene. When used properly, moisture-retentive and occlusive dressings can offer significant advantages over the traditional technique of caring for surgical wounds.[89]

Surgical and Traumatic Non-Sutured Wounds

Examples of surgical and traumatic wounds that are left to heal by secondary intention include: heavily contaminated or dehisced wounds, contaminated traumatic wounds, second-degree burn wounds, skin graft donor sites, dermabrasions as well as some biopsy and surgical excision (i.e., Mohs surgery) wounds. These wounds need a dressing that protects against the environment, is comfortable, and facilitates repair. If the wound is clean and superficial, the dressing should help re-epithelialization. If the wound is clean and deep, it should also facilitate the formation of granulation tissue. In otherwise healthy patients, healing time of these wounds depends mainly on wound depth and the type of dressing used (Table 3-2).

Clean, Surgical, and Traumatic Partial-Thickness Wounds

Controlled clinical studies have shown that skin graft donor sites take anywhere from 7 to 20 days to heal, depending on wound depth and the type of dressing used (see Table 3-2). Fortunately, many different types of dressings have been carefully evaluated in the management of these wounds, thus clinical decisions are a little less difficult to make.[58-60,70,90-129] In general, wounds covered with occlusive dressings heal faster as compared to wounds dressed with conventional gauze, with or without topical antimicrobial ointments. However, differences among the various occlusive and moisture-retentive dressings have been observed. The reason(s) for these differences are, at this time, not fully understood.

Contaminated or Dehisced Surgical Wounds

Heavily contaminated and/or dehisced wounds will either undergo delayed surgical closure or be left to heal by secondary intention. The primary objection to reclosure of dehisced wounds is the risk of repeat infection. However, studies suggest that chances of repeated infection are 1% to 14% depending on various patient- and wound-related variables, and that healing time is significantly reduced when the wound can be surgically closed.[130-132] Unfortunately, surgery is not always an option, and many wounds are left to granulate and re-epithelialize. In

Table 3-2. Prospective, Controlled Clinical Studies on Acute Superficial and Partial-Thickness Wounds Left to Heal by Secondary Intention

Author	Type of Wound	Treatment and Healing	Comment
Barnett (1983)	Skin graft donor sites	Fine mesh gauze: mean 10.5 days Tegaderm film dr: mean 6.7 days OpSite film dr: mean 6.9 days	No statistical analysis
Blight (1991)	Skin graft donor sites	Vaseline impregn. gauze: average 19.4 days Cultured epithelial graft: average 11 days OpSite film dr: average 10.5 days	p<.02 compared to gauze
Hermans (1986)	Superficial second-degree burns	Silver sulfadiazine and gauze: average 11 days Human allografts: average 12 days DuoDERM HCD dr: average 8 days	No statistical analysis
	Partial-thickness second-degree burns	Silver sulfadiazine and gauze: average 19.5 days Human allografts: average 16.5 days DuoDERM HCD dr: average 12.5 days	
Lawrence (1991)	Skin graft donor sites	Scarlet Red dr: 85% of wounds healed on day 10 Kaltostat CaAlg dr: 72% of wounds healed on day 10	p<.04
Nemeth (1991)	Shave biopsies	Bacitracin and gauze: 63% of wounds healed at 2 weeks DuoDERM HCD dr: 100% of wounds healed at 2 weeks	p<.05
Phillips (1993)	Shave biopsies	Bacitracin and gauze: 88% of wounds healed at 1 week Cutinova Hydro HCD dr: 84% of wounds healed at 1 week	p>.05
Porter (1991)	Skin graft donor sites	Kaltostat CaAlg dr: mean 15.5 days DuoDERM HCD dr: mean 10 days	p<.05
Poulsen (1991)	Second-degree out-patient burns	Silver sulfadiazine and gauze: median 7 days OpSite film dressing: median 10 days	p>.05
Rohrich (1991)	Skin graft donor sites	OpSite film dressing: mean 12.7 days DuoDERM CGF HCD dr: mean 11.7 days	p>.05
Tan (1993)	Skin graft donor sites	Zenoderm hydrogel: 75% of wounds healed day 10 DuoDERM CGF HCD dr: 97% of wounds healed day 10	p=.02
Waffle (1988)	Second-degree out-patient burns	Silver sulfadiazine and gauze: average 10.6 days OpSite film dressing: average 9.18 days	p>.05
Wyatt (1990)	Second-degree out-patient burns	Silver sulfadiazine and gauze: mean 15.5 days DuoDERM HCD dr: mean 10.2 days	p<.01

This listing is not complete, rather, it includes a variety of treatment modalities studied in this type of wound. Additional controlled clinical studies are listed in Table 3-4.

addition to following the basic wound management principles related to treating an infection, debridement, and cleansing, these wounds need an environment that protects, prevents secondary complications, is comfortable, and facilitates the formation of granulation tissue. Many patients with dehisced wounds are discharged and the ideal treatment would also facilitate personal hygiene, mobility, and be easy to use. Since these wounds are usually quite deep, several case studies regarding the use of wound-filler products and dressings have reported good results.[133-137] In a controlled study it was found that wounds dressed with a moisture-retentive dressing (a hydrogel, foam, or film dressing) could be surgically closed an average of 3 days earlier as compared to those treated with traditional saline moistened wet-to-dry dressings.[138] Similarly, in a controlled double-blind study of penetrating chest wounds, those dressed with a hydrocolloid were found to heal significantly faster as compared to those dressed with petrolatum impregnated gauze dressing.[139] However, when calcium alginates were compared to gauze dressings, no healing time differences were observed.[47] In another study, aloe vera gel-treated, deshisced wounds healed after a mean of 83 days, and saline/sodium hypochlorite solution impregnated gauze dressed wounds healed after a mean of 53 days.[140]

Very few controlled clinical studies on deshisced and/or contaminated wounds have been published and, with respect to healing, the results are not entirely consistent. However, these wounds are often very painful and in all studies, patients report that the moisture-retentive or occlusive dressings are comfortable (see Figure 3-2).

Clean, Surgical, and Traumatic Full Thickness Wounds

Deep wounds take longer to heal than partial-thickness wounds and they need a dressing to facilitate granulation tissue formation. In a study comparing healing times of biopsy wounds, 100% of partial-thickness shave biopsies and 36% of punch biopsies dressed with a hydrocolloid healed after 2 weeks whereas only 63% of shave biopsies and 7% of punch biopsies treated with a topical antimicrobial and gauze healed after 2 weeks.[54] Similarly, facial excision wounds were reported to heal after a median of 20 days when dressed with a polyurethane film versus 26 days when treated with a topical antimicrobial ointment and gauze dressing.[53] In both controlled clinical studies wounds dressed with conventional treatments were more painful. The number of controlled clinical studies on the management of clean, deep wounds is limited compared to the number of studies on partial-thickness wounds, but the trend is the same: moisture-retentive or occlusive dressings facilitate healing and reduce pain as compared to gauze control.

CHRONIC WOUNDS

When repeated insult interrupts or destroys tissue formation or when one or more chemical or cellular elements of the healing process are deficient, a wound can become chronic. Often, but not always, these events are signaled by renewed or chronic inflammation and the inflamed or swollen wound alerts its caregiver to search for a cause of renewed or chronic tissue breakdown.[3] When the existing imbalance between the underlying etiology and the wound environment can be restored by removing the cause of the wound and improving the wound environment, these wounds will heal.

Pressure Ulcers

The general principles of wound management also apply to pressure ulcers, e.g., necrotic tissue should be removed and the wound cleansed. Theoretically, when the underlying etiology has been addressed, chronic wounds should heal at approximately the same rate as acute wounds. Unfortunately, not all pressure ulcer studies report the time to healing by ulcer depth. When they do, time to healing (or proportion of patients healed during the study) is consistently shown to be related to ulcer depth (Table 3-3).[141-145] When reviewing the data in Table 3-3, it is clear that extrapolation and comparison of study results is difficult. Healing time analysis methods vary from one study to the other, and when proportions of healed patients are calculated, a median or mean time to healing is not always reported. Also, in many studies, patients with multiple ulcers are enrolled and the results are analyzed per ulcer. This violates the assumption of independence upon which the data analysis is based. Other covariates that have been found to influence the healing of pressure ulcers such as nutritional status, use of pressure ulcer relieving measures, incontinence, mobility, and age may further dilute the effect of treatments studied.[143,148-154]

Table 3-3. Reported Healing Rates of Pressure Ulcers

Author	Type of Study/ Number of Wounds (N)	Treatment Result (Healing) by Ulcer Depth (and Dressing Type)	Comment
Berlowitz (1990)	Prospective review of patient records; long-term care hospital (N = 89)	Saline or povidone-iodine gauze dressings, surgical or enzymatic debridement. After 6 weeks, 65% of Stage II, 14% of Stage III, and 0% of Stage IV ulcers were healed.	$p<.001$
Gorse (1987)	Prospective, controlled; acute care facilities (N = 76 wounds, 27 patients)	Dakin's solution/gauze: 63% of Stage II ulcers healed (mean 8.7 days) and 0% of Stage III ulcers healed. DuoDERM HCD dr: 75% of Stage II ulcers healed (mean 8.2 days) and 4% of Stage III ulcers healed.	Statistical analysis by ulcer, not by patient. $p<.05$
Ferrell (1993)	Prospective, controlled; nursing home residents (N = 84)	Gauze with saline or antiseptics, or semi-permeable dressings for both Rx groups. Pat. on foam mattress: median time to healing Stage II ulcer: 53 days. Median for Stages III and IV could not be calculated (<50% healed during 90-day study). Pat. on LAL* bed: median time for Stage II ulcers to heal: 30 days. Median for Stages III and IV ulcers could not be calculated.	$p>.05$
Neill (1989)	Prospective, controlled; tertiary care facility and nursing home (N = 87)	Saline soaked gauze dr: 26% of Stage II and 9% of Stage III ulcers healed after 8 weeks. Tegasorb HCD dr: 44% of Stage II and 12% of Stage III ulcers healed after 8 weeks.	$p>.05$ Statistical analysis by ulcer, not by patient. High drop-out rate.
Sebern (1986)	Prospective, controlled; home health care (N = 77 wounds, 48 patients)	Hydrogen peroxide and saline/gauze: 0% of Stage II and 0% of Stages III and IV ulcers were healed after 6 weeks. Tegaderm PUF dressing: 64% of Stage II and 0% of Stages III and IV ulcers were healed after 6 weeks.	Statistical analysis by ulcer, not by patient. $p<.001$ for stage II only.
Xakellis (1992)	Prospective, controlled; long-term care (N = 39)	Saline moistened gauze: 86% of Stage II** ulcers healed (median 11 days). DuoDERM HCD dr: 89% of Stage II ulcers healed (median 9 days).	$p>.05$

*LAL = Low-air-loss
** 2 of 21 patients had a Stage III ulcer
This listing is not complete, rather, it includes a variety of treatment modalities studied by initial ulcer depth/Stage. Additional controlled clinical studies are listed in Table 3-4.

When reviewing the results of the above mentioned, as well as other controlled and non-controlled studies, the results do not seem to contradict those reported for acute wounds.[143,145-147,155-169] Pressure ulcers will heal more expediently and are less painful when kept moist. However, the number of problems and adverse experiences reported with different types of dressings range from 0% to 18%, suggesting that these dressings should be chosen carefully.

Leg Ulcers

Patients with venous ulcers account for 80% to 90% of all patients with lower-extremity ulceration, arterial disease accounts for another 5% to 10%, and most others are due to neuropathy or combinations of those diseases.[170] Although the exact mechanism of venous ulceration at the cellular level remains controversial, ambulatory venous hypertension leads to tissue trauma, which in turn, results in ulceration. Therefore, compression therapy remains one of the most important components of venous ulcer management. However, it is very important to diagnose these ulcers prior to initiating any type of wound treatment modality since compression therapy is not indicated in patients with arterial or neuropathic ulcers (see Chapter 7).

Like other chronic wounds, leg ulcers present the clinician interested in evaluating the effect of treatments with many covariants that may be difficult to control. Variables found to delay healing include: increased age, deep vein involvement, longer duration of the ulcer, large baseline area, male sex, strong wound odor at baseline, the presence of diabetes mellitus, and the country in which the study is conducted.[171-175] Despite the presence of these variables and the different study and data analysis methods employed, results of the controlled clinical studies available do show a trend. First, pain, which is a significant problem for leg ulcer patients, is reduced when moisture-retentive dressings are used, and second, most of these dressings facilitate the healing process.[174-181]

However, the results are not always consistent. A few studies involving the use of film, foam, or hydrocolloid dressings report no difference in time to healing as compared to traditional gauze type dressings. Whether these results are related to the treatment modalities studied or an unequal distribution of confounding variables is unknown. However, in a few studies the treatment group did not receive compression therapy.[173,174,182,183] Also, differences in healing rates and the number of adverse experiences and allergic reactions between different types of hydrocolloid dressings have been observed.[184-186] It has been postulated that one reason for the observed difference in healing is related to fibrin, since the fibrin cuffs that are present in the skin surrounding venous ulcers may contribute to impaired tissue oxygenation, nutrient exchange, and/or trap growth factors and other stimulatory or homeostatic substances necessary for tissue repair.[36,37,187] Specifically, it has been shown that following 1 week of treatment

patients with venous ulcers randomized to hydrocolloid dressing (DuoDERM) and compression therapy were significantly more likely to have a reduction in the number of fibrin cuffs as compared to patients who received compression treatment only.[188] Even though the exact role of fibrin cuffs in venous disease is not completely understood, further studies into the capability of dressings to influence the pathophysiology of the wounds appear warranted and may help answer the many remaining questions.

In summary, leg ulcer patients need a dressing that reduces pain and facilitates the healing process. Clinical studies have shown that most moisture-retentive dressings do reduce pain and also that 50% to 80% of patients heal when these dressings are used. However, in the case of venous ulcers, occlusive dressings should not replace the use of compression therapy.

CLINICAL DECISIONS

Chances are that every time one reads a journal or attends a conference new dressings are added to the multitude of products available today. Treatment decisions should be based not only on what the patient and the wound need, but also on the results of the controlled clinical studies available for the product intended to be used (Figure 3-3). Table 3-4 contains a listing of commonly used wound dressings, their features, benefits, and indications, as well as references to the controlled clinical studies on different types of wounds published in peer-reviewed journals.

Once a treatment modality has been selected, careful monitoring of the healing process is warranted. Refer to Tables 3-2 and 3-3 for data on time of wound healing. The importance of measuring wounds frequently, and carefully recording their depth and size, as well the presence of granulation and necrotic tissue, cannot be overemphasized. First, it will provide a permanent record of the status of the wound at different times and encourage other caregivers to adopt the same evaluation method

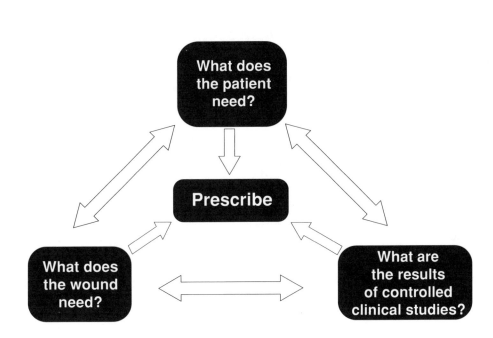

Figure 3-3. Treatment prescription based on controlled clinical studies.

when they are changing the dressings. Second, frequent measurements may reduce unnecessary suffering. Recent studies have shown that reduction in ulcer area after 2 or 4 weeks of treatment is a predictor of treatment outcome and time to healing of deep pressure ulcers as well as venous leg ulcers.[153,154,172,175,189] In general, if an ulcer does not exhibit a 30% reduction in area after 2 weeks of treatment, extra efforts to diagnose and treat additional causes of tissue breakdown and/or a change in the treatment modalities are indicated. Also, the possibility of carcinomatous degeneration in wounds of long duration, such as pressure ulcers, pilonidal sinuses, and leg ulcers, should always be considered if a wound fails to respond to treatment.[170,190,191]

Another part of the clinical decision equation, treatment cost, deserves attention. When discussing treatment cost, one tends to focus on product price. However, product cost is almost always lower than the cost of nursing or medical care.[192,193] As a result, treatment methods that reduce the amount of time it takes to care for wounds have consistently been found to be cost-effective.[146,147,160,164,166,194,195]

CONCLUSION

It is the clinician's responsibility to help patients deal the best they can. Clinicians must continuously monitor procedures and compare them to the outcomes reported in the literature. "We need to make every effort to look for scientific support for the things we do clinically and to insist that our successors, today's students and residents, are imbued with a spirit of critical inquiry rather than with the passing of the torch the way we have always done it."[1]

REFERENCES

1. Silen W. Veritas, dogma, and numbers. *Arch Surg.* 1993;128:12-14.
2. ICWM consensus statement: wound management. *Ostomy Wound Manage.* 1993;39:80-84.
3. Bolton L, van Rijswijk L. Wound dressings: meeting clinical and biological needs. *Derm Nurs.* 1991;3:146-161.
4. Kessler DA, Pape SM, Sundwall DN. The federal regulation of medical devices. *N Engl J Med.* 1987;317:357-366.
5. *Dorland's Illustrated Medical Dictionary.* 26th ed. Philadelphia, PA: WB Saunders Co; 1985.
6. Altemeier W, Burkerts F, Pruitt B, Sandusky W. *Manual on Control of Infection in Surgical Patients.* 2nd ed. Philadelphia, PA: JB Lippincott; 1984.

Table 3-4. Controlled Clinical Trials Published in Peer-Reviewed Journals by Dressing Type

Material Description/Agent	Trade Name	Manufacturer	References, Controlled Clinical Studies
Nonsynthetic dressings: Not impregnated **Indications: All wound sites** **General features: Cover wound/absorb exudate**			
Woven gauze	Kling Kerlix Generic	Johnson & Johnson Medical Kendall Healthcare Products Several	159 47, 50, 53, 83, 88, 101, 140, 143, 146, 147, 158, 161, 166, 169, 194, 204, 205, 208
Gauze packing wound/strips	Nu-gauze packing	Johnson & Johnson Medical	
Fine mesh gauze*	Generic	Several	48, 90, 99, 106, 108, 124, 114, 124
Coarse mesh gauze* *Differentiated by number threads per square inch	Generic	Several	
Nonsynthetic dressings: Impregnated **Indications: All wound sites** **General features: Cover wound, absorb exudate, some are non-adherent**			
Soft paraffin, vegetable oil	Several	Several	52, 55, 91, 95, 96, 98, 103, 105, 119, 120, 126, 173, 176, 180, 201
Petrolatum	Vaseline gauze	Sherwood Medical	106, 139
Hydrophylic petrolatum	Adaptic gauze	Johnson & Johnson Medical	182, 202
Furacin	Furacin Soluble Dressing	Norwich Eaton Pharm	112, 117, 124
Sodium chloride	Mesalt	Scott Health Care	197
Bismuth tribromophenate	Xeroform	Sherwood Medical	70, 82, 106, 109, 115, 125, 127
Scarlet Red	Scarlet Red gauze	Chesebrough-Ponds	94, 100, 102, 111, 116, 118
Saline	Dermagran	Dermasciences	
Zinc oxide, calamine, gelatin (compression bandage)	Unna Boot double layer bandage (generic)	Several	56, 174, 175, 177, 179, 181, 188, 198, 199

7. Pasteur L. De l'attenuation virus du cholera des poules. *Compte Rendus de l'Academic des Sciences.* 1880;91:673-680.
8. Cruse PJE, Foord R. The epidemiology of wound infection: a 10 year prospective study of 62,939 wounds. *Surg Clin N Am.* 1980;60:27-40.
9. Hutchinson JJ, McGuckin M. Occlusive dressings: a microbiologic and clinical review. *Am J Inf Control.* 1990;18:257-268.
10. Meakins JL. Guidelines for prevention of surgical site infection. In: Wilmore DW, Brenna MF, Harken AH, Holcorft JW, Meakins JL. *Care of the Surgical Patient. IX Infection.* New York, NY: Scientific American; 1993:3-12.
11. Kunin CM. Resistance to antimicrobial drugs: a worldwide calamity. *Ann Int Med.* 1993;118:557-561.
12. Thomson PD, Taddonio TE, Tait MJ, Rice T, Prasad J, Smith DJ. Correlation between swab and biopsy for the quantification of burn wound microflora. *Proc Int Cong Burn Inj.* 1990;8:381.
13. Levine NS, Lindberg RB, Mason AD, Pruitt BA. The quantitative swab culture and smear: a quick, simple method for determining the number of viable aerobic bacteria on open wounds. *J Trauma.* 1976;16:89-94.
14. Rudensky B, Lischits M, Isaacsohn M, Sonnenblick M. Infected pressure sores: comparison of methods for bacterial identification. *Southern Med J.* 1992;85:901-903.

Table 3-4. **Controlled Clinical Trials Published in Peer-Reviewed Journals by Dressing Type (Continued)**

Material Description/Agent	Trade Name	Manufacturer	References, Controlled Clinical Studies
Synthetic and semisynthetic dressings **Indications: All wound sites** **General features: Cover wound, absorb exudate, some are non-adherent**			
Polyamide	Owens Surgical dressing Cover-Roll	David & Geck Beiersdorf Inc.	
Polyester/cellulose	Nu-Gauze	Johnson & Johnson Medical	
Cellulose with aquaphor	Aquaphor	Beiersdorf Inc.	124
Cellulose/combination	Sofsorb	DeRoyal Industries	
Non-woven polymer	N-Terface	Winfield Lab	125
Cellulose-polyester combination	Telfa Release Coverlet/Coverpad® Band-Aid dressings Curad bandages Medipore Dress-it Exu-Dry Covaderm	Kendall Healthcare Johnson & Johnson Medical Beiersdorf Inc. Johnson & Johnson Medical Kendall Healthcare 3M Health Care Frastec wound care products DeRoyal Industries	201 54, 97
Synthetic and semisynthetic dressings, polymers, and polymer composites **Indications: IV sites, acute and chronic superficial wounds** **General features: Moist wound environment, some provide bacterial barrier, translucent or transparent, conform to wound/adhesive, may foster autolytic debridement, reduce pain**			
Polyurethane film	Bioclusive HydroDerm OpSite	Johnson & Johnson Medical Willshire Med Prod. Smith & Nephew United	53, 85, 122 48, 51, 52, 58, 59, 68, 85, 86, 98, 99, 102, 121, 122, 126, 128, 129, 156, 158, 164, 203, 204
	ACU-Derm Tegaderm Polyskin II Uniflex	Acme United Corp. 3M Health Care Kendall Healthcare Smith & Nephew United	83, 85, 99, 147, 205, 207
Polyester film	Blisterfilm	Sherwood Medical	

15. Lipsky BA, Pecoraro RE, Larson SA, Hanley ME, Ahroni JH. Outpatient management of uncomplicated lower extremity infections in diabetic patients. *Arch Int Med.* 1990;150:790-797.
16. *Physicians' Desk Reference.* Montvale, NJ: Medical Economics Co; 1992.
17. Berger SA, Barza M, Haher J, et al. Penetration of antibiotics in decubitus ulcers. *J Antimicrob Chemother.* 1981;7:193-195.
18. Bränemark PI, Albrektsson B, Linstrom J, Lundborg G. Local tissue effects of wound disinfectants. *Acta Chir Scand.* 1966;357(suppl):166-167.
19. Bränemark PI, Ekholm R. Tissue injury caused by wound disinfectant. *J Bone Joint Surg.* 1967;49A:48-61.
20. Stevenson TR, Thacker JG, Rodeheaver GT, et al. Cleansing the traumatic wound by high pressure syringe irrigation. *J Am Coll Phys.* 1976;5:17-21.
21. Wheeler CB, Rodeheaver GT, Thacker JG, Edgerton MT. Side effects of high pressure irrigation. *Surg Gynecol Obstet.* 1976;143:775-778.
22. Elek SD. Experimental staphylococcal infections in the skin of man. *Ann NY Acad Sc.* 1956;65:85-90.
23. Daltrey DC, Rhodes B, Chattwood JG. Investigation into the microbial flora of healing and non-healing decubitus

Table 3-4. **Controlled Clinical Trials Published in Peer-Reviewed Journals by Dressing Type (Continued)**

Material Description/Agent	Trade Name	Manufacturer	References, Controlled Clinical Studies
Synthetic and semisynthetic dressings, polymers, and polymer composites Indications: Abrasions, blisters, donor sites, chronic wounds, minor burns General features: Provide moist or partially moist environment, some provide bacterial barrier, may foster autolytic debridement, some are adhesive or become adhesive over time			
Polyurethane foam/composite	Mitraflex Allevyn	Calgon Vestal Smith & Nephew United	138, 181, 183
Polyurethane foam	Synthaderm Lyofoam Epi-lock	Armour Pharm Co. Acme United Corp. Calgon Vestal	179, 180, 197 108, 207 101
Gauze/polyurethane foam and film	Ventex Covaderm Plus	Kendall Healthcare Prod. DeRoyal Industries	200
Silastic foam	Silastic foam	Dow Corning Corp.	57
Polyacrylate	Hydron	Allergan Pharm	
PTFE Teflon/PDMS Silastic	Silon	BioMed Sciences	125
Polyethylene film/ polyurethane foam	Epigard	Ormed Med. Techn.	
Crosslinked polymer/polyethylene oxide (hydrogels) with or without polyethylene film backing	Vigilon Geliperm Spenco 2nd skin Intrasite Gel Clear Site Nu-Gel Royl-Derm Biofilm Aquasorb	Bard Altana Inc. Spenco Medical Corp. Smith & Nephew United New Dimensions in Med. Johnson & Johnson Medical Acme United Corp. BF Goodrich Co. DeRoyal Industries	121, 122 123 138 167,173
Hydrogel/polyurethane or gauze combination	Carrington hydrogel dr. Viasorb Elastogel Plus	Carrington Sherwood Medical Southwest Technologies	140

ulcers. *J Clin Pathol.* 1981;34:701-705.

24. Keighley MRB, Burdon DW. Aetiology of surgical infection. In: Keighley MRB, Burdon DW. *Antimicrobial Prophylaxis in Surgery.* Kent, UK: Pitman Medical Publishing Co Ltd; 1979:1-22.

25. Constantine B, Bolton L. A wound model for ischemic ulcers in the guinea pig. *Arch Derm Res.* 1986;278:429-431.

26. Evans AJ. Experiences of the burns unit: a review of 520 cases. *BMJ.* 1957;1:547-551.

27. Demling RH. Improved survival after massive burns. *J Trauma.* 1983;23:179-184.

28. Sorensen B, Thomsen M. The burns unit in Copenhagen. III: treatment and mortality. *Scan J Plast Reconstr Surg.* 1968;2:16-23.

29. Holm J, Andren B, Grafford K. Pain control in the surgical debridement of leg ulcers by the use of a topical lidocaine-prilocaine cream, Emla. *Acta Derm Venereol (Stockh).* 1990;70:132-136.

Table 3-4. Controlled Clinical Trials Published in Peer-Reviewed Journals by Dressing Type (Continued)

Material Description/Agent	Trade Name	Manufacturer	References, Controlled Clinical Studies
Synthetic and semisynthetic dressings, polymers, and polymer composites (hydrocolloids) Indications: Abrasions, blisters, donor sites, minor burns, chronic wounds (check labeling for depth and wound type) General features: Moist wound environment, some provide bacterial barrier and lyse fibrin, adhesive, foster autolytic debridement, reduce pain, protect against re-injury.			
Hydrocolloid (formulations vary)/foam and/or film combination	Comfeel Ulcer dr.	Coloplast Inc.	37, 169, 184
	Comfeel Transp. dr.	Coloplast Inc.	96
	Comfeel Extra abs. dr.	Coloplast Inc.	186
	Cutinova Hydro	Beiersdorf Inc.	97
	DuoDERM Hydroactive dr.	ConvaTec	37, 48-50, 54, 59, 88, 90, 91, 110, 113, 119-122, 139, 143, 145, 146, 160, 162, 165, 166, 168, 174-176, 178, 182, 183, 185, 188, 199, 202, 208-210
	DuoDERM CGF dr.	ConvaTec	56, 58, 92, 93, 95, 100, 177, 184, 194, 200
	DuoDERM Extra Thin CGF dr.	ConvaTec	82
	RepliCare	Smith & Nephew United	
	Restore	Hollister	37, 162, 165, 209
	Restore Extra-Thin dr.	Hollister	
	Sween-A-Peel	Sween	
	Tegasorb	3M Health Care	145, 209
	Ultec	Sherwood Medical	
Other dressing types			
Alginates (absorb exudate)	Algosteril	Johnson & Johnson Medical	
	Curasorb	Kendall Healthcare Prod.	
	Kaltostat	Calgon Vestal	47, 93, 94, 104, 107, 120, 186
	Sorbsan	Dow B. Hickam, Inc.	201
Starch copolymer (absorb exudate)	Hydragran	Baxter Healthcare Corp.	161

This table has been adapted, with permission, from: Bolton LL, van Rijswijk L. Wound dressings: meeting clinical and biological needs. *Dermatology Nursing.* 1991;146-161.

Note: This table does not provide a complete listing of all dressing available, nor does inclusion imply endorsement. Wound fillers/beads/powders and pastes have not been listed.

Information sources: *Medical Device Register United States and Canada.* Vols 1 and 2. Stamford, CT: Medical Device Register Inc; 1992. *Physicians Desk Reference.* 46th ed. Oradell, NJ: Medical Economics Company Inc; 1992. Medlars Elhill Database (Medline) and Health Database, 1966-August 1993, National Library of Medicine's Online Network. Bethesda, MD: Department of Health and Human Services. Bennett RG. *Fundamentals of Cutaneous Surgery.* St. Louis, MO: CV Mosby; 1988:Chapter 9.

30. Glenchur H, Patel BS, Pathmarajah C. Transient bacteremia associated with debridement of decubitus ulcers. *Milit Med.* 1981;146:432-433.

31. Witkowski J, Parish L. Debridement of cutaneous ulcers. In: Shear NH. *Clincal Dermatology: Dermatologic Pharmacology 2.* 1992;9:585-591.

32. Constantine B, Monte K. Burn debridement under occlusion. *Proc American Burn Association.* Las Vegas, NV; 1990.

33. van Rijswijk L, Cuzzell JC. Managing full-thickness wounds. *Am J Nurs.* 1991;6:18-22.

34. Chen WY, Rogers AS, Lydon MJ. Characterization of biologic properties of wound fluid collected during early stages of wound healing. *J Invest Derm.* 1992;99:559-564.

35. Grinnell F, Ho CH, Wysocki A. Degradation of fibronectin and vitronectin in chronic wound fluid: analysis by cell blotting, immunoblotting, and cell adhesion assays. *J Invest Derm.* 1992;98:410-416.

36. Lydon M, Hutchinson J, Rippon M, et al. Dissolution of wound coagulum and promotion of granulation tissue under DuoDERM. *Wounds.* 1989;1:95-106.

37. Mulder G, Walker A. Preliminary observations on clotting under three hydrocolloid dressings. *J Royal Soc Med.* 1989;82:739-740.

38. Gilje O. On taping, adhesive tape treatment of leg ulcers. *Acta Derm Venereol (Stockh).* 1948;28:454-467.

39. Winter GD. Formation of scab and the rate of epithelialization on superficial wounds in the skin of the domestic pig. *Nature.* 1962;193:293-294.

40. Hinman CD, Maibach HI, Winter GD. Effect of air exposure and occlusion on experimental human skin wounds. *Nature.* 1963;200:377-378.

41. Winter GD, Scales JT. Effects of air drying and dressings on the surface of a wound. *Nature.* 1963;197:91-92.

42. Linsky CB, Rovee DT, Dow T. Effect of dressings on wound inflammation and scar tissue. In: Dineen P, Hildick-Smith G. *The Surgical Wound.* Philadelphia, PA: Lea & Febiger; 1981:191-205.

43. Alvarez OM, Mertz PM, Eaglstein WH. The effect of occlusive dressings on collagen synthesis and epithelialization in superficial wounds. *J Surg Res.* 1983;35:142-148.

44. Bolton L, Pirone L, Chen J, Lydon M. Dressing's effect on wound healing. *Wounds.* 1990;2:126-134.

45. Leipziger LS, Glushko V, DiBernardo B, et al. Dermal wound repair: role of collagen matrix implants and synthetic polymer dressings. *J Am Acad Derm.* 1985;12(suppl):409-419.

46. Barnett SE, Varley SJ. The effects of calcium alginate on wound healing. *Ann Royal Coll Surg.* 1987;69:153-155.

47. Dawson C, Armstrong MWJ, Fulford SCV, Fauqi RM, Galland RB. Use of calcium alginate to pack abscess cavities: a controlled clinical trial. *J Royal Coll Surg.* 1992;37:177-179.

48. Madden M, Nolan E, Finkelstein J, et al. Comparison of an occlusive and a semi-occlusive dressing and the effect of the wound exudate upon keratinocyte proliferation. *J Trauma.* 1989;29:924-931.

49. Wyatt D, McGowan DN, Najarian MP. Comparison of a hydrocolloid dressing and silver sulfadiazine cream in the outpatient management of second-degree burns. *J Trauma.* 1990;30:857-865.

50. Hermans MHE, Hermans RP. DuoDERM, an alternative dressing for smaller burns. *Burns.* 1986;12:214-219.

51. Waffle C, Simon RR, Joslin C. Moisture-vapour-permeable film as an outpatient burn dressing. *Burns.* 1988;14:66-70.

52. Poulsen TD, Freund KG, Arendrup K, Nyhuus P, Pedersen OD. Polyurethane film (OpSite) vs. impregnated gauze (Jelonet) in the treatment of outpatient burns: a prospective, randomized study. *Burns.* 1991;17:59-61.

53. Hien N, Praver S, Katz H. Facilitated wound healing using transparent film dressing following Mohs micrographic surgery. *Arch Derm.* 1988;124:903-906.

54. Nemeth AJ, Eaglstein WH, Taylor JR, Peerson LJ, Falanga V. Faster healing and less pain in skin biopsy sites treated with an occlusive dressing. *Arch Derm.* 1991;127:1679-1683.

55. Hermans MHE. Hydrocolloid versus Tulle Gauze in the treatment of abrasions in cyclists. *Int J Sports Med.* 1991;12:581-584.

56. Cordts PR, Hanrahan LM, Rodriguez AA, et al. A prospective, randomized trial of Unna's boot versus DuoDERM CGF hydroactive dressing plus compression in the management of venous leg ulcers. *J Vasc Surg.* 1992;15:480-486.

57. Macfie J, McMahon MJ. The management of the open perineal wound using a foam elastomer dressing: a prospective clinical trial. *Br J Surg.* 1980;67:85-89.

58. Rohrich RJ, Pittman CE. A clinical comparison of Duo-DERM CGF and OpSite donor site dressings. *Wounds.* 1991;3:221-226.

59. Tejerina RA, Codina J, Hidalgo J, Mirabet V. Application of a new cictrization dressing in treating second-degree burns and donor sites. *Ann Med Burn Soc.* 1991;4:174-176.

60. Hedman LA. Effect of a hydrocolloid dressing on the pain level from abrasions on the feet during intensive marching. *Milit Med.* 1988;153:188-190.

61. Levy AM, Barnes R, van Rijswijk L. Evaluation of a new dressing in the treatment of sports-related skin lesions. *Cutis.* 1987;39:161-164.

62. Hermans MHE, van Wingerden S. Treatment of industrial wounds with DuoDERM bordered: a report on medical and patient comfort aspects. *J Soc Occup Med.* 1990;40:101-102.

63. Bannon M. Healing the whole person. *Nurs Times.* 1993;89:62-68.

64. AHCPR. Acute Pain Management Panel. Acute pain management: operative or medical procedures and trauma. *Clinical Practice Guideline #92-0032.* Rockville, MD: Agency for Health Care Policy and Research, Public Health Services, US Dept of Health and Human Services; 1992.

65. Zawacki BE. Reversal of capillary stasis and prevention of necrosis in burns. *Ann Surg.* 1974;180:98-102.

66. Zawacki BE. The natural history of reversible burn injury. *Surg Gynecol Obstet.* 1974;139:867-871.

67. Witkowski JA, Parish LC. Cutaneous ulcer therapy. *Int J*

Derm. 1986;25:420-426.

68. Varghese MC, Balin AK, Carter DM, Caldwell D. Local environment of chronic wounds under synthetic dressings. *Arch Derm.* 1986;122:52-57.

69. Hutchinson JJ, McGuckin M. Occlusive dressings: a microbiologic and clinical review. *Am J Inf Control.* 1990;18:257-268.

70. Smith DJ, Thomson PD, Bolton LL, Hutchinson JJ. Microbiology and healing of the occluded skin-graft donor site. *Plast Reconstr Surg.* 1993;91:1094-1097.

71. Mertz P, Marshall D, Eaglstein W. Occlusive wound dressings to prevent bacterial invasion and wound infection. *J Am Acad Dermatol.* 1985;12:662-668.

72. Wilson P, Burroughs D, Dunn LJ. Methicillin-resistant Staphyloccus aureus and hydrocolloid dressings. *Pharm J.* 1988;17:787-788.

73. Lawrence JC, Lilly HA, Kidson A. Wound dressings and airborne dispersal of bacteria "letter." *Lancet.* 1992;339:807.

74. Nishijima S, Namura S, Mitsuya K, Asasa Y. The incidence of isolation of Methicillin-resistant staphyloccus aureus (MRSA) strains from skin infections during the past three years. *J Derm.* 1993;20:193-197.

75. Bowler P, Delargy H, Prince D, Fondberg L. The viral barrier properties of some occlusive dressings and their role in infection control. *Wounds.* 1993;5:1-8.

76. Cherry GW, Ryan TJ, Cameron J. Blueprint for the treatment of leg ulcers and the prevention of recurrence. *Wounds.* 1991;3:2-15.

77. van Rijswijk L. Gloves and other rubber based devices: benefits, problems and guidelines. *Wounds.* 1992;4:65-73.

78. Weber BB, Speer M, Swartz D, et al. Irritation and stripping effects of adhesive tapes on skin layers of coronary artery bypass graft patients. *Heart Lung.* 1987;16:567-572.

79. Kessler DA. Introducing medwatch: a new approach to reporting medication and device adverse effects and product problems. *JAMA.* 1993;269:2765-2768.

80. Brunius U, Zederfeldt B. Suture materials in general surgery: a comment. *Prog Surg.* 1970;8:38-44.

81. Ordman LJ, Gilman T. Studies in the healing of cutaneous wounds. I. The healing of excisions through the skin of pigs. *Arch Surg.* 1966;93:857-882.

82. Michie DD, Hugill JV. Influence of occlusive and impregnated gauze dressings on incisional healing: a prospective, randomized, controlled study. *Ann Plast Surg.* 1993;32:57-64.

83. Moshakis V, Fordyce MJ, Griffiths JD, McKinna JA. Tegaderm versus gauze dressing in breast surgery. *Br J Clin Pract.* 1984;38:149-152.

84. Shah M, Foreman DM, Ferguson MWJ. Control of scarring in adult wounds by neutralising antibody to transforming growth factor ß. *Lancet.* 1992;339:213-214.

85. Rubio PA. Use of semiocclusive, transparent film dressings for surgical wound protection: experience in 3637 cases. *Int Surg.* 1991;76:253-254.

86. Eaton AC. A controlled trial to evaluate and compare a sutureless skin closure technique (OpSite skin closure)

with conventional skin suturing and clipping in abdominal surgery. *Br J Surg.* 1980;67:857-860.

87. Hermans MHE. Clinical benefit of a hydrocolloid dressing in closed surgical wounds. *J ET Nurs.* 1993;20:68-72.

88. Rasmussen H, Jojer Larsen MJ, Skeie E. Surgical wound dressing in outpatient podiatric surgery. *Dan Med Bull.* 1993;40:252-254.

89. Wheeland RG. The newer surgical dressings and wound healing. *Dermatol Clinics.* 1987;5:393-407.

90. Roberts LW, McManus WF, Mason AD, Pruitt BA. Duo-DERM in the managment of skin graft donor sites. In: Hall CW. *Surgical Research: Recent Developments.* Proceedings Academy of Surgical Research: Pergamon Press; 1985:55-58.

91. Perrot J, Carsin H, Gilbaud J. Use of DuoDERM dressing in the healing of graft donor sites in burned patients. Apropos of 20 cases. *Ann Chir Plast Esthet.* 1986;31:279-282.

92. Tan ST, Roberts RH, Sinclair SW. A comparison of Zenoderm with DuoDERM E in the treatment of split skin graft donor sites. *Br J Plast Surg.* 1993;46:82-84.

93. Porter JM. A comparative investigation of re-epithelialization of split skin graft donor areas after application of hydrocolloid and alginate dressings. *Br J Plast Surg.* 1991;44:333-337.

94. Lawrence JE, Blake GB. A comparison of calcium alginate and scarlet red dressings in the healing of split thickness skin graft donor sites. *Br J Plast Surg.* 1991;44:247-249.

95. Demetriades D, Psaras G. Occlusive versus semi-open dressings in the management of skin graft donor sites. *S Afr J Chir.* 1992;30:40-41.

96. Andersson AP, Puntervold T, Warburg FE. Treatment of excoriations with a transparent hydrocolloid dressing: a prospective study. *Injury.* 1991;22:429-430.

97. Phillips TJ, Kapoor V, Provan A, Ellerin T. A randomized prospective study of a hydroactive dressing vs conventional treatment after shave biopsy excision. *Arch Derm.* 1993;129:859-860.

98. Blight A, Fatah MF, Datubo-Brown DD, Mountford EM, Cheshire IM. The treatment of donor sites with cultured epithelial grafts. *Br J Plast Surg.* 1991;44:12-14.

99. Barnett A, Berkowitz RL, Mills R, Vistnes LM. Comparison of synthetic adhesive moisture vapor permeable and fine mesh gauze dressings for split-thickness skin graft donor sites. *Am J Surg.* 1983;145:379-381.

100. Tan ST, Roberts RH, Blake GB. Comparing DuoDERM E with scarlet red in the treatment of split skin graft donor sites. *Br J Plast Surg.* 1993;46:79-81.

101. Stair TO, D'Orta J, Altieri MF, Lippe MS. Polyurethane and silver sulfadiazene dressings in treatment of partial-thickness burns and abrasions. *Am J Emerg Med.* 1986;4:214-217.

102. Morris WT, Lamb AM. Painless skin donor sites: a controlled double-blind trial of Opsite, scarlet red and bupivacaine. *Aust NZ J Surg.* 1990;60:617-620.

103. Healy CMJ, Boorman JG. Comparison of E-Z Derm and Jelonet dressings for partial skin thickness burns. *Burns.*

1989;15:52-54.

104. Vanstraelen P. Comparison of calcium sodium alginate (Kaltostat) and porcine xenograft (E-Z Derm) in the healing of split-thickness skin graft donor sites. *Burns.* 1992;18:145-148.

105. Wright A, MacKechnie DWM, Paskins JR. Management of partial thickness burns with Granuflex E dressings. *Burns.* 1993;19:128-130.

106. Gemberling RM, Miller TA, Caffee H, Zawacki BE. Dressing comparison in the healing of donor sites. *J Trauma.* 1976;16:812-814.

107. Attwood AI. Calcium alginate dressing accelerates split skin graft donor site healing. *Br J Plast Surg.* 1989;42:373-379.

108. Freshwater MF, Su CT, Hoopes JE. A comparison of polyurethane foam dressing and fine mesh gauze in the healing of donor sites. *Plast Reconstr Surg.* 1978;61:275-276.

109. Hart NB, Lawrence JC. Tulle-gras dressings. *Burns.* 1984;11:26-30.

110. Hermans MH. Hydrocolloid dressing (DuoDERM) for the treatment of superficial and partial thickness burns. *Scan J Plast Rec Surg & Hand Surg.* 1987;21:283-285.

111. Hirschowitz G, Moscona R, Dvir E, et al. A new polymer-iodine combination (iodoplex) for treatment of donor sites: a preliminary controlled study. *Ann Plast Surg.* 1979;2:84-88.

112. Johansen AM, Sorensen B. Treatment of donor sites: a controlled trial with fucidin gauze. *Scand J Plast Rec Surg.* 1972;6:47-50.

113. Leicht P, Siim E, Sorensen B. Treatment of donor sites—DuoDERM or Omiderm? *Burns.* 1989;15:7-10.

114. Levine NS, Lindberg RA, Salisbury RE, et al. Comparison of coarse mesh gauze with biologic dressings on granulating wounds. *Am J Surg.* 1976;131:727-729.

115. Salisbury RE, Bevin AG, Dingeldein GP, Grisham J. A clinical and laboratory evaluation of a polyurethane foam: a new donor site dressing. *Arch Surg.* 1979;114:1188-1192.

116. Zapata-Sirvent R, Hansbrough JF, Carroll W, Johnson R, Wakimoto A. Comparison of biobrane and scarlet red dressings for treatment of donor site wounds. *Arch Surg.* 1985;120:743-745.

117. Sagi A, Walter P, Walter MH, et al. "Dermodress," a new temporary skin substitute: pilot study on donor sites. *Int J Tis React.* 1986;8:153-156.

118. Prasad JK, Feller I, Thompson PD. A prospective controlled trial of Biobrane versus scarlet red on skin graft donor areas. *J Burn Care Rehab.* 1987;8:384-386.

119. Afilalo M, Dankoff J, Guttman A, Lloyd J. DuoDERM hydroactive dressing versus silversulphadiazine/bactigras in the emergency treatment of partial skin thickness burns. *Burns.* 1992;18:313-316.

120. Basse P, Siim E, Lohmann M. Treatment of donor sites: calcium alginate versus paraffin gauze. *Acta Chir Plast.* 1992;34:92-98.

121. Pinski JB. Dressings for dermabrasion: occlusive dressings and wound healing. *Cutis.* 1986;38:471-476.

122. Eaglstein WH. Experiences with biosynthetic dressings. *J Am Acad Derm.* 1985;12:434-440.

123. Fulton JE. The stimulation of post-dermabrasion wound healing with stabilized aloe vera gel-polyethylene oxide dressing. *J Dermatol Surg Oncol.* 1990;16:460-467.

124. Waymack PJ, Nathan P, Robb EC, Plessinger J, et al. An evaluation of aquaphor gauze dressing in burned children. *Burns.* 1986;12:443-448.

125. Dillon ME, Okunski WJ. Silon non-adherent film dressings on autograft and donor sites. *Wounds.* 1992;4:203-207.

126. Neal DE, Whalley PC, Flowers MW, Wilson DH. The effects of an adherent polyurethane film and conventional absorbent dressing in patients with small partial thickness burns. *Br J Clin Pract.* 1981;35:254-257.

127. Feldman DL, Rogers A, Karpinski RHS. A prospective trial comparing Biobrane, DuoDERM and Xeroform for skin graft donor sites. *Surg Gynecol Obstet.* 1991;173:1-5.

128. Fong PH, Wong KL. Opsite, a synthetic burns dressing. *Ann Acad Med Singapore.* 1985;14:387-390.

129. Alling R, North AF. Polyurethane film for coverage of skin graft donor sites. *J Oral Surg.* 1981;39:970-971.

130. Walters MD, Dombroski RA, Davidson SA, Mandel PC, Gibbs RS. Reclosure of disrupted abdominal incisions. *Obstet Gynecol.* 1990;76:597-602.

131. Hermann GC, Bagi P, Christofferson I. Early secondary suture versus healing by second intention of incisional abscesses. *Surg Gynecol Obstet.* 1988;167:16-18.

132. Dodson MK, Magann EF, Meeks GR. A randomized comparison of secondary closure and secondary intention in patients with superficial wound dehiscence. *Obstet Gynecol.* 1992;80:321-324.

133. Jeter KF, Chapman RM, Tintle T, Davis A. Comprehensive wound management with a starch-based copolymer dressing. *JET.* 1986;13:217-225.

134. Brown-Etris M, Myers RB, Rideout BK. A non-traditional approach to abdominal wound closure. *Ostomy Wound Manage.* 1991;34:37-43.

135. Butterworth R, Bale S. Treating open perineal wounds. *Nurs Standard.* 1991;5:29-30.

136. Krasner D. Treating postoperative wounds with an amorphous hydrogel. *J Wnd Care.* 1993;2:148-150.

137. Latham W, Steiner I, Lefkowitz H. Hydrocolloid for deep wound dehiscence. *J Am Pod Med Assoc.* 1989;79:74-76.

138. Gates JL, Holloway GA. A comparison of wound environments. *Ostomy Wound Manage.* 1992;38:34-37.

139. Alsbjörn BJ, Ovesen H, Walther-Larsen S. Occlusive dressing versus petroleum gauze on drainage wounds. *Acta Chir Scand.* 1990;156:211-213.

140. Schmidt JM, Greenspoon JS. Aloe vera dermal wound gel is associated with a delay in wound healing. *Obstet Gynecol.* 1991;78:115-117.

141. Berlowitz DR, Van B, Wilking S. The short-term outcome of pressure sores. *J Am Geriatr Soc.* 1990;38:748-752.

142. Gentzkow GD, Pollack SV, Kloth LC, Stubbs HA. Improved healing of pressure ulcers using dermapulse, a new

electrical stimulation device. *Wounds.* 1991;3:158-169.

143. Gorse GJ, Messner RL. Improved pressure sore healing with hydrocolloid dressings. *Arch Derm.* 1987;123:766-771.

144. Ferrell BA, Osterweil D, Christensen P. A randomized trial of low-air-loss beds for treatment of pressure ulcers. *JAMA.* 1993;269:494-497.

145. Neill KM, Conforti C, Kedas A, Burris JF. Pressure sore response to a new hydrocolloid dressing. *Wounds.* 1989;1:173-184.

146. Xakellis GC, Chrischillis EA. Hydrocolloid versus saline-gauze dressings in treating pressure ulcers: a cost-effectiveness analysis. *Arch Phys Med Rehab.* 1992;73:463-468.

147. Sebern MD. Pressure ulcer management in home health care: efficacy and cost effectiveness of moisture vapor permeable dressing. *Arch Phys Med Rehab.* 1986;67:726-729.

148. Allman RM, Laprade CA, Noel LB, et al. Pressure sores among hospitalized patients. *Ann Int Med.* 1987;107:641-643.

149. Allman RM, Walker JM, Hart MK, et al. Air-fluidized beds or conventional therapy for pressure sores. *Ann Int Med.* 1987;107:641-643.

150. Bergstrom N, Braden B. A prospective study of pressure sore risk among institutionalized elderly. *J Am Geriatr Soc.* 1992;40:747-758.

151. Pinchofsky GD, Kaminski MV. Correlation of pressure sores and nutritional status. *J Am Geriatr Soc.* 1986;34:435-440.

152. Robson MC, Phillips LG, Lawrence WT, et al. The safety and effect of topically applied recombinant basic fibroblast growth factor on the healing of chronic pressure sores. *Ann Surg.* 1992;216:401-406.

153. van Rijswijk L. Full-thickness pressure ulcers: patient and wound healing characteristics. *Decubitus.* 1993;6:16-21.

154. van Rijswijk L, Polansky M. Predictors of time to healing deep pressure ulcers. *Wounds.* 1994;6:159-165.

155. Yarkony GM, Kramer E, King R, Lukane C. Pressure sore managment: efficacy of a moisture reactive occlusive dressing. *Arch Phys Med Rehab.* 1984;65:597-600.

156. Smietanke MA, Opit LJ. A trial of a transparent adhesive dressing (OpSite) in ten treatment of decubitus ulcers. *Austr Nurs J.* 1981;10:40-42.

157. Tudhope M. Management of pressure ulcers with a hydrocolloid occlusive dressing: results in twenty-three patients. *JET.* 1984;11:102-105.

158. Oleske DM, Smith XP, White P, Pottage J, Donavan MI. A randomized clinical trial of two dressing methods for the treatment of low-grade pressure ulcers. *JET.* 1986;13:90-98.

159. Sheridan CA, Jackson BS. Clinical safety and efficacy evaluation of a hydroactive hydrocolloid dressing in the care of cancer patients. *JET.* 1989;16:213-219.

160. Shannon ML, Miller B. Evaluation of hydrocolloid dressings on healing of pressure ulcers in spinal cord injury patients. *Decubitus.* 1988;1:29-30.

161. Saydak SJ. A pilot test of two methods for the treatment of pressure ulcers. *JET.* 1990;17:139-142.

162. Myers RB, Moore K, Mulder GD, Pike RA, Kissil MT. Report of a multicenter clinical trial on the performance characteristics of two occlusive hydrocolloid dressings in the treatment of noninfected, partial-thickness wounds. *JET.* 1988;15:158-161.

163. McMullen D. Clinical experience with a calcium alginate dressing. *Derm Nurs.* 1991;3:216-219,270.

164. Kurzuk-Howard G, Simpson L, Palmieri A. Decubitus ulcer care: a comparative study. *West J Nurs Res.* 1985;7:58-75.

165. Watts C, Shipes E. A study to compare the overall performance of two hydrocolloid dressings on partial thickness wounds. *Ostomy Wound Manage.* 1988;21:28-31.

166. Brady SM. Management of pressure sores with occlusive dressings in a select population. *Nurs Manage.* 1987;18:47-50.

167. Darkovich SL, Brown-Etris M, Spencer M. Biofilm hydrogel dressing: a clinical evaluation in the treatment of pressure sores. *Ostomy Wound Manage.* 1990;29:47-60.

168. Brod M, McHenry E, Plasse TF, Fedorczyk D, Trout JR. A randomized comparison of Poly-hema and hydrocolloid dressings for treatment of pressure sores. *Arch Derm.* 1990;126:969-970.

169. Alm A, Hornmark AM, Fall PA, et al. Care of pressure sores: a controlled study of the use of a hydrocolloid dressing compared with wet saline gauze compresses. *Acta Dermatol Venereol (Stockh).* 1989;149(suppl):1-10.

170. Phillips TJ, Dover JS. Leg ulcers. *J Am Acad Derm.* 1991;25:965-987.

171. Skene AI, Smith JM, Dore CJ, Charlett A, Lewis JD. Venous leg ulcers: a prognostic index to predict time to healing. *BMJ.* 1992;305:1119-1121.

172. van Rijswijk L. Full-thickness leg ulcers: patient demographics and predictors of healing. *J Fam Pract.* 1993;36:625-632.

173. Smith JM, Dore CJ, Charlett A, Lewis JD. A randomized trial of biofilm dressing for venous leg ulcers. *Phlebologie.* 1992;7:108-113.

174. Kikta MJ, Schuler JJ, Meyer JP, et al. A prospective randomized trial of Unna's boots versus hydroactive dressing in the treatment of venous stasis ulcers. *J Vasc Surg.* 1988;7:478-483.

175. Arnold TE, Stanley JC, Sellows EP, et al. Prospective, multicenter study of managing lower-extremity venous ulcers. *Ann Vasc Surg.* 1994;8:356-362.

176. Handfield-Jones SE, Grattan CEH. Comparison of a hydrocolloid dressing and paraffin gauze in the treatment of venous ulcers. *Br J Derm.* 1988;118:425-427.

177. Cordts PR, Hanrahan LM, Rodriquez AA, Woodson J, LaMorte WW, Menzoian JO. A prospective, randomized trial of Unna's boot versus DuoDERM CGF hydroactive dressing plus compression in the management of venous leg ulcers. *J Vasc Surg.* 1992;15:480-486.

178. Friedman SJ, Daniel SU WP. Management of leg ulcers

with hydrocolloid occlusive dressing. *Arch Derm.* 1984;120:1329-1336.

179. Rubin JR, Alexander J, Plecha EJ, Marman C. Unna's boot vs. polyurethane foam dressings for the treatment of venous ulceration. *Arch Surg.* 1990;125:489-490.

180. Banerjee AK, Levy DW, Raslinson D. Leg ulcers: a compartive study of Synthaderm and conventional dressings. *Care Elderly.* 1990;2:123-125.

181. Loiterman DA, Byers PH. Effect of a hydrocellular polyurethane dressing on chronic venous ulcer healing. *Wounds.* 1991;3:178-181.

182. Blackhouse CM, Blair SD, Savage AP, Walton J, McCollum CN. Controlled trial of occlusive dressings in healing chronic venous ulcers. *Br J Surg.* 1987;74:626-627.

183. Zuccarelli FA. A comparative study of the hydrocellular dressing Allevyn and the hydrocolloid dressing Duo-DERM in the treatment of leg ulcers. *Phlebologie.* 1992;45:529-533.

184. Burgess B. An investigation of hydrocolloids. *Prof Nurse.* 1993;8(suppl):3-6.

185. Brandrup F, Menne T, Agren M, et al. A randomized trial of two occlusive dressings in the treatment of leg ulcers. *Acta Derm Venereol (Stockh).* 1990;70:231-235.

186. Rainey J. A comparison of two dressings in the treatment of heavily exuding leg ulcers. *J Wnd Care.* 1993;2:199-200.

187. Falanga V, Eaglstein WH. The "trap" hypothesis of venous ulceration. *Lancet.* 1993;341:1006-1007.

188. Mulder G, Jones R, Cederholm-Williams S, Cherry G, Ryan T. Fibrin cuff lysis in chronic venous ulcers treated with a hydrocolloid dressing. *Int J Derm.* 1993;32:304-306.

189. Margolis DJ, Gross EA, Wood CR, Lazarus GS. Planimetric rate of healing in venous ulcers of the leg treated with pressure bandage and hydrocolloid dressing. *J Am Acad Derm.* 1993;28:418-421.

190. Harris B, Eaglstein WH, Falanga V. Basal cell carcinoma arising in venous ulcers and mimicking granulation tissue. *J Derm Surg Oncol.* 1993;19:150-152.

191. Stankard CE, Cruse CW, Wells KE, Karl R. Chronic pressure ulcer carcinomas. *Ann Plast Surg.* 1993;30:274-277.

192. Frantz RA. Pressure ulcer costs in long-term care. *Decubitus.* 1989;2:56-57.

193. Wood CR, Margolis DJ. The cost of treating venous leg ulcers to complete healing using an occlusive dressing and a compression bandage. *Wounds.* 1992;4:138-141.

194. Colwell J. A comparison of the efficacy and cost effectiveness of two methods of managing pressure ulcers. *Decubitus.* 1993;6:28-36.

195. Fellin R. Managing decubitus ulcers. *Nurs Manage.* 1984;15:29-30.

196. Brown-Etris M, Myers RB, Pasceri P. A new generation of gauze dressings. *Ostomy Wound Manage.* 1991;34:57-59.

197. Martin A, Virby NG, Tabone Vassallo M, et al. Synthaderm in the management of pre-tibial lacerations: a controlled study. *Arch Emerg Med.* 1987;4:179-186.

198. Hendricks WM, Swalow RT. Management of stasis leg ulcers with Unna's boots versus elastic support stockings. *J Am Acad Derm.* 1985;12:90-98.

199. Ericksson G. Comparison of two occlusive bandages in the treatment of venous leg ulcers. *Br J Dermatol.* 1986;114:227-230.

200. Phillips TJ, Provan A, Colbert DA. A comparative trial of a vented adhesive two part dressing with a hydrocolloid in the treatment of chronic leg ulcers. *Wounds.* 1993;5:57-61.

201. Thomas S. Sorbsan in the management of leg ulcers. *Pharm J.* 1989;243:706-709.

202. Eisenberg M. The effect of occlusive dressings on re-epithelialization of wounds in children with epidermolysis bullosa. *J Pediatr Surg.* 1986;21:892-894.

203. Williamson DM, Sherman KP, Shakespeare DT. The use of semipermeable dressings in fingertip injuries. *J Hand Surg.* 1987;4:413-418.

204. Alper JC, Welch EA, Ginsberg M, et al. Moist wound healing under a vapor permeable membrane. *J Am Ac Derm.* 1983;8:347-353.

205. Moshakis V, Fordyce MJ, Griffiths JD, et al. Tegaderm versus gauze dressing in breast surgery. *Br J Clin Pract.* 1984;38:149-152.

206. Shell JA, Stanutz F, Grimm J. Comparison of moisture vapor permeable (MVP) dressings to conventional dressings for management of radiation skin reactions. *Oncol Nurs Forum.* 1986;13:11-16.

207. Kaletsch B. Foam-gel film and gel film in trauma surgery. *Unfallchir.* 1986;12:204-207.

208. Milburn PB, Zinger JC, Milburn MA. Treatment of scleroderma skin ulcers with a hydrocolloid membrane. *J Am Acad Derm* (Part 1). 1989;21:200-204.

209. Payne RL, Martin ML. Skin tears: the epidemiology and management of skin tears in older adults. *Ostomy Wound Manage.* 1990;26:27-37.

210. Apelqvist J, Larsson J, Stenstrom A. Topical treatment of necrotic foot ulcers in diabetic patients: a comparative trial of DuoDERM and MeZinc. *Br J Derm.* 1990;123:787-792.

Chapter 4

Topical Medications and Pharmacological Agents in Wound Healing

*Laura L. Bolton, PhD, Carole L. Johnson, PhD, PT, and
Ann-Jeanette Fattu*

Topical wound medications have been applied through the centuries for a variety of real or imagined reasons, from driving out evil spirits or evoking "laudable pus" to promoting healing. In early history, wound care changed with each new theory that was in vogue. More recently, wound infections and other complications have been vastly reduced as wound care decisions were based increasingly on scientific evidence. The purpose of this chapter is to review the scientific literature supporting topical wound care treatment decisions in eight key areas of wound management: hemostasis, wound cleansing, reducing infection, limiting inflammation, pain relief, removing necrotic tissue, tissue glues to assist wound closure, and fostering healing. The literature is reviewed with the goal of giving wound care professionals a scientific basis for their choices of topical wound care medications as recommended by the International Committee on Wound Management.[1] Without this scientific basis, the wound care professional has little rationale for the choice of treatment, and is left with scant basis for planning a treatment program, justifying reimbursement, or responding to administrative or legal queries. With scientific backing, choices among the once confusing array of medications become clear, and the variety of scientifically supported claims become valued tools in planning patient care.

SCIENTIFIC LITERATURE

Wound care professionals need quantitative, controlled clinical results supporting efficacy to guide their decisions in the use of these topical wound medications. Without this scientific basis, wound care is largely a matter of trial and error. With the goal of giving the wound care professional a head start in clinical wound management, published controlled studies, which support the clinical efficacy of medications in each of these key areas of wound care, are summarized here. Wound care professionals are encouraged to choose their medications based on science rather than anecdotal evidence, and to exercise their right to know the scientific evidence for efficacy of any medication they use. In the spirit of networking for the benefit of patients, readers are encouraged to build upon this database so that it can serve as a continuously improving tool for wound management.

Within this chapter, scientific support is defined as objective, measurable, reliable, clinically relevant results of an unbiased comparison of a test treatment with an appropriate control treatment. Quality science has the following seven hallmarks. It is:

- *Prospective*: done with each progressive step unfolding according to a study plan, which addresses a previously stated objective.
- *Controlled*: test group(s) is(are) compared to appropriate controls so that the researcher knows the source of the effects observed.
- *Objective*: results are reliably measured in a way that others can replicate.
- *Unbiased*: treatments are assigned by randomization, or objective criteria which prevent treatment bias and initially equate groups on criteria likely to affect the outcome.
- *Blinded*: results are measured without knowledge of treatment given.
- *Statistically sound*: the simplest statistics are used appropriate to the data being analyzed.
- *Clinically relevant*: the measured outcome pertains to the desired clinical outcome.

All the studies reviewed here meet at least two of these criteria: those of being controlled and clinically relevant. The latter criterion occasionally includes animal studies in vivo, particularly if clinical studies were scant, on the premises that tissue repair in animals and man has much in common and that controlled studies in real tissue are a better basis for wound care decisions than no data. No in vitro data on responses of either microbes or tissue cells in culture are included here because, in our hands, these results have not generalized well to wounds in animals or humans. Two possible reasons for this are:

- In vivo or in the clinic cytokines (molecules affecting cells) and cells are continually entering wounds. These may interact with topically applied substances in ways not predicted in vitro.
- The dilution factors in clinical wounds vary widely with amount and type of exudate.

For those wishing to generalize from cell studies in culture to clinical effects, a general "rule of thumb" which works for about 80% of topical agents reported is to multiply the effective or toxic doses of the agents in vitro by 1000 to derive their corresponding effective or toxic doses in vivo or in the clinic.

This rule is derived by comparing results of in vitro research, such as that by Teepe[2] with those obtained by testing the same agents in vivo, e.g., Bolton and associates.[3] This does not work for relatively insoluble agents like hexylresorcinol or silver sulfadiazine, which act according to their own gradual dissolution characteristics. Also, it is not a precise rule as active agents differ in their capacity to adhere to or be inactivated by tissue proteins.

The review covers two outcomes of key clinical interest: the efficacy and safety of each treatment. For the purposes of this chapter, efficacy means that the treatment works as it is indicated, and safety means that it does not harm the patient or hinder wound healing. Like the science it summarizes, this chapter is but an attempt to listen to nature and convey current knowledge available to the clinician. Readers are encouraged to build upon it with their own scientific studies and let us know of others not yet included so that together we may strengthen the field of wound care and better serve our patients.

USES OF TOPICAL MEDICATIONS IN WOUND MANAGEMENT

HEMOSTASIS

First aid for bleeding wounds begins with hemostasis. Little can be accomplished for the patient unless the bleeding is stopped. Ideally this should be done in a way that minimizes damage to the tissue and does not impede subsequent healing. The hemostatic agents include thrombin or fibrin preparations, oxidized regenerated cellulose, absorbable gelatin foam or powder, and fibrous collagen or alginate products.[4] The more rapidly effective hemostats reported in the literature are porous materi-

Table 4-1. Safety and Efficacy of Topical Wound Cleansers and Antiseptics

Agent	Efficacy	Safety	Reference
Chlorhexidine	0.05-0.5% solutions bacteriostatic to gram positive	0.26% delayed healing with silver sulfadiazine.	11
		Very little healing in 8 days for >0.05%.	3
Chloramine-T	300 ppm cidal in vitro	Normal incision healing.	8
NaOCl Dakins—0.1% Eusol—2.5%	Cured bowel surgery infections	Normal healing applied daily normal wounds.	12
		In gauze delayed ulcer healing vs. hydrocolloid.	13
		Delayed healing 3.5 days vs. dextranomer.	7
Soap and water	Cleaned grease from rat incisions better than commercial products	Tissue growth better than wounds treated with grease removers.	9

als like oxidized regenerated cellulose, alginates, or collagen sponges, though concerns have been raised that these foreign bodies may compromise host defenses and potentiate infection.[5] However, an appropriate quantity of oxidized regenerated cellulose was found that was hemostatic and did not foster infection[6]; therefore, it may provide more benefit in clinical use.

WOUND CLEANSERS AND ANTISEPTICS

For most chronic wounds, care begins with cleansing so that the clinician can assess the wound accurately; remove loose necrotic tissue, debris, or bacteria; and minimize the chances of subsequent infection. Efficacy of cleansers has usually been measured with respect to microorganisms left in the wound after cleansing and mainly in vivo.[3,7-9] Though their true goal is broader, they often contain antiseptics with this goal in mind. Cleansing should be performed gently, and if a syringe or other water focusing device is used, the water pressure impinging on the wound surface should not exceed 8 psi. Table 4-1 summarizes the safety and efficacy of some common wound cleansers. Commercial grease removers, chlorhexidine concentrations of more than 0.05%, and sodium hypochlorite appear effective in removing bacteria or debris, but healing can be impaired when they are used.[3,7-9] For transient reduction of wound bacterial content without adversely affecting healing, chlorhexidine 0.05%,[3] chlorazine,[3] or propylene glycol[3] were effective. For grease removal, soap and water was deemed more beneficial than commercially available preparations, accomplishing similar results without delaying repair.

ANTIMICROBIALS

Antimicrobials are used to prevent or cure bacterial, fungal, or viral infection. Efficacy is measured in terms of their spectrum of activity, which is usually limited to particular types or groups of organisms, and their duration of antimicrobial activity or substantivity. Antibiotics are antimicrobials derived from cell fermentation products, while other antimicrobials are usually synthesized chemically. Readers are cautioned that most of the studies reviewed define efficacy in terms of reductions of target organism colony-forming units (CFUs), but the real measure of clinical efficacy of an antimicrobial should be in terms of its capacity to prevent or cure infection, as indicated by the presence of the commonly accepted clinical signs of erythema, edema, heat, pain, odor, and purulence.[10] Conversely, invasive infection may not be present even when more than 10^5 pathogenic organisms are cultured from a wound, especially in the absence of the clinical signs. Also if necrotic tissue or debris is present or the patient's host defense mechanisms are compromised, broad spectrum antimicrobials are usually preferable to narrow spectrum ones because the latter may kill the organism causing the initial infection, but leave the wound prey to other opportunistic organisms.

The antibiotics have the most scientific support information, followed closely by silver sulfadiazine and by chlorhexidine preparations which are discussed above as cleansers. Topical antibiotics are usually used in combination for a broad spectrum of activity against gram positive and gram negative organisms in ointment or spray formulations. These have proven safe and effective on blisters,[15] burns,[16,18,21,27,30,31] dermatitis,[20,29] dermal excisions,[33] impetigo,[28,29,32] superficial acute and chronic wounds,[34,35] pyoderma,[20,35] surgical incisions,[18,19,26,36,37] tape-stripped wounds,[17,22] open[24] and closed[25] traumatic wounds, and venous ulcers.[23] Their use at venous catheter insertion sites has yielded mixed results, with reports of fewer colonized catheter tips,[40,41] but no reduction in phlebitis[38] or pathogens colonizing the sites.[39] Interpretation of these results is complicated by the observation that some venous catheter insertion sites appeared infected, but yielded sterile cultures.[41] Silver sulfadiazine also has broad-spectrum, antimicrobial activity lasting for more than 24 hours in a 1% cream formulation which has been reported to permit normal healing.[3] Table 4-2 summarizes the safety and efficacy of some common topical antimicrobial agents.

ANTI-INFLAMMATORY AGENTS

Inflammation presents a clinical paradox. While early inflammation after wounding triggers repair, too much may excessively destroy local tissue. Correspondingly, longer inflammation may increase scarring. Moreover, the pain caused by inflammation may reduce patient mobility and function, increase the need for analgesia, delay resumption of normal activities, and limit quality of life. To address inflammation, anti-inflammatory agents are usually given systemically, where they have been reported to inhibit healing. The scant research on their topical effects (Table 4-3) suggests that they may[42,45] or may not[44] delay ocular healing, and that this delay can be counteracted by simultaneous application of retinoic acid[45] or epidermal growth factor.[42] No healing delay was seen on shallow skin wounds on swine.[43]

ANESTHETICS AND ANALGESICS

Anesthetics and analgesics may also help reduce patient pain and restore normal activities. They, too, have few controlled studies (Table 4-4) on their topical safety and efficacy, usually being injected in clinical use. When topically applied to surgical incisions before closure[46-48] or to pediatric traumatic wounds[50] or tooth extraction sockets in monkeys,[57] they generally appear safe and effective. However, high concentrations of lignocaine, especially when combined with epinephrine, were reported to delay wound healing in rats.[49]

DEBRIDING ENZYMES

Of the debriding enzymes, sutilains formulations have been the subject of the most scientific research (Table 4-5). They have proven effective on clinical[69-76] and animal burns,[54,77,79] and on ischemic ulcers in guinea pigs,[80] with occlusive coverings reportedly fostering debridement activity. Hospital stays and time to autografting have been reduced by 10 to 17 days in burn patients treated with sutilains ointment, though treatment is reportedly accompanied by some wound pain and dermatitis[60,69,71-73,76] or conjunctivitis if the enzyme contacts the eyes. Inoculated burns in rabbits[77] or rats[60,78] treated with sutilains ointment have respectively been accompanied by positive bacterial blood cultures[60,78] or unchanged resistance to infection,[79] but this has not been reported in clinical burns. Other debridement agents with controlled clinical studies of efficacy include streptokinase/streptodornase with 8-day earlier preparation of infected laparotomy incisions for secondary suture,[63] and 1 to 3 week debridement reported on traumatic,[66] venous, or arterial[67] ulcers, though treatment may be accompanied by mild transient pain. This enzyme combination was no more effective than zinc oxide

Table 4-2. **Safety and Efficacy of Topical Antimicrobial Agents**

Agent	Efficacy	Safety	Reference
(Silver compounds) Nitrate	Equal infection rate for silver nitrate and mafenide acetate	More burn pain; healing delayed vs. film dressing with silver	14
Sulfadiazine	Silver sulfodiozine had broad spectrum antimicrobial activity for >24 hours in guinea pig excisions	No significant healing delay	3
3Benzalkonium Cl	Not as good as triple antibiotic on S.aureus inoculated blisters	No adverse effects	15
Camphorphenol	Not as good as triple antibiotic on S.aureus inoculated blisters	No adverse effects	15
Double antibiotic	Not as good as triple antibiotic on S.aureus inoculated blisters	No adverse effects	15
	Better than penicillin against S.aureus with chlorhexidine added	No adverse effects	16
	Less effective than oral erythromycin in impetigo	No adverse effects	17
	0-1% infections in high-risk incisions vs. 3.5-5.7% with controls	No adverse effects	18
	More zero bacterial cultures than with iodophor in incisions	No adverse effects	19
Erythromycin	10 mg/g ointment 100% effective in pyogenic skin infections	No adverse effects	20
Framycetin	As effective in burn infection as gentamycin	No adverse effects	21
Gentamycin	As effective in burn infection as neomycin/bacitracin	No adverse effects	21
Herbromin	Not as good as triple antibiotic on S.aureus inoculated blisters	No adverse effects	15
Hydrogen peroxide	Not as good as triple antibiotic on S.aureus inoculated blisters	No adverse effects	15
Iodine	Not as good as triple antibiotic on S.aureus inoculated blisters	Stinging in 71% and contact allergy or irritation in 42%	15
	Iodophor spray reduced appendectomy infections	No adverse effects	26

ointment[64] or dextranomer[65] in debriding pressure ulcers. Bromelain has been shown effective in debriding full-thickness burns on rats[79] and swine.[53] Collagenase has been shown to debride arterial or venous ulcers in 1 to 4 weeks,[50,57,90,93] and pressure ulcers in 7 days.[56] Fibrinolysin/desoxyribonuclease combinations have also been reported to debride more venous or mixed leg ulcers than a placebo control treatment, though healing was not improved. Papain-treated pressure ulcers, arteriosclerotic ulcers, and burns were reportedly debrided in 3 to 4 days without side effects.[61] Though trypsin preparations were not studied for efficacy, in safety studies, they reduced rat incision tensile strength.[82] In contrast, healing of clinical pressure ulcers was not delayed by one tenth the concentration of

Table 4-2. **Safety and Efficacy of Topical Antimicrobial Agents (Continued)**

Agent	Efficacy	Safety	Reference
Neomycin	1% cream reduced organisms colonizing chronic dermatoses vs. placebo cream	No adverse effects	17
	5 mg with 5 mg/g chlorhexidine reduced burn colonization vs. penicillin 10,000 U/g	No healing difference	120
	0.5% cream + dexamethasone had same effect on infected dermatoses as dexamethasone alone	Neomycin-resistant staphylococci emerged	121
	0.5% cream + fluocinolone acetonide more remission of dermatitis than steroid alone	Mild burning in 2 patients treated with antibiotic	122
	Three times as many dermatitis cleared in 3 weeks with above combination than with steroid alone	1 sensitivity to neomycin	21
	0.25% with gramicidin reduced CFUs, clinical signs of infection on tape stripped wounds	No adverse effects	18
	0.5% ointment reduced severity, seeded tape stripped site infection	No adverse effects	22
	0.5% ointment healed more venous ulcers than vehicle at 16 weeks	No adverse effects	23
Oxytetracyclin	10 mg/mL spray reduced trauma infection	No adverse effects	24
Penicillin	Solution irrigation decreased infection rate of sutured trauma	No adverse effects	25
Thimersol	Not as good as triple antibiotic on S.aureus inoculated blisters	Stinging in 71% of patients	15

trypsin used in the rat study.[89] More recently, a krill enzyme debrided venous ulcers 3 days faster than control treatment with acetic acid/povidone iodine, without reported toxicity.[59] In general, enzymatic debridement has been reported effective on a variety of clinical and animal wounds, with transient pain reported as a mild side effect.

TISSUE GLUES

Few controlled studies (Table 4-6) have explored safety or efficacy of the two main tissue glues, which have been used to assist wound closure:
- cyanoacrylates, available in Canada and Europe but not in the United States, and
- fibrin glues, derived from heterologous or homologous blood products.

Cyanoacrylates were reportedly effective in closing 100% of 178 surgical incisions without any infections versus a 19% infection rate observed in the 32 control incisions closed with fibrin glue.[83] The one side effect observed with the cyanoacrylate, local heating, was alleviated by distributing applications more widely in time or space. Surgical incisions treated with fibrin sealant were reported to have reduced anastomotic bursting pressure[85] and increased abscess formation.[83,85] Defect filling with fibrin sealant treatment was more pronounced when auxiliary treatment included Endothelial Cell Growth Factor.[84]

Agent	Efficacy	Safety	Reference
Table 4-2. Safety and Efficacy of Topical Antimicrobial Agents (Continued)			
Terramycin	30 mg/g killed bacteria in burns, trauma sites	No effect of agent or bacteria on healing	27
	<7 days to clear impetigo	No adverse effects	28
	<7 days to clear sycosis barbae	No adverse effects	9
Triple antibiotic	Better healing of S.aureus inoculated blister wounds than double antibiotic, benzalkonium chloride, merbromin, thimerosal, 3% hydrogen peroxide, iodine, or camphorphenol	Contact allergy in 4% of patients	11
	22% bacteria free swabs vs. 2% for penicillin or no treatment		
	Slightly more (88%) survived major burns than if treated with gentamycin ointment	No adverse effects	30
	Impetigo cured 3 days earlier with oral erythromycin than with triple antibiotic	No adverse effects	31
	Spray formulation permitted fewer excision infections than no treatment		
	Cleared infected wounds more often in 10 days than vehicle	No side effect related to treatment	32
	100% pyoderma cured in 2-20 days by triple antibiotic vs. 16% cured by vehicle at 24 days	No adverse effects	33
	Slightly fewer clinical infections in surgical wounds	No adverse effects	34
	0.9% infection rate in powder treated surgical incisions vs. 3.8% in no-spray controls	No adverse effects	35
	Lower infection rate in trauma wounds than no spray	No adverse effects	36
	More sterile venous catheters antibiotic than vehicle	No adverse effects	37
	More sterile venous catheters; no effect on infection rate	No adverse effects	24
	Fewer colonized venous catheter tips than placebo	No adverse effects	38
	Fewer colonized venous cut-down sites	More pathogens in antibiotic group	41

WOUND HEALING AGENTS

Though cellular effects of growth factors have been promising, effects have not always generalized to clinical improvement of healing.[118] As can be seen from Table 4-7, combinations of growth factors may be more effective than single growth factors applied topically, and a growing number of studies have revealed the rich broth of growth factors in wound fluid sequestered beneath occlusive or moisture-retentive dressings.[119] In view of these findings, occlusive dressings may serve as a valuable control for clinical growth factor studies.

The most widely studied growth factors include EGF, PDGF and related mixtures, and TGF and basic FGF. Epidermal growth factor (EGF) has produced mixed results both on animal and clinical wounds, primarily on epithelization. Plate-

Table 4-3. Safety and Efficacy of Anti-Inflammatory Agents

Agent	Anti-Inflammatory Efficacy	Safety	Reference
Corticosteroids	Not measured	Delayed repair of canine keratectomies was improved by concomitant vitamin A	45
Dexamethasone	Not measured	Reduced rabbit ocular incision tensile strength	42
Hydrocortisone	Not measured	Swine donor site epithelization progressed normally	43
Ibuprofen	Not measured	Swine donor site epithelization progressed normally	43
Indomethacin	Not measured	Swine donor site epithelization progressed normally	43
Meclofenamate	Not measured	Swine donor site epithelization progressed normally	43
Prednisolone acetate	Not measured	Keratoplasty healing time unchanged	44
Triamcinolone acetonide	Not measured	Swine donor site epithelization progressed normally	43

Table 4-4. Safety and Efficacy of Topical Anesthetics and Analgesia

Agent	Efficacy	Safety	Reference
Bupivacaine	Surgical incision pain reduced by perfusion with 0.5% solution	No adverse effects	46
EMLA cream (lidocaine, prilocaine)	Not measured	Rat incision healing equivalent to 1% lidocaine topical treatment	47
Lidocaine	100 mg/mL spray on incision before closure reduced post-op pain and systemic analgesia need in hernia	No adverse effects	48
Lignocaine	Not measured	0.5-1% normal healing; 2% delayed healing of rat biopsy excisions, further delayed by addition of epinephrine	49
Tetracaine/cocaine	Pediatric trauma pain reduced equally with or without addition of tetracaine to cocaine	Normal wound healing	50

let derived growth factor (PDGF) effects range from reported efficacy in increasing granulation tissue or reversing adriamycin-impaired healing in animals to sporadic efficacy in clinical wounds. TGFα and bFGF, both members of the heparin-binding growth factor family, increase collagen deposition and are associated with occasional reports of inflammation.

Many topical wound treatments have not been covered in this chapter, such as combination antibiotic-steroid preparations,[120,121] which by synergistic action, may improve clinical outcomes more than either component alone. Other agents reported to promote healing include the "liquid dressings," like polyethylene glycol,[122] or agents with specialized effects on capillaries or blood cells, such as lazeroids which preserve blood flow.[123] Readers are encouraged to watch the literature for

Table 4-5. **Safety and Efficacy of Topical Debriding Enzymes**

Agent	Debriding Efficacy	Safety	Reference
Acids: citric, hydrochloric, lactic, phosphoric, pyruvic	Ointment of pH 2, but not 4 or 6 accelerated sloughing of full-thickness burns on guinea pigs	No adverse effects	51
Bromelain	Rapid debridement of full-thickness burns in rats, enhanced by addition of nacetylcystein	No adverse effects	52
	50% bromelain debrided full-thickness swine burns in 1 day; 2.5% in 12 days vs. 20 days for vehicle	Skin grafts did not take	53
Collagenase arterial	Collagenase did not debride scald burns on rats as well as sutilains did	Petrolatum vehicle increased mortality from 0 to 60%, not reduced by addition of enzymes	54
	0.5% ointment debrided arterial, pressure, and venous ulcers in 1-3 weeks vs. no debridement for vehicle	No adverse effects	55
	Pressure ulcer granulation in 7 days vs. none in 30 days for vehicle	No adverse effects	56
	Dermal ulcers treated with 250 U/mL ointment had less pus, odor, necrosis, inflammation than placebo	Reversible erythema on surrounding skin in 1 patient.	57
Fibrinolysin (F) + deoxyribonuclease (D)	F 25 U+D 15, 000 U debrided mixed and venous leg ulcers more, but in a week longer time than placebo powder, dressed with saline gauze	Healing to graftable wound bed of debrided ulcers equalled control	58
Hyaluronidase	No debridement of full-thickness guinea pig burns	No adverse effects	51
Krill enzyme	Debrided venous ulcers in 7 days vs. 10 days for acetic acid/iodine/saline gauze control	No adverse effects	59
Papain	12.5-50% ointment debrided full-thickness scald burns in rats in 1-6 days vs. 14 days for vehicle	Skin excoriation	60
	10, 000/g in 10% urea ointment debrided pressure or arteriosclerotic ulcers and burns in 3-4 days.	No adverse effects	61
	Debrided full-thickness burns on guinea pigs in 8 vs. 19 days for control ointment	No adverse effects	51

advances in clinical evidence on such promising agents or to perform appropriate controlled studies of their own to evaluate clinical efficacy.

CONCLUSION

A variety of topical wound treatment agents have been described in this chapter, each with clearly defined outcome measures of efficacy. Few

Table 4-5. **Safety and Efficacy of Topical Debriding Enzymes (Continued)**

Agent	Debriding Efficacy	Safety	Reference
Streptokinase (SK)/ Streptodornase (SD)	Full-thickness burns readied for grafting 3-4 days before controls	No adverse effects	62
	No effect on debridement of full-thickness guinea pig burns	No adverse effects	51
	Readied infected laparotomy incisions for suture after 5 days of treatment vs. 13 days for saline	No adverse effects	63
	No greater debriding effect than zinc oxide during 8 weeks on pressure ulcers	Larger ulcers took longer to debride	64
	Dextranomer produced better clinical pressure ulcer assessments at 7 days than SK/SD	Pain and irritation reported with SK/SD	65
	Less pus and debris in traumatic wounds after 1 week treatment with SK/SD than with trypsin	Mild transient pain with SK/SD	66
	More venous or arterial ulcers debrided after 3 weeks treatment with SK/SD than with trypsin 50 mg	More pain with trypsin than SK/SD	67
Sutilains	100% amputation sites debrided with sutilains after mechanical debridement with wet/dry gauze failed	Pain in 2 of 7 patients. No allergic reactions	68
	Third-degree burns treated with sutilains with or without silver sulfadiazine (SSD) ready for grafting 6-13 days earlier, hospital stay reduced by 10-21 days vs. SSD gauze	Mild wound pain, mild dermatitis. Fat was unaffected. Conjunctivitis with eye contact. Hemostasis needed for necrotic vessels.	69-75
	If treatment started more than 4 days post burn, no effect of sutilains on full-thickness burns	Pain	76
	Rabbit full-thickness burns debrided 7-9 days vs. 18 days for controls with or without SSD	Positive bacterial blood cultures (all groups inoculated with Pseudomonas aeruginosa)	77
	Rats with third degree burns inoculated with pathogens needed additional antimicrobial to survive, but those that survived healed 1 week earlier than untreated	Without added antimicrobial, enzyme increased mortality	78, 79
	Sutilains debrided third degree scald burns better than collagenase	Petrolatum vehicle increased mortality, op cit.	54
	Sutilains debrided in 1 day under occlusion, but not under saline gauze	No harm to surrounding intact skin also treated	80
	No effect on resistance to infection	No effect on rat incision breaking strength	81
Trypsin	Trypsin debrided third-degree guinea pig burns in 6 days, faster than papain (8 days) or SK/SD (ineffective)	No adverse effects	51
	Incisions on rats treated with trypsin	Reduced rat incision tensile strength	82
	Slower debridement of chronic wounds with trypsin than with SK/SD	More pain with trypsin than with SK/SD	66, 67

Table 4-6. Safety and Efficacy of Tissue Glues

Agent	Efficacy	Safety	Reference
Cyanoacrylate	100% of 178 incisions stayed closed without infection vs. 81% of 32 incisions closed with fibrin glue	Exothermic polymerization causes heating which was alleviated by spacing application	83
Fibrin glue	Fibrin sealant with endothelial cell growth factor was more effective in filling meniscal defects than fibrin sealant alone	No adverse effects	84
	Fibrin sealant reduced anastomotic bursting pressure, and did not improve same in steroid-impaired rats	Increased abscess formation with fibrin sealant	85

Table 4-7. Safety and Efficacy of Growth Factors and Other Wound Healing Agents

Agent	Efficacy	Safety	Reference
Acidic Fibroblast Growth Factor (aFGF)	Transient increase in incision tensile strength in rats	Increased cellular content and collagen deposition	86
Angiotropin	Less necrosis in rabbit full-thickness skin flaps injected with 5 ng/mL angiotropin in buffered serum	No adverse effects	87
	Increased new dermis formation in rabbit grafts treated with 0.5 ng angiotropin		
Basic Fibroblast, Growth Factor (bFGF)	More contraction, fibroblasts, and capillaries at 10-21 days in full-thickness excisions on diabetic mice treated with 0.4 mg bFGF daily	No adverse effects	88
	Sustained release of 5 ug bFGF/mL in red blood cell ghosts increased rat incision tensile strength. Collagen or saline delivery decreased it below control levels	Increased cellularity	89
	5 ug/mm^2 of wound area increased rabbit full-thickness ischemic excision mononuclear cells, angiogenesis, and epithelization over collagen vehicle	Increased mononuclear cells which can reflect inflammation	90,91
	1-10 ug/cm^2 of pressure ulcer area increased fibroblasts and capillaries over placebo control	No significant serum absorption or antibody formation	92
Carbopol 93 UP	No effect on swine donor site healing	No adverse effects	93
Collagen	Sponge accelerated swine donor site healing	No adverse effects	93
	With TGFβ increased breaking strength of adriamycin-impaired rat full-thickness incisions	Not explored	94, 95
	Faster healing of mixed ulcers using various forms of lyophilized type I collagen	Increased inflammation	96

Table 4-7. **Safety and Efficacy of Growth Factors and Other Wound Healing Agents (Continued)**

Agent	Efficacy	Safety	Reference
Epidermal Growth Factor (EGF)	5 ug/mL saline 0.1 mL did not affect blister healing	No adverse effects	97
	10 ug/mL silver sulfadiazine 1% cream accelerated donor site healing by 1.5 days vs. vehicle control	No adverse effects Healing delayed at 0.005 or 1 mg/mL	98
	0.01-0.1 mg/mL increased rabbit corneal incision strength; 0.001 and 1.0 mg/mL had no effect	Alone EGF had no effect	99
	100 ng/mL with TGFß + PDGF increased collagen concentrations in adriamycin impaired rat incisions	No adverse effects	
	10 ug EGF in liposomes but not in hydrogel or saline increased rat full-thickness incision tensile strength	No adverse effects	100
	3.7 ug/mL EGF injections into rat wound cylinders increased collagen content	No adverse effects	101
	No effect of daily 300 ng/mL EGF in 2 mL Ringer's lactate on swine full-thickness incision healing	No adverse effects	102
	EGF 5 ug/mm^2 increased epithelization in ischemic rabbit ear excisions vs. collagen vehicle	No adverse effects	103
	EGF 10 ug/g 3 times daily in silver sulfadiazine cream healed 8 of 9 ulcers of mixed depth and etiology in 34 days vs. none for vehicle	No adverse effects	104
	10 ug/mL twice daily in water had no significant effect on healing of venous ulcers	No adverse effects	111
Growth Factors Combined	500 ng each of PDGF, IGF, FGF, and TGF were ineffective except for TGFα + PDGF which increased granulation tissue thickness in swine donor sites	TGFß inhibited keratinocyte growth and increased inflammation	105
	EGF, TGFß, and PDGF combinations improved healing in adriamycin-impaired rats	No adverse effects	100
Ketanserin	Ketanserin increased formation of granulation tissue and epithelization of chronic ulcers at 2 weeks	No adverse effects	106
Lazeroids	Lazeroids preserved healthy blood flow in rat burns	No adverse effects	107

choices for clinical treatment are clear or simple. Results have often varied from study to study as important patient, wound, and care factors such as wound etiology, top dressings, treatment regimens, and associated preventive measures were rarely comparable for any two studies. Still, science begins with a summary of the state of available knowledge. We hope that the reader will use this knowledge to form new hypotheses and do the much-needed science on which to base treatment choices.

Table 4-7. Safety and Efficacy of Growth Factors and Other Wound Healing Agents (Continued)

Agent	Efficacy	Safety	Reference
Live Yeast Cell Derivative (LYCD)	LYCD 2000 u/g in ointment base accelerated donor site healing	Mild stinging pain in 7 of 9 patients	108
Placental Growth Factor(s) (PGF)	PGF 26 ug/cm² of Geliperm Gel dressing subjectively increased granulation of venous ulcers	No adverse effects	109
Platelet Derived Growth Factor (PDGF)	PDGF 1 ug/day increased fibroblasts and capillaries in full-thickness excision tissue in diabetic mice	No adverse effects	88
	PDGF with or without EGF had no effect on wound chamber repair in adriamycin-impaired rats	No adverse effects	100
	5 ug/mm² increased epithelization of and matrix proteins in rabbit full-thickness is-chemic excisions	No adverse effects	90, 91
	1 ug/mL enhanced healing of pressure ulcers vs. placebo	No adverse effects	110
Platelet Derived Wound Healing Factors (PDWHF)	PDWHF reduced chronic ulcer area 94% vs. 73% for placebo	No adverse effects	112
	PDWHF + 1% silver sulfadiazine cream dressing healed mixed chronic ulcers faster than historic control	No adverse effects	113
Polyethylene Glycol	Polyethylene glycol acclerated epithelization of swine donor sites vs. gauze	No adverse effects	93
Socoseryl	20% gel accelerated healing of partial-thickness wounds in rats vs. placebo gel	No adverse effects	114
Transforming Growth Factor ß (TGFß)	100 ng/mL or more of TGFß reversed adri-amycin impairment of rat full-thickness inci-sion healing and improved normal incision healing and collagen content	No adverse effects	95, 100, 115
	4 ug/mL TGFß in 1 mL PBS widened granu-lating zones in swine full-thickness incisions	Inflammatory response not as-sessed	116
	TGFß1 0.1-2 ug increased collagen deposi-tion in ischemic rabbit ear excisions	No adverse effects	91
Tumor Necrosis Factor (TNF)	In phosphabe buffered saline, TNF did not affect rat full-thickness incision strength, but combined with collagen, 5-500 ng TNF/dose increased tensile strength	No adverse effects	117

One important piece which is missing from the wound healing story for each of these agents is cost effectiveness, i.e., the cost for each agent to heal each square centimeter of wound area. Healing, pain, quality of life, and cost-effectiveness are all clinical outcomes which need to be factored into the effectiveness of any wound treatment. All wound care professionals are encouraged to perform prospective, randomized, controlled, blind evaluation trials versus "best available treatment," measuring each of these key outcomes to determine the most promising topical agents described here.

REFERENCES

1. ICWM consensus statement: wound management. *Ostomy Wound Manage.* 1993;39:80-84.
2. Teepe RG. Cytotoxic effects of topical antimicrobial and antiseptic agents on human keratinocytes in vitro. *J Trauma.* 1983;35:8-19.
3. Bolton L, Oleniacz W, Constantine B, et al. Repair and antibacterial effects of topical antiseptic agents in vivo. In: Maibach H, Lowe N. *Models in Dermatology.* Vol 2. Basel: Karger; 1985:145-158.
4. Edlich R, Rodeheaver G, Thacker J. *Surgical Devices in Wound Healing Management: Wound Healing Biochemical and Clinical Aspects.* Philadelphia, PA: WB Saunders; 1992.
5. Cippola AF, Naraf JK. Effect of absorbable sponges on infection: an experimental study. *Surgery.* 1948;24:828-834.
6. Hait MR, Robb CA, Baxter CR, et al. Comparative evaluation of Avitene microcrystalline collagen. *Am J Surg.* 1973;125:284-834.
7. Goode A. Infected wounds. *Care: Science and Practice.* 1982;1:3-7.
8. Henderson JD, Leming JT, Melon-Niksa D. Chloramine-T solutions: effect on wound healing in guinea pigs. *Arch Phys Med Rehabil.* 1989;70:628-631.
9. Thompson W, Herschman B, Unthank P, Pieper D, Hawtof D. Toxicity of cleaning agents for removal of grease from wounds. *Ann Plast Surg.* 1990;24:40-44.
10. Altemeier W, Burkerts F, Pruitt B, Sandusky W. *Manual on Control of Infection in Surgical Patients.* Philadelphia, PA: JB Lippincott; 1984.
11. Stern HS. Silver sulphadiazine and the healing of partial thickness burns: a prospective clinical trial. *Br J Plast Surg.* 1989;42:581-585.
12. Fotherby Y, Spanwick A, Gibbs S, Barclay C, Potter J, Castleden M. Effect of various dressings on wound healing in healthy volunteers. *J Tissue Viability.* 1991;3:68-70.
13. Gorse GJ, Messner RL. Improved pressure sore healing with hydrocolloid dressing. *Arch Derm.* 1987;123:766-771.
14. Stair T, D'Orta J, Altieri M, Lippe M. Polyurethane and silver sulfadiazene dressings in treatment of partial thickness burns and abrasions. *Am J Emerg Med.* 1986;4:214-217.
15. Leyden JL, Bartelt NM. Comparison of topical antibiotic ointments, a wound protectant, and antiseptics for the treatment of human blister wounds contaminated with Staphylococcus aureus. *J Fam Pract.* 1987;6:601-604.
16. Cason JS, Lowbury EJ. Prophylactic chemotherapy for burns: studies on the local and systemic use of combined therapy. *Lancet.* 1960;2:501-507.
17. Marples RR, Kligman AM. Limitations of paired comparisons of topical drugs. *Br J Dermatol.* 1973;88:61-67.
18. Belzer FO, Salvatierra O, Schweizer RT, Kountz SL. Prevention of wound infections by topical antibiotics in high risk patients. *Am J Surg.* 1973:126:180-185.
19. Saik RP, Walz CA, Rhoads JE. Evaluation of a bacitracin-neomycin surgical skin preparation. *Am J Surg.* 1971:121:557-560.
20. Miller JL, Jennings RG, Weschler HL, Langamfelter CS, Johnson BA. Topical therapy with antibiotics: effectiveness of erythromycin, erythromycin-neomycin, and oxytetracycline contrasted with placebo. *NY State J Med.* 1955;55:2179-2184.
21. Proctor DSC. The treatment of burns: a comparative trial of antibiotic dressings. *S Afr Med J.* 1971;45:231-236.
22. Panzer JD, Atkinson WH. Final report: neomycin. Effectiveness of neomycin on the topical treatment of superficial pyodermas-part B. Therapy of experimental S. aureus infections: (1) infection of stripped skin and (2) therapy of established S. aureus infections of normal skin. Unpublished; 1970.
23. Cochrane GM. A practical domiciliary method for the treatment of varicose ulcers. *Practitioner.* 1961;187:787-789.
24. Heisterkamp C, Vernick J, Simmons RL, Matsumoto T. Topical antibiotics in war wounds: a re-evaluation. *Milit Med.* 1969;134:13-18.
25. Lindsey D, Nava C, Marti M. Effectiveness of penicillin irrigation in control of sutured lacerations. *J Trauma.* 1982;22:186-192.
26. Gilmore OJ, Martin TD, Fletcher BN. Prevention of wound infection after appendicectomy. *Lancet.* 1973;1:220-222.
27. Reiss F, Pulaski EJ, Anderson V. Over the counter topical antibiotic products: data on safety and efficacy. *Int J Dermatol.* 1976;15:1-118.
28. Reiss F. Terramycin in the treatment of skin diseases. *NY State J Med.* 1952;52:1031-1033.
29. Lloyd KM. The value of neomycin in topical corticosteroid preparations. *South Med J.* 1969;62:94-96.
30. Lowbury EJL, Babb JR, Brown VI, Collins BJ. Neomycin-resistant Staphylococcus aureus in a burn unit. *J Hyg.* 1964;62:221-228.
31. Bush CA, Stone HH. Care of the burn wound with topical neosporin. *South Med J.* 1972;65:1083-1087.
32. Hughes WT, Wan RT. Impetigo contagiosa: etiology, complications and comparison of therapeutic effectiveness of erythromycin and antibiotic ointment. *Am J Dis Child.* 1967;113:449-453.
33. Purssey BS. The use of an aerosol antibiotic in minor surgery. *Med J Aust.* 1970;1:989-992.

34. Mack RM, Cantrell JR. Quantitative studies of the bacterial flora of open skin wounds: the effect of topical antibiotics. *Ann Surg.* 1967;166:886-895.

35. Stubenrauch GO, Dalton JE, Armstrong B, Starcs H. Clinical evaluation of therapeutic effects of a combined antibiotic ointment in pyodermas. *J Indiana State Med Assn.* 1956;49:1063-1065.

36. Jackson DW, Pollock AV, Tindal DS. The effect of an antibiotic spray in the prevention of wound infection: a controlled trial. *Br J Surg.* 1971;58:565-566.

37. Fielding G, Rao A, Davis NC, Wernigk N. Prophylactic topical use of antibiotics in surgical wounds: a controlled clinical trial using polybactrin. *Med J Aust.* 1965;2:159-161.

38. Norden CW. Application of antibiotic ointment to the site of venous catheterization: a controlled trial. *J Infect Dis.* 1969;120:611-615.

39. Zinner SH, Denny-Brown BC, Braun P, Burke JP, Toala P, Kass EH. Risk of infection with intravenous in dwelling catheters: effect of application of antibiotic ointment. *J Infect Dis.* 1969;120:616-619.

40. Levy RS, Goldstein J, Pressman RS. Value of a topical antibiotic ointment in reducing bacterial colonization of percutaneous venous catheters. *J Albert Einstein Med Cent.* 1970;18:67-70.

41. Moran JM, Atwood RP, Rowe MI. A clinical and bacteriological study of infections associated with venous cutdowns. *N Engl J Med.* 1965;272:554-560.

42. Calel B, Fagerholm P. Human epidermal growth factor: the influence on the healing of surgically closed corneal wounds. *Acta Ophthalmol Suppl (Copenh).* 1987;182:58-61.

43. Alvarez OM, Levendorf KD, Smerbeck RV, Mertz PM, Eaglstein WH. Effect of topically applied steroidal and nonsteroidal anti-inflammatory agents on skin repair and regeneration. *Federation Proceedings.* 1984;43:2793-2798.

44. Sugar A, Bokosky JE, Meyer RF. A randomized trial of topical corticosteroids in epithelial healing after keratoplasty. *Cornea.* 1984;3:268-271.

45. Martin CL. Effect of topical vitamin A, antibiotic, mineral oil, and subconjunctival corticosteroid on corneal epithelial wound healing in the dog. *J Am Vet Med Assoc.* 1971;159:1392-1399.

46. Thomas DFM, Lambert WG, Williams KL. The direct perfusion of surgical wounds with local anaesthetic solution: an approach to postoperative pain? *Ann Royal Col Surg Engl.* 1983;65:226-229.

47. Nykanen D, Kissoon N, Rieder M, Armstrong R. Comparison of a topical mixture of lidocaine and prilocaine (EMLA) versus 1% lidocaine infiltration on wound healing. *Ped Emerg Care.* 1991;7:15-17.

48. Sinclair R, Cassuto J, Högström S, et al. Topical anesthesia with lidocaine aerosol in the control of postoperative pain. *Anesthesiology.* 1988;68:895-901.

49. Morris T, Tracey J. Lignocaine: its effects on wound healing. *Br J Surg.* 1977;64:902-903.

50. Bonadio WA, Wagner V. Efficacy of TAC topical anesthetic for repair of pediatric lacerations. *ADJC.* 1988;142:203-205.

51. Oey FT, Bonnet J. Experimental investigations into the pharmacotherapy of necrosis of the skin. *Arch Chir Neerl.* 1957;9:274-288.

52. Levenson SM, Gruber DK, Gruber C, Lent R, Seifter E. Chemical debridement of burns: mercaptans. *J Trauma.* 1981;81:632-644.

53. Levine N, Seifter E, Connerton C, Levenson SM. Debridement of experimental skin burns of pigs with bromelin, a pineapple-stem enzyme. *Plast Reconstr Surg.* 1973;52:413-424.

54. Dugan RC, Nance FC. Enzymatic burn wound debridement in conventional and germ-free rats. *Surg Forum.* 1977;28:33-34.

55. Boxer AM, Gottesman N, Berstein H, Mandl I. Debridement of dermal ulcers and decubiti with collagenase. *Geriatrics.* 1969;24:75-86.

56. Barrett D, Klibanski A. Collagenase debridement. *Am J Nurs.* 1973;73:849-851.

57. Varma AO, Bugatch E, German F. Debridement of dermal ulcers with collagenase. *Surg Gynecol Obstet.* 1973;136:281-282.

58. Westerhof W, Jansen F, de Wit F, Cormane R. Controlled double-blind trial of fibrinolysin-desoxyribonuclease (Elase) solution in patients with chronic leg ulcers who are treated before autologous skin grafting. *J Am Acad Dermatol.* 1987;17:32-39.

59. Westerhof W, van Ginkel CJW, Cohen EB, Mekkes JR. Prospective randomized study comparing the debriding effect of krill enzymes and a non-enzymatic treatment in venous leg ulcers. *Dermatologica.* 1990;181:293-297.

60. Baliarsing S, Krishna G. Evaluation of chemicals and enzymes in the debridement of experimental burns. *Indian J Med Res.* 1968;56:1670-1674.

61. Piana M. An economical enzymatic debriding agent for chronic skin ulcers. *Psychiatr Q.* 1968;42(suppl):98-101.

62. Connell JF, Rousselot LM. The use of enzymatic agents in the debridement of burn and wound sloughs. *Surgery.* 1951;30:43-55.

63. Poulsen J, Kristensen VN, Brygger HE, Delikaris P. Treatment of infected surgical wounds with Varidase. *Acta Chir Scand.* 1983;149:245-248.

64. Ågren MS, Strömberg HS. Topical treatment of pressure ulcers: a randomized comparative trial of Varidase and zinc oxide. *Scand J Plast Reconstr Surg.* 1985;19:97-100.

65. Hulkko A, Holopainen VO, Orava S. Comparison of dextranomer and streptokinase-streptodornase in the treatment of venous leg ulcers and other infected wounds. *Ann Chir Gynecol.* 1981;70:65-70.

66. Suomalainen O. Evaluation of two enzyme preparations: Trypure and Varidase in traumatic ulcers. *Ann Chir Gynecol.* 1983;72:62-65.

67. Hellgren L. Cleansing properties of stabilized trypsin and streptokinase-streptodornase in necrotic leg ulcers. *Eur J Clin Pharmacol.* 1983;24:623-628.

68. Kerstein MD. Management of amputation-stump break-down. *Am J Surg.* 1975;41:581-583.

69. Levick PL, Brough MP, Vasilescu CT, Laing JE. Treatment of full-thickness burns with Travase: results of a clinical trial. *Burns.* 1978;4:281-284.

70. Muller FE. Debridement of burns with proteolytic enzymes from Bacillus subtilis. *Z Plast Chir.* 1979;3:197-206.

71. Pennisi V, Capozzi A. Travase: observations and controlled study of the effectiveness in burn debridement. *Burns.* 1975;1:247-278.

72. Pennisi VR, Abril F, Cappozzi A. The combined efficacy of Travase and silver sulphadiazine in the acute burn. *Burns.* 1975;2:169-172.

73. Dimick AR. Experience with the use of proteolytic enzyme (Travase) in burn patients. *J Trauma.* 1977;17:948-955.

74. Levick PL, Brough MD, Vasilescu CT, Laing JE. Treatment of full-thickness burns with Travase: results of a clinical trial. *Burns.* 1978;4:281-284.

75. Krizek T, Robson M, Koss M, Heinriech J, Fichandler B. Emergency nonsurgical escharotomy in the burned extremity. *Ortho Rev.* 1975;4:53-55.

76. Singh GB, Snelling CFT, Hogg GR, Waters WR. Debridement of the burn wound with sutilains ointment. *Burns.* 1980;7:41-48.

77. Harris NS, Compton JB, Larson DL. The relationship of Travase debridement and the development of bacteraemia in a rabbit burn model. *Burns.* 1976;2:261-266.

78. Krizek TJ, Robson MC, Groskin MG. Experimental burn wound sepsis: evaluation of enzymatic debridement. *J Surg Res.* 1974;17:219-227.

79. Silverstein P, Helmkamp GM, Walker HL, McKeel DW, Pruitt BA. Laboratory evaluation of enzymatic burn wound debridement in vitro and in vivo. *Surg Forum.* 1972;23:31-33.

80. Constantine BE, Monte, K. Burn debridement under occlusion. *Proceedings of the American Burn Association.* Las Vegas, NV; 1990.

81. Rodeheaver G, Wheeler CB, Rye DG, Vensko J, Edlich RF. Side-effects of topical proteolytic enzyme treatment. *Surg Gynecol Obstet.* 1979;148:562-566.

82. Hagelbäck B, Lundborg H. Studies on the cytotoxic effect of enzyme preparations. *Eur Surg Res.* 1982;14:386-392.

83. Ellis D, Shaikh A. The ideal tissue adhesive in facial plastic and reconstructive surgery. *J Otolaryngol.* 1990;19:68-72.

84. Hashimoto J, Kurosaka M, Yoshiya S, Hirohata K. Meniscal repair using fibrin sealant and endothelial cell growth factor: an experimental study in dogs. *Am J Sports Med.* 1992;20:537-541.

85. Houston KA, Rotstein OD. Fibrin sealant on high-risk colonic anastomoses. *Arch Surg.* 1988;123:230-234.

86. Mellin T, Mennie R, Cashen D, et al. Acidic fibroblast growth factor accelerates dermal wound healing. *Growth Factors.* 1992;7:1-14.

87. Höckel M, Burke JF. Angiotropin treatment prevents flap necrosis and enhances dermal regeneration in rabbits. *Arch Surg.* 1989;124:693-698.

88. Greenhalgh DG, Sprugel KH, Murray MJ, Ross R. PDGF and FGF stimulate wound healing in the genetically diabetic mouse. *Am J Pathol.* 1990;136:1235-1246.

89. Slavin J, Hunt JA, Nash JR, Williams DF, Kingsnorth AN. Recombinant basic fibroblast growth factor in red blood cell ghosts accelerates incisional wound healing. *Br J Surg.* 1992;79:918-921.

90. Mustoe TA, Pierce GF, Morishma C, Deuel TF. Growth factor-induced acceleration of tissue repair through direct and inductive activities in a rabbit dermal ulcer model. *J Clin Invest.* 1991;87:694-703.

91. Pierce GF, Tarpley JE, Yanagihara D, Mustoe TA, Fox GM, Thomason A. Platelet-derived growth factor (BB homodimer), transforming growth factor-α1, and basic fibroblast growth factor in dermal wound healing: neovessel and matrix formation and cessation of repair. *Am J Pathol.* 1992;140:1375-1388.

92. Robson MC, Phillips LG, Lawrence WT, et al. The safety and effect of topically applied recombinant basic fibroblast growth factor on the healing of chronic pressure sores. *Ann Surg.* 1992;216:401-408.

93. Chvapil M, Holubec H, Chvapil T. Inert wound dressing is not desirable. *J Surg Res.* 1991;51:245-252.

94. Curtsinger JL, Pietsch JD, Brown GL, von Fraunhofer A, Ackerman D, Schultz GS. Reversal of adriamycin-impaired wound healing by transforming growth factor-beta. *Surg Gynecol Obstet.* 1989;168:517-522.

95. Pierce GF, Mustoe TA, Deuel TF. Transforming growth factor beta induces increased directed cellular migration and tissue repair in rats. *Prog Clin Biol Res.* 1988;266:93-102.

96. Mian E, Mian M, Beghe F. Lyophilized type-I collagen and chronic leg ulcers. *Int J Tiss Reac.* 1991;13:257-269.

97. Greaves MW. Lack of effect of topically applied epidermal growth on man in vivo. *Clin Exp Dermatol.* 1986;5:1-103.

98. Brown GL, Nanney LB, Griffen J, et al. Enhancement of wound healing by topical treatment with epidermal growth factor. *N Engl J Med.* 1989;321:76-79.

99. Mathers WD, Sherman M, Fryczkowski A, Jester JV. Dose-dependent effects of epidermal growth factor on corneal wound healing. *Invest Ophthalmol Vis Sci.* 1989;30:2403-2406.

100. Lawrence WT, Sporn MB, Gorschboth C, Norton JA, Grotendorst GR. The reversal of an adriamycin induced healing impairment with chemoattractants and growth factors. *Ann Surg.* 1986;203:142-147.

101. Brown GL, Curtsinger LJ, White M, et al. Acceleration of tensile strength of incisions treated with EGF and TGF-ß. *Ann Surg.* 1988;208:788-794.

102. Hennessey PJ, Nirgiotis JG, Shinn MN, Andrassy RJ. Continuous EGF application impairs long-term collagen accumulation during wound healing in rats. *J Pediatr Surg.* 1991;26:362-366.

103. Jijon AJ, Gallup DG, Behzadian A, Metheny WP. Assessment of epidermal growth factor in the healing process of clean full-thickness skin wounds. *Am J Obstet Gynecol.* 1989;161:1658-1662.

104. Brown GL, Curtsinger L, Jurkiewicz MJ, Nahai F, Schultz G. Stimulation of healing of chronic wounds by epidermal growth factor. *Plast Recontr Surg.* 1991;88:189-194.

105. Lynch SE, Colvin RB, Antoniades HN. Growth factors in wound healing: single and synergistic effects on partial thickness porcine skin wounds. *J Clin Invest.* 1989;84:640-646.

106. Janssen P, Janssen H, Cauwenbergh G, et al. Use of topical ketanserin in the treatment of skin ulcers: a double-blind study. *J Am Acad Dermatol.* 1989;21:85-90.

107. Choi M, Ehrlich P. U75412E, a lazaroid, prevents progressive burn ischemia in a rat burn model. *Am J Pathol.* 1993;142:519-528.

108. Kaplan JZ. Acceleration of wound healing by a live yeast cell derivative. *Arch Surg.* 1984;119:1005-1008.

109. Burgos H, Herd A, Bennett JP. Placental angiogenic and growth factors in the treatment of chronic varicose ulcers: preliminary communication. *J Roy Soc Med.* 1989;82:598-599.

110. Robson MC, Phillips LG, Thomason A, et al. Recombinant human platelet-derived growth factor-BB for the treatment of chronic pressure ulcers. *Ann Plast Surg.* 1992;29:193-201.

111. Falanga V, Eaglstein WH, Bucalo B, Katz MH, Harris B, Carson P. Topical use of human recombinant epidermal growth factor (h-EGF) in venous ulcers. *J Dermatol Surg Oncol.* 1992;18:604-606.

112. Steed DL, Malone JM, Goslen JB, Bunt TJ, Holloway GA, Webster MW. Randomized prospective double-blinded trial in healing chronic diabetic foot ulcers: CT-102 activated platelet supernatant, topical versus placebo. *Diabetes Care.* 1992;15:1598-1604.

113. Atri SC, Misra J, Bisht D, Misra K. Use of homologous platelet factors in achieving total healing of recalcitrant skin ulcers. *Surgery.* 1990;108:508-512.

114. Isler H, Bauen A, Hubler M, Oberholzer M. Morphometric assessment of wound healing in rats treated with a protein-free haemodialysate. *Burns.* 1991;17:99-103.

115. Mustoe TA, Pierce GF, Thomason A, Gramates P, Sporn MB, Deuel TF. Accelerated healing of incisional wounds in rats induced by transforming growth factor-ß. *Science.* 1987;237:1333-1336.

116. Quaglino D, Nanney LB, Ditesheim JA, Davidson JM. Transforming growth factor-beta stimulates wound healing and modulates extracellular matrix gene expression in pig skin: incisional sound model. *J Invest Dermatol.* 1991;97:34-42.

117. Mooney DP, O'Reilly M, Gamelli RL. Tumor necrosis factor and wound healing. *Ann Surg.* 1990;221:124-129.

118. Howell R, Ksander G. Animal models of acute wound healing: selection and interpretation in drug development in clinical trial issues of topical wound healing biologics. *Proceedings of CBER/FDA Workshop.* Bethesda, MD; April 22-23, 1993.

119. Chen WYJ, Rogers AA, Lydon MJ. Characterization of biological properties of wound fluid collected during early stages of wound healing. *J Invest Dermatol.* 1992;99:559-564.

120. Lowbury EJL, Miller RWS, Cason JS, Jackson DM. Local prophylactic chemotherapy for burns treated with tulle gras and by the exposure method. *Lancet.* 1962;2:958-963.

121. Davis CM, Fulghum DD, Taplin D. The value of neomycin-steroid cream. *JAMA.* 1968;203:298-300.

122. Clark RF. The case for corticosteroid-antibiotic combinations. *Cutis.* 1974;14:737-741.

123. Lee LK, Ambrus JL. Collagenase therapy for decubitus ulcers. *Geriatrics.* 1975;30:91-93,97-98.

Chapter 5

Nutritional Considerations in Wound Management

Saroj M. Bahl, PhD, RD, LD

Cellular and tissue growth are complex processes. Continuation and maintenance of such processes, which are characteristic of all living organisms, require the presence of several essential nutrients. These nutrients range from the energy-producing macronutrients such as carbohydrates, fat, and protein, all required in relatively large amounts, and a broad spectrum of micronutrients, including several vitamins and minerals needed in smaller amounts.

The processes of cell division, multiplication, and differentiation are ongoing and continuous throughout life. Each cell develops and adapts its structure and function according to its designated function in the bodily tissue or organ. While one cannot generalize the various activities underlying these complex processes, it is commonly agreed that certain principles apply to all cells, regardless of their specific function. A cell constitutes the metabolically active unit of the body. Further, it is well known that the cell obtains its nutrition from the surrounding extracellular fluid. This extracellular fluid serves as the medium for exchange of nutrients and removal of waste products. Replenishment of the nutrient supply in the extracellular fluid, which in turn, is dependent upon the absorption of essential nutrients from the digestive tract, is crucial for the health of the cells. Consequently, it can be concluded that the nutritional status of an individual is a primary factor influencing the growth and maintenance of all tissues in a healthy state.

From this discussion, it is logical to assume that the role of nutrition may also be vital in the repair of tissue that has been damaged by trauma, injury, or surgery such as that which occurs in the formation of wounds. A wound is defined as: "a bodily injury caused by physical means, with disruption of the normal continuity of structures."[1] Several types of wounds are known to occur. These range from minor superficial scrapes, incisions, and lacerations, to deep, penetrating, or perforating wounds, sometimes involving several underlying tissues and organs. However, all wounds are characterized by broken, traumatized tissue which needs to repair itself. This repair or healing process occurs in three phases: inflammatory, fibroplastic, and remodeling. Detailed activities underlying these phases have been described in Chapter 1. Nutrition is closely linked with all of these phases. The purpose of this chapter is to describe the metabolic changes that occur with wounds, roles of various nutrients for effective wound management, and nutritional needs for specific types of wounds.

METABOLIC CHANGES

STATE OF PHYSIOLOGICAL STRESS

Before one can address the specific roles of various nutrients in wound management, it is important to understand the metabolic changes that accompany any state of trauma or stress. Surgery, extensive burns, and traumatic injuries initiate a state of physiological stress in the body. The result is several neurohormonal changes which, in turn, cause many metabolic effects. These include lower blood pressure, decreased cardiac output, low body temperature, and decreased oxygen consumption in the initial stages. In the later "adaptive" stage, a state of hypermetabolism and hypercatabolism is created. The purpose of this state is to facilitate wound healing and protect the integrity of the nervous system.

However, the hypermetabolic state necessitates an increased intake of energy as well as other nutrients. Appropriate nutrition intervention strategies, following an adequate nutritional assessment, can prevent further tissue degeneration and enhance the wound healing process.

ENERGY METABOLISM IN THE HYPERMETABOLIC STATE

The intensity of the "stress response" created by the physiological stress varies with the magnitude of the stressful event. However, there are many similarities between the various responses. Generally, there is a significant increase in basal energy expenditure (BEE) caused by severe physiological stress. This increase in BEE can vary from 15% to 25% in fractures of the long bones to 100% in extensive burns.[2] Increased blood flow and oxygen consumption in the wound area accompany the hypermetabolic state. Net result of all these changes is enhanced energy needs for the individual affected.

SOURCES OF ENERGY

In order to meet the increased energy requirements created by the state of physiological stress, endogenous energy reserves are rapidly mobilized. Breakdown of glycogen stores and lipids occurs rapidly; amino acids are released from body proteins and used for gluconeogenesis. Glucose is the preferred fuel source for the brain, nervous system, and red blood cells. Wound repair is also dependent upon a continuous supply of glucose. Amino acids are derived from the extensive muscle tissue and these provide substrate for hepatic gluconeogenesis.

ESTIMATION OF ENERGY AND PROTEIN REQUIREMENTS

As one may assume, energy requirements increase significantly during periods of physiological stress. Generally, the increase in energy and protein needs is proportional to the degree of trauma. Energy requirements can be estimated by several methods; however, the most commonly used formula was developed by Harris-Benedict and includes allowances for activity and injury factors suggested by Long.[3] For most patients, 30 to 35 kcal/kg ideal body weight (IBW) is adequate to maintain nitrogen balance (a state of protein homeostasis). But, in severely stressed, critically ill patients (such as those with extensive burns), provision of 40 to 45 kcal/kg IBW or more may become necessary to achieve an anabolic, rehabilitative state. Adequate energy intake is essential to ensure that protein will not be used as a source of energy. Approximately 14% to 20% of total daily calories should be obtained from protein. In the presence of adequate energy levels, such as those mentioned earlier, this level of protein should promote positive nitrogen balance and restoration of protein reserves. However, as the rate of nitrogen excretion varies with different trauma states, it is necessary to conduct regular monitoring of nitrogen balance to assess adequacy of energy and protein consumption. The goal of nutritional planning and support is to achieve an anabolic state. This facilitates closing of wounds and burns, thereby permitting early recovery and rehabilitation.

While there is general agreement regarding increased energy and protein needs during periods of physiological stress, the quantitative requirements of other essential nutrients have not been determined. Yet, it is well recognized that several nutri-

Table 5-1. **Role of Energy-Producing Nutrients in the Maintenance of Healthy Tissue and Wound Healing**

Nutrient	Role in the Maintenance of Healthy Tissue	Specific Role in Wound Healing
I. Energy-Yielding Nutrients A. Carbohydrates	Source of energy for normal growth and tissue health Formation of ground substance	Glucose is the preferred energy source for wound repair Formation of ground substance (during fibroplastic phase)
B. Fats/Fatty acids	Source of energy Fatty acids are essential constituents of cell membranes Synthesis of prostaglandins	Prostaglandins may mediate the activities underlying the inflammatory phase (prerequisite to wound healing)
C. Proteins	Essential for cellular and tissue growth Synthesis of connective tissue Production of enzymes and hormones	Support cellular multiplication (fibroblastic proliferation) required for wound healing Synthesis of connective tissue/collagen necessary for wound repair
D. Specific Amino Acids 1. Cysteine	Tissue growth Source of sulfur for body tissues	Essential for fibroblastic proliferation Critical component of the terminal peptide of the intracellular procollagen molecule
2. Methionine	Essential amino acid; source of cysteine	Fibroblastic proliferation
3. Arginine	Semi-essential amino acid; required for normal tissue synthesis	Stimulates secretion of insulin and growth hormones Formation of collagen

ents perform specific roles in wound repair. The role of some of these nutrients, including the energy-producing nutrients (carbohydrates, fatty acids, proteins/amino acids, vitamins, and minerals) are summarized in Tables 5-1 through 5-3.

ENERGY-YIELDING NUTRIENTS

GLUCOSE

Glucose is the preferred fuel source during wound repair. It is well accepted that more amino acids, carbohydrates, and lipids are utilized during tissue repair than in the process of normal tissue maintenance.[4] Extensive consumption of glucose occurs in the process of wound healing. Energy requirements of cells such as leukocytes and fibroblasts that are actively involved in the process of wound repair cannot be met without adequate amounts of glucose. Delayed or poor healing of wounds related to defective carbohydrate and fat metabolism has been documented in diabetics.[5] Diabetes, and the consequent hyperglycemic state, are also associated with decreased phagocytosis and decreased function of leukocytes.[6] Glucose contributes to wound repair by its relationship to the synthesis of ground substance in the connective tissue. It is well known that glucose is an integral constituent of mucopolysaccharides such as glycosaminoglycans, which in turn, form an essential component of the ground substance.[7]

FATS/FATTY ACIDS

Fats, in the form of fatty acids, serve as an important source of energy to all bodily tissues. The role of fatty acids in wound healing requires further research. However, fatty acids are essential constituents of cell membranes; hence, their deficiency may affect wound repair in an adverse manner. Fatty acids may influence wound healing in other ways as well. The essential fatty acid, arachidonic acid, is a precursor of prostaglandins. These compounds mediate several important physiological and biochemical processes in the body. Some of the prostaglandins (those of the E-series) cause vasodilation, exudation, and increased sensitivity to painful stimuli (tenderness). Thus, inflammation, a prerequisite for the wound healing process, may be modulated by prostaglandins. Interrelationships of antibody-producing cells and the action of suppressor T-cells may also be mediated by prostaglandins.[8] Experimental animals maintained on a diet deficient in essential fatty acids indicated a significant reduction in primary and secondary immune responses.[9] From this discussion, it can be concluded that essential fatty acids may exert a significant influence on wound healing by their link with prostaglandins.

PROTEIN

Severe trauma has an adverse influence on protein metabolism. It generally manifests its effect by shifting the nitrogen balance (a measure of protein homeostasis) to the negative state. Excretion of urinary nitrogen is increased significantly in this situation. Studies have indicated that there is an impairment of fibroblastic proliferation, neoangiogenesis, collagen synthesis, and wound remodeling in protein deficiency.[10] Hypoalbuminemia, which is a characteristic feature of protein deficit, may lead to edema and this further impairs fibroplasia in long-term situations. Undernutrition and protein deficiency may also influence cell-mediated immune mechanisms and certain leukocyte functions such as phagocytosis. The net result of these effects in protein deficient subjects may be a greater risk of infections and hence delayed wound healing.[11,12]

SPECIFIC AMINO ACIDS

While efficient wound repair requires a good mixture of all amino acids, certain members appear to make specific contributions to wound healing. In particular, the sulfur-containing amino acids methionine and cysteine have been shown to support collagen formation and fibroblastic proliferation.[13] The terminal peptide of the intracellular procollagen molecule contains cysteine. Hence, these amino acids may make significant contributions to wound repair.

Arginine, a semi-essential amino acid, is another nutrient that may influence wound healing. This amino acid is a precursor for collagen-bound proline and also stimulates the secretion of insulin and growth hormone. Deficiency of arginine has a deleterious effect upon the T-cells and macrophages, thereby delaying wound healing. Protein catabolism that results from injury or trauma is favorably affected by arginine administration. By reducing urinary nitrogen losses, arginine enhances post-traumatic nitrogen retention. As a result, wound healing, as assessed by breaking strength and reparative collagen synthesis, shows significant improvement. It has been demonstrated that incorporation of hydroxyproline in collagen synthesis may be significantly enhanced with administration of arginine in pharmacologic doses.[14]

VITAMINS

Table 5-2 summarizes the functions of vitamins in maintenance of healthy tissue and wound healing. Several vitamins are involved in support of healthy tissue. The needs of these vitamins are probably enhanced in situations of surgical stress or others accompanied by open wounds. However, while the qualitative roles of these vitamins are well appreciated, quantitative requirements have not been established.

Vitamin A

Several studies conducted with experimental animals have supported the role of vitamin A in wound healing. Processes such as wound closure, epithelization, rate of collagen synthesis, and cross linkages in newly generated collagen are adversely affected in experimentally induced vitamin A defi-

Table 5-2. Role of Vitamins in the Maintenance of Healthy Tissue and Wound Healing

Nutrient	Role in the Maintenance of Healthy Tissue	Specific Role in Wound Healing
I. Fat-Soluble Vitamins A. Vitamin A	Maintenance of healthy epithelial tissue Synthesis of mucopolysaccharides	Epithelialization; rebuilding of damaged tissue Enhances collagen synthesis (during fibroplastic phase) Synthesis of glycoprotein and proteoglycans Suppresses action of certain infections
B. Vitamin K	Synthesis of prothrombin and clotting factors	Promotes normal clotting; important role in inflammatory phase of wound healing
C. Vitamin D	Maintenance of calcium homeostasis Essential for bone formation	Calcium homeostasis affects action of tissue collagenases
II. Water-Soluble Vitamins A. Vitamin C	Collagen synthesis (hydroxylation of proline and lysine) Builds resistance to infections	Essential for normal fibroblastic function Enhanced collagen synthesis during fibroplastic phase requires this vitamin Essential for neutrophil formation
B. Vitamin B-complex	Several B-complex vitamins serve as cofactors in a variety of enzyme systems	Specific effects unknown; deficiencies associated with impaired wound healing

ciency.[15] Other investigations have also suggested that wounds heal more rapidly if supplemental dietary vitamin A is provided.[16]

Vitamin A is often referred to as an "anti-infective" vitamin and this may yet be another way in which it supports wound healing. The vitamin is known to suppress certain infections and this effect is possibly mediated by the thymus gland. It has been suggested that patients who have suffered severe injury or are at risk for vitamin A deficiency due to malabsorption should receive daily supplements (5000 IU/day). In order to be most effective, supplements should be given at the time of occurrence of the wound or within 3 to 4 days.[17]

Vitamin K

Vitamin K is essential for the synthesis of prothrombin and several blood clotting factors.

Deficiency of this vitamin may cause excessive bleeding and formation of hematomas. By virtue of its important role in blood clotting, the vitamin can make a significant contribution to wound healing in the early inflammatory phase (see Chapter 1). Patients suffering from intestinal malabsorption, who may be at risk for deficiency of this vitamin, should therefore receive supplements.

Vitamins D and E

Vitamin D contributes to bone health by its effect on calcium metabolism. The vitamin stimulates absorption of calcium and phosphorus which facilitates the normal mineralization of bone. It also maintains homeostasis of calcium which may affect the action of tissue collagenases. Thus, vitamin D may have an indirect effect on wound healing.

The role of vitamin E (fat-soluble vitamin) in

wound healing is mostly speculative; it is well accepted that this vitamin functions as an antioxidant and hence, may contribute to cell-membrane integrity. Animal studies have indicated that the breaking strength of wounds following radiotherapy may be enhanced with supplemental vitamin E.[18] However, further research is needed to understand the precise role of vitamin E in wound repair.

Water-Soluble Vitamins

Table 5-2 also summarizes the relationships of water-soluble vitamins such as vitamins C and B-complex with the maintenance of healthy tissue and wound healing. Further research in this direction is necessary however.

Vitamin C

The role of vitamin C in the synthesis of collagen is well understood and accepted. This synthesis requires hydroxylation of lysine and proline amino acids that form an integral component of the collagen molecule. In addition to vitamin C or ascorbic acid, this hydroxylation reaction also requires oxygen, alpha-ketoglutarate, and iron. These cofactors act in conjunction with lysyl and prolyl hydroxylases, the enzymes that catalyze these reactions. In the absence of vitamin C, collagen formation is impaired. Scurvy or vitamin C deficiency is characterized by abnormal wound healing and fragility of capillaries.

Vitamin C is also needed for immune function and building resistance to infection. The vitamin is essential for phagocytosis and normal neutrophil function. Critically ill patients may be extremely susceptible to vitamin C deficiency; supplements ranging from 100 to 2000 mg/day may become necessary, depending upon the extent of the injury.[19]

Vitamin B-Complex

Several members of the B-complex group of vitamins act as co-enzymes or cofactors in the intermediary metabolism of carbohydrate, protein, and fat. Disturbances in energy production and other adverse effects may thus occur during deficiency states of these vitamins. Studies exploring the relationships of these vitamins with wound healing are scanty.

However, there is sufficient evidence to indicate that wound repair may be adversely affected during deficiency states. For example, one study indicated that wound healing is markedly delayed in pyridoxine- and riboflavin-deficient animals.[20] Several B-complex vitamins have been linked with antibody formation; hence, this may be another mechanism through which wound healing may be influenced.

Specific roles for some B-complex vitamins in wound management have been postulated. For example, the combined effect of pantothenic acid (member of B-complex group) and ascorbic acid in the wound healing process was studied. Parameters such as growth of fibroblasts, cell proliferation, and protein synthesis were evaluated. Results suggested that these two vitamins were more effective in combination than alone. Hence, the combined use of these two vitamins might be quite valuable in postsurgical therapy and in wound healing.[21]

MINERALS

In recent years, considerable attention has been focused on the relationship of minerals, macro and micro, with wound healing. Some of these roles have been summarized in Table 5-3. Particularly noteworthy are the roles of trace minerals, iron and zinc. However, macrominerals such as sodium, potassium, calcium, chloride, and phosphorus perform important functions related to cellular health and hence, wound repair.

Sodium, Potassium, and Chloride

As a major constituent of the extracellular fluid, sodium contributes to electrolyte and water balance which, in turn, affects cell health. More than 95% of body potassium occurs within the cells. Plasma concentrations of both sodium and potassium are maintained within narrow limits by the combined action of some hormones and renal excretion. Along with these two minerals, chloride, another extracellular element, also contributes to water balance, acid-base equilibrium, and normal muscular irritability.

Following surgery or other forms of trauma, significant amounts of potassium are lost and high concentrations occur in the urine.[22] Debilitated,

Table 5-3. **Role of Minerals in the Maintenance of Healthy Tissue and Wound Healing**

Nutrient	Role in the Maintenance of Healthy Tissue	Specific Role in Wound Healing
I. Macrominerals A. Calcium	Principal component of skeletal tissue Maintenance and function of cell membrane Influences blood clotting	Required for the action of tissue collagenases Promotes normal clotting that occurs in the inflammatory phase
B. Magnesium	Protein synthesis Cofactor in the energy release cycle Maintenance of muscle and nerve tissue	Due to its involvement with several enzymes, its presence is essential in all phases of wound healing
II. Trace Minerals A. Iron	Affects the health of all bodily tissues by its central role in hemoglobin formation Required for effective collagen synthesis (hydroxylation of lysine and proline)	Formation of collagen/connective tissue (fibroplastic phase) Anemia may interfere with wound healing
B. Zinc	Constituent of DNA/RNA polymerases Protein synthesis Collagen formation	Wound repair requires additional protein which is synthesized with the help of zinc Enhanced collagen synthesis
C. Copper	Erythropoiesis (affects all bodily tissues) Component of lysyl oxidase	Cross-linkages in collagen synthesis Strengthening of scar tissue
D. Manganese	Activation of several enzymes including those involved in energy production Glycosylation of procollagen molecules	Collagen synthesis (glycosylation of procollagen molecules in the fibroplastic phase of wound healing)

hyponatremic patients demonstrate an enhanced manifestation of this response. Dietary intakes of sodium and potassium are thus very significant at such times. While there is very little chance of a deficiency of these nutrients in a healthy person's diet, there is a greater likelihood of a serious deficit occurring in traumatized individuals following excessive utilization and excretion.

Calcium and Phosphorus

Two minerals that are present in significant amounts in the body are calcium and phosphorus. Ninety-nine percent of calcium, which is the most abundant mineral in the body, is present in bones and teeth. Serum extracellular fluid and the cells of soft tissue contain the remaining calcium, and here it modulates many important physiological and bio-

chemical functions. These include cell membrane stabilization, maintenance of muscle tone, nerve excitation, activation or release of several enzymes, and blood clotting, to name just a few. Several of these functions influence tissue repair and thus wound healing. For example, calcium is known to regulate the function of tissue collagenases which perform a crucial role in remodeling of collagen fibers. The remodeling phase, which is the final stage of wound healing, may be affected by dietary calcium.

Phosphorus represents the second largest element in human tissues. The skeletal tissue contains 80% of the phosphorus, where it occurs as a component of calcium phosphate crystals. The remaining 20% of the phosphorus occurs in the extracellular fluid and every cell in the body tissues. This nutrient is very active metabolically and performs many important functions. As part of high-energy compounds, adenosine triphosphate (ATP) and adenosine monophosphate (AMP), phosphorus participates in the energy production cycle. Phospholipids, which contain phosphorus, are crucial components of the structure of cell membranes. The role of phosphorus in the energy release cycle is of vital importance to cellular health and has widespread consequences for all bodily tissues. Deficiency of phosphorus is accompanied by neuromuscular, skeletal, hematologic, and renal abnormalities.

Magnesium

As an intracellular cation, magnesium ranks second in abundance to potassium. The majority of total body magnesium is found in bone (60%) and the remainder is distributed in the muscle, soft tissues, and body fluids. Like phosphorus, magnesium is an essential cofactor in the energy release cycle. In addition, it is also required for protein synthesis and maintenance of muscle and nerve tissue. Since the action of several enzymes is influenced by magnesium, its presence is essential for all phases of wound healing. Formation of collagen during the translation phase also requires magnesium. Deficiency of this nutrient may be precipitated in several conditions such as pancreatitis, protein-calorie malnutrition, diabetes, parathyroid gland disorders, and postsurgical stress.[23]

Iron

By its central role as a component of hemoglobin, iron facilitates oxygen and electron transport, thereby affecting all body tissues. Hydroxylation of lysine and proline and hence, effective collagen synthesis, requires the presence of divalent ionic iron. Some investigators have suggested that iron deficiency anemia may interfere with wound healing.[24] Others have counteracted this claim and state that there are no differences in healing rates of wounds in anemic and control animals.[25] In an attempt to resolve this controversy, Hunt and Zederfeldt[4] hypothesize that factors such as hypovolemia, trauma, increased blood viscosity, and vasoconstriction, rather than anemia, impair oxygen transport.

Zinc

The role of zinc in wound healing has been extensively documented.[26-28] Delayed wound healing has been associated with low plasma zinc levels in experimental animals. It is well known that zinc performs several important biological functions in the body. It is an essential constituent of several metalloenzymes. Specifically, DNA and RNA polymerases, which contain zinc, are essential for protein synthesis. Cell mitosis and proliferation, which are very active during the fibroblastic phase of wound healing, are dependent upon adequate amounts of zinc. However, additional zinc, in the presence of adequate zinc, does not hasten the healing process.[29] Non-steroidal anti-inflammatory drugs (NSAIDs) are known to have a suppressant effect on the breaking strength and the inflammatory response in wound healing. Administration of zinc sulfate, in doses of 220 mg twice a day, may be helpful in reversing these effects.[30,31] The metabolism of vitamin A requires zinc in several stages; hence, deficiency of zinc may have an adverse influence on wound healing by reducing the availability of vitamin A.

Zinc is also essential for collagen synthesis. In zinc-deficient experimental animals, synthesis of collagen and non-collagenous protein has been shown to be depressed. Deficiency of zinc may occur in patients suffering from malabsorption, infections, and severe injury. Critically ill patients who are maintained on prolonged, unsupplemented, intravenous hyperalimentation may be at risk for developing zinc deficiency. This can be corrected readily with administration of oral zinc sulfate.

Copper

Copper is well noted for certain of its biochemical functions which contribute to normal tissue health. It is a component of several metalloenzymes such as ceruloplasmin (ferroxidase I), ferroxidase II, monoamine oxidase, and lysyl oxidase. The oxidation of the ferrous to the ferric ion, which constitutes an essential step in iron metabolism, is catalyzed by ferroxidases. Through this role, copper contributes to erythropoiesis in the mammalian systems. As a component of lysyl oxidase, it influences the formation of the covalent cross linkages that strengthen scars.[32] Copper deficiency may occur in critically ill patients who have been maintained on long-term, intravenous alimentation which has not included supplements of this nutrient.

Manganese

Activation of several enzymes such as phosphatases, kineses, glycosyltransferases, and decarboxylases requires manganese. Energy production in the cells is related to the action of some of these enzymes. Manganese is thus essential for cellular and tissue health. Specifically, it influences wound healing through its activation of the enzymes responsible for glycosylation of procollagen molecule. Hence, it can be inferred that synthesis of connective tissue would possibly suffer during manganese deficiency.

NUTRITIONAL STATUS AND WOUND HEALING

While all these nutrients have been specifically associated with various aspects of wound healing, they also work synergistically and interrelate with each other for utilization, absorption, and transport. Hence, a generally good nutritional status constitutes the cornerstone of success in wound management. Whether a wound has been acquired as a result of surgery (elective or non-elective) or sustained accidentally, the dietary goal should be to provide sufficient calories to maintain weight or prevent weight loss. Additionally, the protein intake should be quite generous providing between 15% to 20% of the total calories. As discussed earlier, vitamins and minerals should meet or exceed the recommended dietary allowances (RDA) for a healthy

state. In certain cases, supplements of certain nutrients may be desirable.

MALNUTRITION AND WOUND HEALING

A wide array of metabolic changes that occur consequent to malnutrition may influence wound repair. These include physiological, biochemical, and endocrinological changes associated with stress, and these cause aberrations in energy and protein metabolism. Delayed wound healing has been reported in malnourished animals. It is believed that wounds in malnourished animals could possibly be weaker due to a slower rate of healing as well as the formation of a structurally inferior scar tissue. Protein-calorie malnutrition (PCM) is associated with delayed wound healing and the impairment occurs quite early in the course of PCM. Available evidence indicates that adequate nutritional support, whether provided enterally or parenterally, may significantly improve the prognosis for wound repair. Nutritional status prior to surgery (preoperative nutrition) may be a significant factor in wound healing as well.

HIGH-RISK SURGICAL PATIENTS

Surgical patients who are at increased operative risk, such as those with diabetes, cirrhosis, heart disease, obesity, renal disease, and substance abuse problems, require carefully planned nutritional interventions. Preoperative nutritional support should be provided, particularly if the patients are malnourished.

Poor wound healing and high incidence of infections are associated with diabetes mellitus. The attendant hyperglycemia in this condition is linked with decreased phagocytosis, decreased chemotaxis, and diminished leukocyte function.[6] Adequate control of blood sugar through rigid dietary intervention and other wound management procedures such as wound debridement, adequate dressings, etc., may be helpful in wound repair in diabetics.

The high-risk surgical patient often faces wound dehiscence as a major complication.[33] Energy and protein requirements are significantly enhanced in these patients, possibly because massive inflammation and infection are associated with wound disruption. Adequate nutritional assessment, utilizing current parameters such as anthropometrics, albumin, transferrin, and immune status could assist in determining specific nutrient deficiencies. Following this assessment, appropriate nutritional repletion could be achieved with enteral or parenteral support.[34]

MANAGEMENT OF SPECIFIC TYPES OF WOUNDS

BURNS

Energy expenditure is generally proportional to the degree of burns. A markedly increased metabolic rate has been documented in burn victims.[35] Several other metabolic aberrations such as increased rate of protein anabolism and catabolism, decreased rate of lipid metabolism, and increased rate of glucose production and utilization have also been reported. Administration of large amounts of calories and protein are necessary to achieve positive nitrogen balance. Estimation of energy and protein requirements is based upon a number of factors including the total body surface area (TBSA) that is burned. Generally, calories at twice the resting energy expenditure and protein at 2.5 gm/kg/day based on ideal body weight is considered adequate.[36] However, nutritional planning and intervention strategies in burn patients are highly individualized. Enteral and parenteral nutritional support is generally necessary. Multivitamin supplements and supplemental vitamin C (1000 to 2000 mg) may be helpful.

PRESSURE ULCERS

These generally occur with a high degree of prevalence in the elderly. These ulcerated skin lesions commonly occur in bedbound patients. However, they may also occur in active youths

with spinal cord injury and other immobile or demented patients. While appropriate wound care is essential, the underlying malnutrition must be identified and corrected to ensure rapid healing of the pressure ulcers. Adequate energy intake, ranging from 25 to 35 kcal/kg body weight, and protein, 1.5 to 2.5 gm/kg body weight, may be necessary in these situations. Stressed and traumatized patients may require higher amounts. Tube feedings, enteral formulas, and in certain cases, total parenteral nutrition (TPN) may become necessary to supply adequate nutrition.

VALUE OF NUTRITIONAL SUPPLEMENTS IN WOUND HEALING

From the aforementioned discussion of nutrient interrelationships with wound healing, it can be logically inferred that an adequate nutritional status is essential for wound repair. Protein, amino acids, and several vitamins and minerals influence the synthesis of collagen which in turn affects wound healing. Several investigators have reported the beneficial effects of nutritional supplements. There is no general agreement on this subject, however. While some have supported the value of pharmacological doses of certain nutrients such as arginine,[13] vitamins such as vitamin C,[19] and minerals such as zinc,[30-31] others do not promote supplements unless the dietary levels of these nutrients are well below the RDA.[10] Further research on the quantitative roles of essential nutrients in wound management is necessary before specific recommendations can be made.

CONCLUSION

Wound healing is a complex process that is affected by several factors. When wounds do not heal adequately, the physical and financial burden of hospitalization is increased tremendously. This poses a difficult challenge for health care providers. Addressing nutritional needs, including energy and protein intake, vitamin and mineral supplements as required, and other wound management techniques, such as tissue perfusion, oxygenation, wound dressing, and sanitation can promote a more rapid and complete recovery.

REFERENCES

1. *Dorland's Illustrated Medical Dictionary.* Philadelphia, PA: WB Saunders Co; 1974.
2. Williamson J. Physiological stress: trauma, sepsis, burn and surgery. In: Mahan LK, Arlin M. *Krause's Food Nutrition and Diet Therapy.* Philadelphia, PA: WB Saunders Co; 1992:491-506.
3. Long CL, Schaffel N, Geiger JW, Schiller WR, Blakemore WS. Metabolic response to injury and illness: estimation of energy and protein needs from indirect calorimetry and nitrogen balance. *J Paren Enter Nutr.* 1979;3:452-456.
4. Hunt TK, Zederfeldt B. Nutritional and environmental aspects of wound healing. In: Dunphy JE, van Winkle W. *Repair and Regeneration: The Scientific Basis for Surgical Practice.* New York, NY: McGraw Hill; 1969:217-228.
5. Hunt TK. *Fundamentals of Wound Management in Surgery.* South Plainfield, NJ: Chirurgecom; 1976.
6. Ehrlichman RJ, Seckel BR, Bryan DJ, Moschella CJ. Common complications of wound healing: prevention and management. *Surg Clin North Am.* 1991;71:1323-1351.
7. Stryer L. *Biochemistry.* New York, NY: Freeman and Co; 1988.
8. Goodwin JS, Webb DR. Review: regulation of the immune response by prostaglandins. *Clin Immun Immunopath.* 1980;15:106-122.
9. Ziff M. Diet in the treatment of rheumatoid arthritis. *Arth Rheum.* 1984;26:457-471.
10. Pollack SV. Wound healing: a review. *J Dermatol Surg Oncol.* 1979;5:615-619.
11. Howard RJ, Simmons RL. Acquired immunologic deficiencies after trauma and surgical procedures. *Surg Gynecol Obstet.* 1974;139:771-782.
12. Smythe PM, Brereton-Stiles GG, Grace HH. Thymolymphatic deficiency and depression of cell-mediated immunity in protein-calorie malnutrition. *Lancet.* 1971;2:939-943.
13. Williamson MB, Fromm HJ. The incorporation of sulfur amino acids into the proteins of regenerating wound tissue. *J Biol Chem.* 1955;212:705-712.
14. Barbul A, Lazarou SA, Efron DT, Wasserkrug ML, Efron G. Arginine enhances wound healing and lymphocyte immune responses in humans. *Surgery.* 1990;108:331-337.
15. Seifter E, Crowley LV, Rettura G. Influence of vitamin A on wound healing in rats with femoral fracture. *Ann Surg.* 1975;181:836-841.
16. Greenwald DP, Sharzer LA, Ladawer J, Levenson SM, Seifter E. Zone II flexor tendon repair: effects of vitamins A, E and beta-carotene. *J Surg Res.* 1990;49:98-102.
17. Hunt TK. Vitamin A and wound healing. *J Am Acad Dermatol.* 1986;15:817-821.
18. Taren DL, Chvapil M, Weber CW. Increasing the breaking strength of wounds exposed to preoperative irradiation using vitamin E supplementation. *Int J Vitam Nutr Res.* 1987;57:133-137.
19. Levenson SM, Seifter E. Dysnutrition, wound healing and resistance to infection. *Clin Plast Surg.* 1977;4:375-388.
20. Bosse MD, Axelrod AE. Nutrition and wound healing. In: Levenson SM, Seifter E, Van Winkle W. *Fundamentals of Wound Management in Surgery.* South Plainfield, NJ: Chirurgecom; 1977.
21. Lacroix B, Didier E, Grenier JF. Role of pantothenic acid and ascorbic acid in wound healing processes: in vitro study on fibroblasts. *Int J Vitam Nutr Res.* 1988;58:407-413.
22. Shils ME, Young VR. *Modern Nutrition in Health and Disease.* Philadelphia, PA: Lea and Febiger; 1988.
23. Czajka-Narins DM. Minerals. In: Mahan LK, Arlin M. *Krause's Food Nutrition and Diet Therapy.* Philadelphia, PA: WB Saunders Co; 1992:109-140.
24. Sandblom P. The tensile strength of healing wounds. *Acta Chir Scand.* 1944;84(suppl):71-85.
25. Jurkiewicz MJ, Garrett LP. Studies on the influence of anemia on wound healing. *Am J Surg.* 1964;30:23-25.
26. Sandstead HH, Shepard GH. The effect of zinc deficiency on the tensile strength of healing surgical incisions in the integument of the rat. *Proc Soc Exp Biol Med.* 1968;128:687-689.
27. Hallmans G. Wound healing with adhesive zinc tape: an animal experimental study. *Scand J Plast Reconstr Surg.* 1976;10:177-184.
28. Orgill D, Demling RH. Current concepts and approaches to wound healing. *Crit Care Med.* 1988;16:899-908.
29. Cumming C. Nutrition for the patient with a chronic wound. In: Rudolph R, Noe JM. *Chronic Problem Wounds.* Boston, MA: Little Brown & Co; 1983:53-63.
30. Rao CM, Kumar A, Kulkarni DR. Effects of enfenamic acid and its zinc salt on wound healing. *Ind J Physiol Pharmacol.* 1988;32:61-66.
31. Pories WJ, Henzel JH, Rob CG. Acceleration of healing with zinc sulfate. *Ann Surg.* 1967;165:432-436.
32. Prockop DJ, Guzman NA. Collagen diseases and the biosynthesis of collagen. *Hosp Pract.* 1977;12:61-68.
33. Hunt TK. Wound healing. In: Way LW. *Current Surgical Diagnoses and Treatment.* 6th ed. Los Altos, CA: Lange Medical Publications; 1983:109-121.
34. Trujillo EB: Effects of nutritional status on wound healing. *J Vascul Nurs.* 1993;11:12-18.
35. Waymack JP, Herndon DN. Nutritional support of the burned patient. *World J Surg.* 1992;16:80-86.
36. Pasulka PS, Wachtel TL. Nutritional considerations for the burned patient. *Surg Clin North Am.* 1987;67:109-131.

Chapter 6

Pressure Ulcers

Diane Krasner, MS, RN, CETN, and Jan Cuzzell, MA, RN

In a typical clinical practice, many of the patients have chronic wounds such as leg or diabetic ulcers. Chronic wounds do not follow the expected path of healing, despite adequate and appropriate care. Patients may also present with pressure ulcers. Pressure ulcers are also chronic wounds that are due primarily to sustained pressure and are exacerbated by a variety of medical conditions. Given the right conditions, these wounds can either develop quickly, in just hours, or slowly over several days. The purpose of this chapter is to describe the clinician's role in pressure ulcer management. Clinicians can participate in the continuum of care from pressure ulcer prevention and early intervention to treatment, such as debridement or removal of devitalized tissue. Collaborations between health care professionals during care planning and implementation is essential for successful pressure ulcer management.

OVERVIEW OF THE PROBLEM

Pressure ulcers have been defined as "localized areas of tissue necrosis that tend to develop when soft tissue is compressed between a bony prominence and an external surface for a prolonged period of time."[1] They are commonly referred to as bedsores, decubitus ulcers, or pressure sores, with pressure ulcer currently being the most acceptable term since it most accurately reflects the cause and condition according to the experts. Based on the definition, it is no surprise that common sites for pressure ulcer development include the sacrum/coccyx, trochanter, ischium, lateral malleolus, and heel. It also follows that persons at risk for pressure ulcer development include those with severe restrictions of mobility, including persons with neurologic impairment (e.g., following CVA, comatose or sedated), with sensory impairment (e.g., following spinal cord injury or due to diabetic neuropathy), and those who are chronically or critically ill.

It has been estimated that pressure ulcer prevalence ranges from 3% to 14% in acute care settings, 15% to 25% in long-term care settings, and 7% to 12% in home care settings.[1] Prevalence includes new and old cases of pressure ulcers and is usually assessed on a cross-sectional, one-time basis. Incidence refers to new pressure ulcer cases occurring over a given period of time. By measuring prevalence and incidence data on a routine basis, clinicians can get a handle on the efficacy of their prevention and intervention efforts. In most settings, data collection is best accomplished by a multidisciplinary team of wound care practitioners dedicated to improving the quality of care, i.e., the Total Quality Management (TQM).

The pressure ulcer problem causes extraordinary amounts of pain, suffering, and disability in over one million patients at any given time in the United States alone. Billions of dollars are spent treating a problem that is largely preventable. Pressure ulcers have serious social and economic consequences, and in the worst case scenario, can result in death due to septicemia. The human tragedy and waste of resources that this problem represents should be a call to arms to all who are in a position to fight the battle against pressure ulcers.

PRESSURE ULCER ETIOLOGIES, RISK FACTORS, AND RISK ASSESSMENT TOOLS

When external pressure is applied to soft tissue over a bony prominence for an extended period of time, blood flow to the area is decreased or diminished altogether, oxygen and nutrients are not carried to the cells, and waste products accumulate. This results in ischemia, followed by reactive vasodilation (hyperemia), edema, tissue necrosis, and eventually the cell death that we recognize as ulceration.

It has been generally accepted that external pressures, or tissue interface pressures, greater than 25 to 32 mmHg cause obstruction to blood flow to the capillaries.[2] Certain tissues, such as muscle and connective tissues, are more susceptible to periods of ischemia than others. Furthermore, it is now recognized that in certain highly susceptible individuals, such as the debilitated elderly, capillary closure pressures may be even lower than 25 mmHg. Other conditions that can compromise blood flow to the tissues and cause ischemia include inadequate cardiac output, low blood pressure, hypovolemia, and vascular disease.

Three other factors besides pressure commonly contribute to pressure ulcer formation. These include shear, friction, and moisture. A shearing force occurs when layers of tissue slide against one another. For example, shearing occurs over the sacrum when the head of the bed is elevated. In response to gravitational forces, the subcutaneous tissue and muscle stretch and angulate while the outer skin layers remain stationary against the bed linens. As a result, this mechanical disruption of tissue causes both superficial and deep tissue destruction. When shear is also a contributing factor, the amount of pressure needed to cause tissue breakdown is greatly reduced. Shear can be minimized by elevating the head of the bed or stretcher no more than 30 degrees whenever possible. Maintaining correct posture and body alignment in a wheelchair for chairbound patients is also an important deterrent to shearing forces.

Friction occurs when the epidermis is rubbed or pulled across a surface, as when the heels are dragged across bed linens. Using lifting rather than sliding techniques to reposition patients can help prevent friction damage. For example, turn sheets and trapeze bars are helpful assistive devices for reducing friction injury. Thin protective dressings, such as transparent films or thin hydrocolloids, can also help prevent friction injury to skin at high risk for mechanical injury. These dressings provide a slick surface that decreases the friction forces to the skin surface. Maceration, or the softening of skin due to moisture, can occur secondary to incontinence, perspiration, or the pooling of secretions or exudate. Macerated skin is prone to breakdown because it is less resistant to mechanical trauma. Careful assessment, the use of skin sealants, the use of moisture barriers, and incontinence management protocols can reduce the maceration component of pressure ulcer formation.

Risk factors for pressure ulcers include extrinsic and intrinsic factors such as: immobility, inactivity, malnutrition, incontinence, impaired sensation, decreased levels of consciousness, fractures, and poor overall physical condition.[1,3] The institutionalized, frail, elderly, and bedbound or chairbound individuals are often at very high risk for pressure ulcer formation. The effects of aging on the skin, such as the thinning of all the skin layers and the flattening of the dermal-epidermal junction, predispose older patients to tissue trauma and skin breakdown. Identification of at-risk status and initiation of preventive strategies, such as regular turning and repositioning schedules, can help to decrease the chance of pressure ulcer formation.

The use of risk assessment tools for determining

at-risk status is recommended by experts in the field and in the Agency of Health Care Policy and Research, *Pressure Ulcers in Adults: Predictions and Prevention, Clinical Practice Guideline No. 3.*[4] Risk assessment tools rate patients on significant predictors for pressure ulcer formation such as immobility and malnutrition. Risk assessment scores, when used to implement prevention and early intervention strategies, can significantly reduce pressure ulcer morbidity and mortality. Risk assessment tools must be reliable and valid, have a high specificity, and be user-friendly. Instruments developed by Abruzzese, Braden and Bergstrom, Gosnell, Norton, and Trelease are commonly used in current clinical practice. Additionally, clinicians should remain alert to less frequently recognized causes of pressure ulcers such as those forming under prostheses, casts, traction, or other devices.

The physical therapist plays a critical role in improving the functional status of immobilized patients, thereby decreasing their risk for pressure ulcers. Mobility should be encouraged whenever possible, especially during or following periods of hospitalization. In an ideal world, all high-risk patients would receive physical therapy consults, and the pressure ulcer prevalence and incidence rates would be nil. Preventive strategies the clinician may institute include:[5]

- Identifying schedules and strategies for turning and repositioning patients
- Instituting range of motion exercises and progressive ambulation to prevent and/or reduce contractures and to increase mobility
- Fitting patients with preventive devices such as chair or wheelchair cushions, wedges, splints, mattress overlays, and mattress replacements or specialty beds
- Identifying ways to decrease friction, shear, and moisture
- Instituting plans for moisturizing dry skin, e.g., after hydrotherapy treatments
- Suggesting moisture/incontinence protocols as necessary
- Recommending dietary consults and nutritional interventions as needed
- Instituting patient and family education programs

PRESSURE ULCER ASSESSMENT

The first step for any clinician evaluating a wound is to determine its etiology. Often a pressure ulcer may mimic other types of chronic wounds, such as leg ulcer or diabetic ulcer. Nonhealing "pressure ulcers" have occasionally turned out to be cancers, pyoderma gangrenosum, or subacute infections. A pressure ulcer is typically found over a bony prominence; if not, some other source of pressure should be identified. A poorly fitting prosthesis, an old, ineffectual wheelchair cushion, urinary catheter, or oxygen cannula tubing are just a few of the less obvious causes. If the etiology is questionable due to concurrent problems with vascular occlusion or neuropathy, further diagnostic testing and/or a consult to a specialist is warranted.

The next step in wound assessment is to stage the ulcer. In the past, many different systems for assessing pressure ulcers were taught and utilized. However, since the Consensus Development Conference sponsored by the NPUAP in 1989,[1] the staging system endorsed at that conference has been widely disseminated, utilized, and accepted (Figures 6-1 through 6-4). This staging system has also been incorporated into the clinical practice guidelines on pressure ulcers that have been published by the AHCPR of the United States Department of Health and Human Services.[4-6] These guidelines will be incorporated extensively throughout the rest of this chapter.

Staging is essentially a description of pressure ulcer depth. Stages I and II pressure ulcers are partial-thickness wounds. Stages III and IV ulcers are full-thickness wounds. Ulcers containing necrotic tissue (eschar or slough) cannot be accurately staged until the necrotic tissue is removed.

In addition to staging, a thorough assessment should include descriptions of surface area (dimensions), depth, color, odor, and other significant characteristics. Surface area and depth are typically measured in centimeters. A disposable paper measuring tape is particularly useful for this purpose (Figure 6-5). A separate tape should be used for each ulcer to avoid cross-contamination. Ulcer depth

Figure 6-1. Stage I: Non-blanchable erythema of intact skin; the heralding lesion of skin ulceration. (NPUAP Pressure Ulcer Staging, Consensus Development Conference Statement, 1989 and NPUAP Slide Set 1, 1992. Used with permission.)

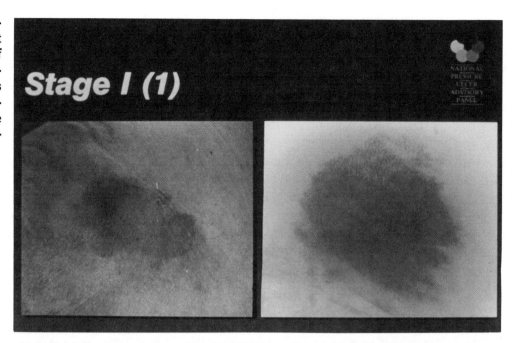

Figure 6-2. Stage II: Partial-thickness skin loss involving epidermis and/or dermis. The ulcer is superficial and presents clinically as an abrasion, blister, or shallow crater. (NPUAP Pressure Ulcer Staging, Consensus Development Conference Statement, 1989 and NPUAP Slide Set 1, 1992. Used with permission.)

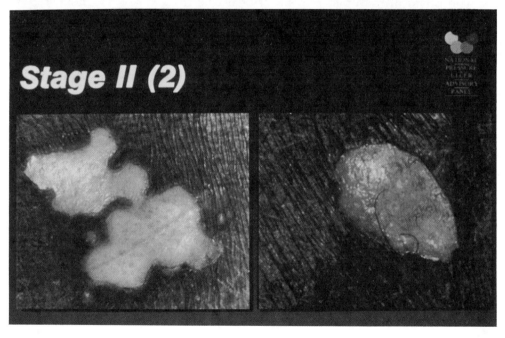

may be determined by gently inserting a sterile cotton swab or gloved finger into the wound base and then comparing the depth against a centimeter rule (see Chapter 2). In certain cases where the ulcer has undermined or tunneled beneath the skin, the depth and location (as indicated by a clock face or compass, e.g., 3 cm of undermining at 10 o'clock) should be noted. Other measures that might be employed are circumference, perimeter, or volume.[7] Regardless of which measuring procedure is used, consistency in measurement is important. Factors such as changes in patient condition and differences in measuring technique between clinicians can result in inaccurate measures of size.

Wound color can be a very important adjunct to the staging and physical descriptors mentioned

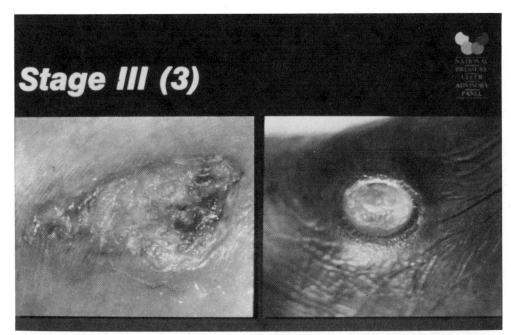

Figure 6-3. Stage III: Full-thickness skin loss involving damage or necrosis of subcutaneous tissue which may extend down to, but not through, underlying fascia. The ulcer presents clinically as a deep crater with or without undermining of adjacent tissue. (NPUAP Pressure Ulcer Staging, Consensus Development Conference Statement, 1989 and NPUAP Slide Set 1, 1992. Used with permission.)

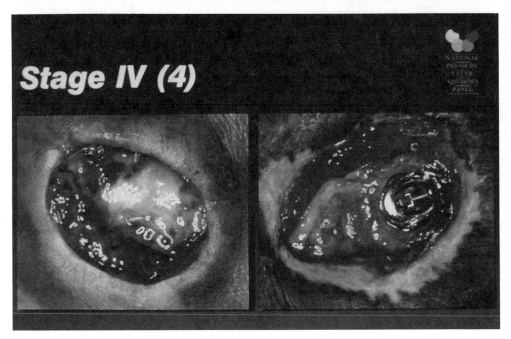

Figure 6-4. Stage IV: Full-thickness skin loss with extensive destruction, tissue necrosis or damage to muscle, bone, or supporting structures, e.g., tendon, joint capsule, etc. (NPUAP Pressure Ulcer Staging, Consensus Development Conference Statement, 1989 and NPUAP Slide Set 1, 1992. Used with permission.)

above. The red-yellow-black system is extremely useful, not only for guiding assessment, but also for determining treatment.[8] According to this system, red wounds are healthy wounds that are in some phase of the wound healing process, such as granulation or remodeling (see Figure 6-5). The goal of treatment for the red wounds is to keep them moist and protected. Yellow wounds are infected wounds or wounds filled with slough. The goal of treatment for the yellow wounds is to control infection and eliminate any necrotic slough (Figure 6-6). Black wounds are wounds covered with eschar. The eschar has to be removed if the wound is going to heal (Figure 6-7). In certain cases where the patient's status is so compromised that healing cannot be an expected outcome, conservative measures may be

Figure 6-5. Red wound (granulating Stage IV pressure ulcer) with measuring tape.

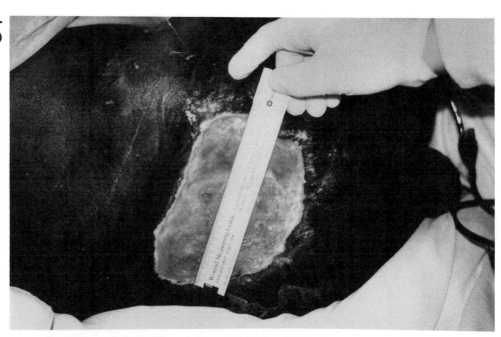

Figure 6-6. Yellow wound (pressure ulcer with slough).

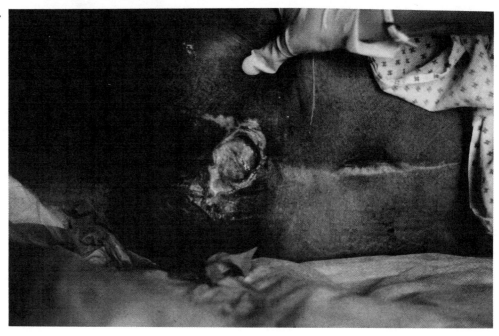

chosen over aggressive debridement. In such cases, careful documentation of a team decision should be noted in the patient's chart. The great advantage of the red-yellow-black assessment system is that it is a universal language. All levels of health care practitioners, as well as caregivers and family members, can easily comprehend a color system and communicate the wound status with accuracy, even by phone.

PREVENTION AND EARLY INTERVENTION

Early pressure ulcer researchers noted that muscle necrosis can occur as quickly as 2 hours after the application of external pressure. Based on this observation and the experience of clinicians, the 2-hour turning schedule has become the gold stan-

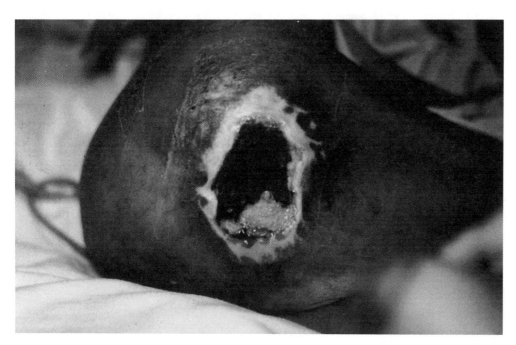

Figure 6-7. Black wound (pressure ulcer with eschar).

dard for intervention. However, it is also recognized that certain high-risk individuals will need even more frequent repositioning and turning, and possibly a specialty bed support surface.

For many at-risk patients, pillows, foam wedges, cushions, and/or socks can be employed quite effectively to augment a turning and repositioning schedule. Placing patients at a 30 degree lateral, side-lying position helps to avoid pressure on the trochanter and the lateral malleolus. Very high-risk patients and patients who are chairbound or sitting for extended periods of time will need special protection to prevent ischial and heel pressure ulcers and sacral shearing. It has long been thought that pressure reduction below 32 mmHg is sufficient to prevent pressure ulcers.[2] It is now recognized that due to the complexity of the pressure ulcer phenomenon, tissue interface pressures of 32 mmHg may not be low enough to prevent tissue trauma in very high-risk patients.

Support surfaces must be selected and the patient's status carefully monitored to see if the pressure reduction is adequate. If reddened areas still appear, a higher end device and/or more frequent turning and repositioning may be required. Under no circumstances should doughnut-type cushions be used, since research suggests that they increase the area of is-

chemia.[4] Two-inch thin, convoluted foam mattress overlays (eggcrates) should only be used as a comfort measure, since they do not adequately reduce pressures.[4] Synthetic sheepskins actually can increase maceration and friction, and should be avoided. Total replacement mattresses may be appropriate for selected patients with long-term needs. For high-risk patients or patients with early stage pressure ulcers, other options for pressure relief include 4-inch foam, air, gel, or water mattress overlays. These devices can substantially reduce pressures over the standard hospital mattress. These devices should always be combined with an individualized turning and repositioning schedule.

If the patient has underlying medical conditions that may contribute to pressure ulcer risk or formation, these conditions must be controlled as effectively as possible. Consultation with the patient's physician may be warranted. Many uncontrolled medical conditions, such as diabetes mellitus and hypertension, will impair the wound healing process.

If malnutrition is a problem, a dietary consult may be needed to improve the patient's nutritional status and potential for wound healing. Nutritional status can be monitored by routine weights, serum pre-albumin or albumin levels, and calorie counts.

TREATMENT OPTIONS

Pressure ulcer treatment must be holistic and multidisciplinary to be successful. Typically, interventions target topical treatments, pressure relief, and nutritional support. These will be discussed in general below as they apply to pressure ulcer patients, and with more detailed discussions following later in selected chapters of this text. Every effort should be made to match the appropriate intervention to the particular patient, to the particular pressure ulcer, and to the particular setting the patient is in.

WOUND CLEANSING

Probably the most frequently forgotten step in pressure ulcer care is wound cleansing. All wounds require routine cleansing before any dressing is applied. Gentle cleansing at low pressures (8 psi or less) with normal saline is the treatment of choice for most pressure ulcers. In certain circumstances (e.g., the home care patient with a clean granulating chronic ulcer), tap water is an appropriate choice.[6] Much research is still needed in this area. Questions remain concerning sterile versus clean technique for chronic wounds, the quantity of cleansing solution needed, and when to discontinue cleansing, especially whirlpool cleansing.

Many of the solutions traditionally used for cleansing pressure ulcers, such as povidone-iodine, acetic acid, Dakins, and hydrogen peroxide, have been shown by researchers to be cytotoxic to fibroblasts in vitro.[9] The research-based recommendation is that these harsh agents be avoided.[6] Don't put in a wound what you wouldn't put into your own eye.[9] Many of these so-called cleansing agents are actually antiseptics that were never intended to be used as wound cleansers. If enhanced wound cleansing is needed, a number of commercial skin and wound cleansers are available. Be sure to distinguish skin cleansers (to be used only on intact skin) from wound cleansers (for open wounds). Also be sure to critically evaluate these products to assure that they do no contain known cytotoxic agents (e.g., preservatives). At the present time FDA approval of these products is not required, so the onus is on the individual practitioner to evaluate them for safety and efficacy. In most cases, the disinfectants added prior to hydrotherapy treatment are diluted enough to minimize cytotoxic effects (see Chapter 8).

Currently, nonionic cleansers (which do not carry an electrical charge) are considered by most wound experts to be the safest cleansing agents in addition to normal saline. Pressures of 8 to 14 psi or less are considered safe and effective. These can be accomplished using a 35 cc syringe and a 19 gauge angiocath, a piston syringe, a bulb syringe, or by pouring straight from the saline bottle. Following cleansing, the wound margins should be patted dry prior to dressing application. For information on dressings see Chapter 9.

DEBRIDEMENT

Pressure ulcers that contain necrotic tissue cannot heal. Furthermore, necrotic tissue harbors bacteria that can cause infection or delay the healing process. Debriding pressure ulcers, therefore, is a basic tenet of modern wound care. Pressure ulcer debridement will be discussed in this section. Further information on debridement in general can be found in Chapter 8.

Full-thickness pressure ulcers are frequently covered with black, hard, leathery, necrotic tissue known as eschar. If desiccated and tough, the eschar will need to be softened (e.g., by hydration with an occlusive dressing) or scored with a sharp blade prior to debridement. Yellow, soft, stringy tissue known as slough is frequently found in the base of an ulcer and must also be removed if the pressure ulcer is going to heal.

For pressure ulcers containing large amounts of necrotic tissue, pressurized irrigation or whirlpool can be used to mechanically debride the wound. The important point to consider is that both of these methods are non-selective forms of debridement, i.e., they remove good tissue as well as necrotic tissue. So, debridement must be discontinued once healthy, granulating tissue is reached, otherwise the treatment will damage newly forming granulation and epithelial tissue, and retard wound healing. Again, pressurized irrigation of 8 to 14 psi has been shown to be safe and effective.[9] Greater pressures cause tissue damage. The best way to obtain 8 psi pressure is with a 30 to 60 cc luer lock syringe and an 18 to 19 gauge angiocath (venous access catheter).

Another common method for mechanically debriding necrotic tissue from a pressure ulcer is by wet-to-dry gauze dressings. While appropriate for ulcers containing large amounts of soft, necrotic tissue, wet-to-dry gauze dressings are also a non-selective form of debridement and should not be used when healthy granulation tissue is present. Cotton mesh gauze with large interstices is best used for wet-to-dry mechanical debridement. With the exception of one new, commercially-available non-woven debriding gauze, most non-woven gauze cannot be effectively used for debridement. Typically, wet-to-dry dressings must be changed at least two or three times a day, making this a very labor intensive and expensive method of debridement.

Other types of debridement include surgical/sharp, high intensity laser, enzymatic, and autolytic. Surgical or sharp debridement can be performed by trained physicians, physicians' assistants, physical therapists, nurses, and other trained health care professionals in accordance with their state professional practice acts. A scalpel and forceps are used to selectively cut and pick away necrotic tissue. With pressure ulcers it is usual for this procedure to be repeated several times before a clean ulcer bed exists. Attention must be paid to pain control and patients may need premedication. Infection control and bleeding are also concerns. Large pressure ulcer debridement should be carried out in a treatment room or the operating room where adequate equipment (e.g., cautery) and infection control is available. High intensity laser debridement is performed by physicians trained in laser use. It is a selective form of debridement, most appropriate for very large pressure ulcers with large amounts of necrotic tissue.

Chemical or enzymatic debridement uses preparations that break down either fibrin or collagen, resulting in semi-selective debridement of necrotic tissue. While slower than other methods, chemical debridement can be cost-effective and practical in many settings. Products have very specific protocols for use, so manufacturers' inserts must be followed religiously. Chemical debriding agents can cause complications, such as cellulitis or pain. They are contraindicated in patients with bleeding disorders.

Autolytic debridement is one of the most popular methods of pressure ulcer debridement in use today because it is relatively painless and can be used easily in a variety of settings. While it may take a little longer than other methods of debridement, autolysis is highly selective. The method uses a moist wound environment to facilitate the breakdown of fibrin and necrotic tissue, using the body's own debriding cells that are trapped in the moist wound environment. Occlusive dressings (e.g., transparent films, hydrocolloids, hydrogels) are extremely efficacious at promoting autolysis. Results are usually seen within 48 hours of instituting treatment. Because occlusive dressings can also harbor silent infections, autolytic debridement should be used with caution in patients who are immunocompromised or have severe neuropathy or vascular impairment.

TOPICAL TREATMENT

The days of heat lamps, dry gauze, and air drying pressure ulcers are over. Desiccated ulcer beds, dehydrated tissue, crust, and eschar are no longer acceptable patient outcomes. Since Winter[10] published his pioneering study on moist wound healing, a revolution in wound care has occurred. It is now known that wound healing is optimized in a moist environment. In a moist environment, collagen synthesis and granulation tissue formation are enhanced, cell migration and epithelial resurfacing occur faster, and there is less pain and reduced scarring. Moist wound dressings allow wound exudate to bathe the wound bed, providing growth factors, leukocytes, and other needed agents and active cells to the healing tissue. The moist wound environment is optimal for cell replication and migration. Moist wound dressings, if used correctly, can be cost-effective and time efficient (see Chapter 9 for further details on wound dressings).

PRESSURE RELIEF

For patients with existing pressure ulcers, special support surfaces for the bed or chair are essential. The support surface should distribute pressure evenly (i.e., as provided by static devices) or provide pressure relief by varying the areas under pressure (i.e., as provided by dynamic devices). Selection of appropriate surfaces from the large number of options now available (Appendix A) is often a complex and challenging task. Patient factors and preferences, pressure ulcer location and status, setting requirements, and economic factors all must be taken into consideration.

NUTRITIONAL SUPPORT

Malnutrition is a key risk factor for pressure ulcer development. One study has shown that hypoalbuminemia is a significant predictor for pressure ulcers.[11] Furthermore, without adequate nutrition, existing pressure ulcers will not heal effectively. Protein, vitamins, and mineral supplements are often required if pressure ulcer patients are to heal. Consults to dieticians are a must for patients with existing pressure ulcers and for high-risk patients (see Chapter 5 for further discussion).

COMPLICATIONS

Infection is the most common complication of pressure ulcers. Signs and symptoms of local infection include erythema, warmth, edema, pain, exudate, odor, cellulitis, and osteomyelitis. Systemic infection (sepsis) may be characterized by fever, malaise, confusion, and elevated white blood cell count. In patients who are immunosuppressed, however, these typical signs of local and systemic infection may be masked. Pressure ulcers not responding to treatment within a reasonable period of time should be assessed further for infection.

Infection can be confirmed by wound or tissue culture or by bone biopsy if osteomyelitis is suspected. Pressure ulcers should be thoroughly cleansed with normal saline without preservative prior to obtaining the culture. Wound exudate and necrotic tissue

should never be sent for culture because they contain common skin contaminants that can give misleading results. Referral to a physician is warranted upon confirmation and isolation of a specific pathogenic organism or organisms so that systemic antibiotic therapy may be initiated. The results of the culture should dictate the selection of systemic and/or topical antibiotics. Most wound experts advocate the use of systemic antibiotics for infected wounds. Additionally, many experts suggest topical treatment with antibiotics (solutions, creams, or ointments) for limited periods of time, with appropriate dressings, for infected pressure ulcers.

Often, a pressure ulcer will get stuck in a particular phase of the healing process, such as the inflammatory phase, and remain a chronic wound. If infection is the cause, and it is not identified and treated, the ulcer will not progress to the other phases of the healing process as noted in Figure 6-8. Radical wound cleansing and debridement, with or without systemic and topical antibiotics, may be needed to "jump start" such a pressure ulcer. Referral to a specialized wound care clinic may be necessary.

OTHER INTERVENTIONS

Various options exist for patients with extensive pressure ulcers, chronic ulcers, or for whom conventional therapy has not resulted in a positive healing outcome. Surgical repair can be performed, provided that the patient is a reasonable surgical candidate. Myocutaneous flap repairs that cover the defect with muscle and bone are often quite successful for pressure ulcers.[12] Selected patients may be candidates for skin grafts, synthetic skin, or primary wound closure, although these methods are more problematic for pressure ulcer repair (for further information see Chapter 15).

PATIENT AND CAREGIVER EDUCATION

Patient and caregiver education should be a major focus of the patient care plan.[13] Whether the

Figure 6-8. Wound healing hierarchy of needs. Copyright 1993 by Diane Krasner.

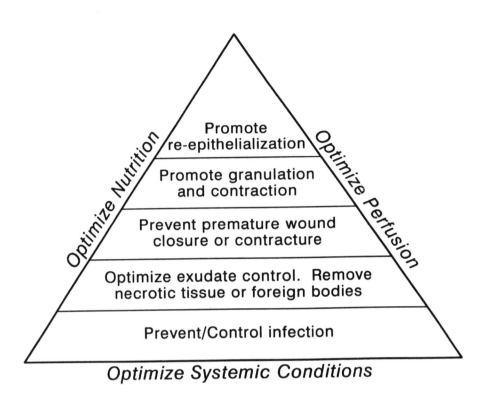

Optimize Nutrition / *Optimize Perfusion*

Promote re-epithelialization

Promote granulation and contraction

Prevent premature wound closure or contracture

Optimize exudate control. Remove necrotic tissue or foreign bodies

Prevent/Control infection

Optimize Systemic Conditions

patient is at risk for, or already has a pressure ulcer, teaching, explaining, and demonstrating interventions are essential. Rate of compliance can be increased when patients and caregivers understand the rationale for topical treatment, pressure relief, and nutritional support. Teaching plans are best designed and implemented using a multidisciplinary approach. By conferring with the physician, nurse, dietician, and physical therapist, the clinician can provide consistent reinforcement of information and important feedback about patient understanding and compliance.

COLLABORATION WITH OTHER HEALTH CARE PROFESSIONALS AND DOCUMENTATION

Based on the most current information about pressure ulcers that has been reviewed above, most authorities advocate the implementation of consistent, multidisciplinary approaches for pressure ulcer care in order to optimize patient outcomes. The responsibilities for carrying out particular interventions can be delegated to any member of the health care team with the expertise and time to carry them out. The crucial point is that someone with the skills and commitment take responsibility for the interventions that are appropriate and necessary for each individual patient. The pressure ulcer problem challenges us to collaborate, to communicate, and to work across professional lines.

Documentation should be performed routinely, at least once a week, and whenever there is a significant change in the status of the pressure ulcer.[14] The location, size, depth, color, and amount of exudate should be noted. Documentation on a multidisciplinary flow sheet facilitates communication and evaluation of pressure ulcer status over time.

RESOURCES AND SOURCES OF INFORMATION

Appendix B lists sources of standards, pressure ulcer information, and teaching materials.

CONCLUSION

While pressure ulcer care is often not glamorous, the pain and suffering that can be alleviated by state-of-the-art wound care is noteworthy. Prevention and early intervention strategies can eliminate many severe pressure ulcer problems. By attending carefully to patient comments and using their professional assessment skills, clinicians are in a unique position to diagnose and treat many pressure ulcer related problems. The role of the physical therapist in helping the multidisciplinary team achieve positive patient outcomes should not be underestimated.

REFERENCES

1. National Pressure Ulcer Advisory Panel. *Pressure Ulcers: Incidence, Economics, Risk Assessment.* Consensus Development Conference Statement. Buffalo, NY; 1989.
2. Landis EM. Microinjection studies of capillary blood pressure in human skin. *Heart.* 1930;15:209-228.
3. Allman RM. Pressure ulcers among the elderly. *N Eng J Med.* 1989;320:850-853.
4. Panel for the Prediction and Prevention of Pressure Ulcers in Adults. *Pressure Ulcers in Adults: Prediction and Prevention. Clinical Practice Guideline, No. 3.* AHCPR Publication No. 92-0047. Rockville, MD: Agency for Health Care Policy and Research, Public Health Service, U.S. Department of Health and Human Services; May 1992.
5. Colburn L. Early intervention for the prevention of pressure ulcers. In: Krasner D. *Chronic Wound Care: A Clinical Source Book for Healthcare Professionals.* King of Prussia, PA: Health Management Publications; 1990:78-88.
6. Bergstrom N, Bennett MA, Carlson CE, et al. *Treatment of Pressure Ulcers. Clinical Practice Guideline, No. 15.* AHCPR Publication No. 95-0652. Rockville, MD: Agency for Health Care Policy and Research, Public Health Service, US Department of Health and Human Services, December 1994.
7. Krasner D. The 12 commandments of wound care. *Nursing 92.* 1992;22(12):34-42.
8. Cuzzell J. The new RYB color code. *Am J Nurs.* 1988;10:1342-1346.
9. Rodeheaver G. Controversies in topical wound management: wound cleansing and wound disinfection. In: Krasner D. *Chronic Wound Care: A Clinical Source Book for Healthcare Professionals.* King of Prussia, PA: Health Management Publications; 1990:282-289.
10. Winter G. Formation of the scab and the rate of epithelialization of superficial wounds in the skin of the young domestic pig. *Nature.* 1962;193:293-294.
11. Allman RM, Laprade CA, Noel LB, et al. Pressure sores among hospitalized patients. *Ann Intern Med.* 1986;105:337-342.
12. Wornum IL. Surgical intervention: grafts and flaps. In: Krasner D. *Chronic Wound Care: A Clinical Source Book for Healthcare Professionals.* King of Prussia, PA: Health Management Publications; 1990:378-390.
13. Maklebust J, Sieggreen M. *Pressure Ulcers: Guidelines for Prevention and Nursing Management.* West Dundee, IL: S-N Publications; 1991.
14. Sussman CA. The role of physical therapy in wound care. In: Krasner D. *Chronic Wound Care: A Clinical Source Book for Healthcare Professionals.* King of Prussia, PA: Health Management Publications; 1990:327-366.

Chapter 7

Ulcers of the Lower Extremities

Gil Micheletti, MD

Lower extremity ulcers are one of the most challenging management problems for health care professionals as well as patients. Leg ulcers, a problem with many causes, affect perhaps half a million Americans.[1] To the patient, leg ulcers are a source of pain, inconvenience, expense, and frustration. There is no quick cure. Successful treatment requires that the patient be kept motivated and included as a vital part of the management team. The team must attend to the many factors involved in healing. These include providing a clean, granulating base to encourage epithelial migration, evaluating and maintaining circulation, preventing and treating edema and infection, and controlling such underlying conditions as diabetes and vasculitis. If the whole team works together in a many-pronged approach, it can usually obtain a satisfactory result.

Leg ulcers are more commonly found in women than men.[2] Although they are seen in patients of all ages, they appear more frequently in the elderly. Many diseases produce leg ulcers (Table 7-1). In discussing leg ulcers, it is convenient to divide them into venous ulcers, arterial ulcers, and diabetic ulcers. Venous ulcers are the most common type, accounting for approximately 80% to 90% of the cases. Arterial ulcers account for another 5% to 10%; most of the remainder are diabetic ulcers.[3,4] The purpose of this chapter is to describe three common types of leg ulcers, their etiology, clinical features, and management.

VENOUS ULCERS

ANATOMY OF LEG VEINS[1,5,6]

Leg ulcers are unique problems because of the peculiar vascular supply of the leg and the influence of gravity. In some ways the veins of the leg are ill equipped for their task of moving a column of blood back to the heart against gravity. Their walls are much thinner than those of arteries, and their muscular layers are much weaker. Three venous systems exist in the leg: deep, superficial, and communicating (Figure 7-1). All are equipped with one-way semilunar valves that prevent retrograde flow.

The deep system, consisting of the tibial and popliteal veins, is part of a closed compartment consisting of massive calf muscles and connective tissue. During walking, the muscles contract leading to increased deep vein pressure and forcing blood towards the heart. As the calf muscle pump empties the deep veins and reduces their pressure, blood is driven from the superficial system through communicating veins into the deep system. Deep vein emptying and the associated fall in pressure is known

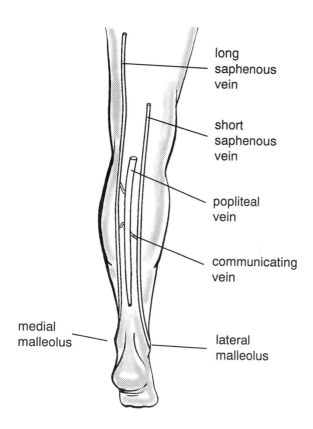

long
saphenous
vein

short
saphenous
vein

popliteal
vein

communicating
vein

medial
malleolus

lateral
malleolus

Figure 7-1. Venous circulation of the lower extremity.

as venous systole, while the filling of veins and the accompanying rise in pressure is called venous diastole. In ambulation, contact with the ground is associated with systole, and non-contact, leg off the ground is associated with diastole.

Between the deep and superficial systems is a system of communicating or perforating veins whose function is to protect the superficial veins from the high pressures generated when the calf muscles contract. Of the approximately 80 communicating veins in a lower extremity, the most important are the internal and external communicating veins of the lower leg.

The superficial veins, consisting of the long and shorter saphenous veins, are a low-pressure system. Coursing through the subcutis, the superficial veins lack the fibromuscular support of the deep venous system. For this reason, they are subject to varicosity and rupture. Like the deep veins, the saphenous veins are equipped with bicuspid, one-

way valves that help prevent retrograde flow. Because of the weight of the column of blood in the leg, the resting venous pressure at the ankle on quiet standing approaches 90 mmHg. When calf muscles contract and the blood flows toward the heart, pressure in the superficial system drops. Elevating the leg in the recumbent position lowers the venous pressure to that of the right atrium. That is why, for those with venous stasis problems, the best posture is recumbent leg elevation (venous pressure 20 mmHg) and the worst is quiet standing (venous pressure 90 mmHg) or sitting with legs in the suspended position (venous pressure 55 mmHg).

ETIOLOGY

Although congenital valvular dysfunction has been described,[6] the vast majority of such dysfunctions are acquired. With aging, the valves, especially in the communicating veins, can become thickened or damaged. Thrombosis, especially at the junction of the communicating veins and the deep veins, can destroy the valves completely. Frequently this event is clinically silent. When valves in the communicating veins become incompetent, blood under high pressure (200 mmHg) reflexes back into the superficial system creating superficial "venous hypertension" and soft tissue trauma. Venous hypertension, then, represents not an absolute increase in pressure, but a failure of the pressure to drop during diastole. Consequently, the tissue hydrostatic pressure rises and triggers a reflex vasoconstriction. Vasoconstriction, in turn, leads to decreased tissue perfusion, epidermal ischemia, and a fibrosing panniculitis. Early on, this valvular dysfunction results in fibrin cuffs around the small blood vessels.[7] Undegraded fibrin, along with tumor necrosis factor alpha and elastase, were found in venous leg ulcers.[8] Although ulcers have been shown to heal despite the persistence of fibrin cuffs, fibrin may be pathogenic by inducing fibrosis which can prolong healing and render the skin hard and vulnerable to breakdown.[9]

CLINICAL FEATURES

Venous ulcers are usually located over the medial malleolus and less frequently over other parts

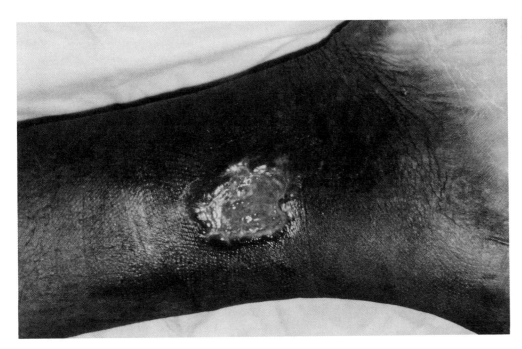

Figure 7-2. Venous ulcer of the leg. *Photo courtesy of Smith & Nephew.*

of the leg. Venous ulcers usually have irregular, "shaggy" borders (Figure 7-2). Most venous ulcers are shallow; the fascia and deep structures are usually not exposed. A non-infected venous ulcer usually has a healthy, pink granulation tissue at the base. Pain, usually mild to moderate, is worst when standing, and is relieved with elevation of the legs. Physical examination may disclose tenderness in the area of valvular incompetence. Because of fluid under high pressure, a brawny edema develops. Patients may complain their shoes feel tight at the end of the day. Unlike the edema of liver, heart, or kidney disease, the edema of venous stasis responds poorly to diuretics. Venous ulcers are usually accompanied by substantial amounts of drainage.

Hydrostatic pressures are greatest in the medial malleolar area, and early changes of venous stasis syndrome are often seen there. Extravasation from rupture of venules and capillaries produces showers of Cayenne pepper macules and purpuric lesions that have been described as Schamberg's Progressive Pigmentary Dermatosis,[10] Majocchi's Purpura Annularis Telangiectoides, and Pigmented Purpuric Lichenoid Dermatitis of Gougerot-Blum.[11] Because of the chronic nature of venous stasis, one sees crops of purpura intermingled with brown or golden-brown hemosiderin pigmentation left as the lesions resolve. As the skin reacts to decreased perfusion, one sees appendage loss manifested by alopecia, asteatosis, and a dry stasis eczema. With worsening chronic panniculitis, the medial malleolar areas show increased fibrosis, decreased elasticity, and tender nodules—the changes known as lipodermosclerosis. Fibrosis encircles the leg leaving edema above and below, resulting in a "champagne-bottle leg" appearance. Repeated episodes of thrombophlebitis and cellulitis occur. Even with minor trauma, the skin breaks down. The name "postphlebitic syndrome" has been given to these end-stage changes. While the majority of these changes are indeed postphlebitic, other factors such as ischemia, neurologic insult, leakage of immune complexes, and precipitation of cryoproteins can have a role in some venous ulcers. Perhaps a better term would be end-stage venous stasis syndrome.

DIAGNOSIS

The diagnosis of venous ulcers can usually be made clinically by the presence of stasis changes. Intact sensations to cotton swab rule out neuropathy. Thorough history and review of symptoms will rule out most of the entities in Table 7-1. Persistent

Table 7-1. **Causes of Leg Ulcers**

Vascular Diseases
  Arterial (hypertensive atherosclerotic, vasospastic)
  Venous Stasis Syndrome
  Congenital Absence of Veins
  A-V Anastomosis (congenital vs. traumatic)

Metabolic Disorders
  Diabetes Mellitus
  Porphyria Cutanea Tarda
  Gout
  Prolidase Deficiency[12]
  Pancreatitic (pancreatitis, carcinoma)

Infections
  Bacterial (desert sore, qas gangrene, Meleny's ulcer,
    tuberculosis, Buruli ulcer, leprosy, swimming pool
    granuloma)
  Spirochetal (syphilis, yaws)
  Mycotic
  Nocardial[13]
  Viral

Vasculitis
  Leukocytoclastic Vasculitis
  Polyarteritis
  Systemic Lupus Erythematosus
  Rheumatoid Vasculitis
  Wegner's Granulomatosis
  Pyoderma

Lymphedema
  Congenital
  Postinfectious
  Postsurgical

Drugs
  Bromides/Iodides
  Ergotism
  Coumadin/Heparin Necrosis
  Vasopressin[14]

Hematological
  Hypercoagulable States
  Sickle Cell Anemia
  Thalassemia
  Polycythemia Vera
  Leukemia
  Dysproteinemia (cryoglobulinemia/
    macroglobulinemia)
  Spherocytosis

Tumors
  Basal Cell Epithelioma
  Squamous Cell Carcinoma
  Sarcoma
  Melanoma
  Kaposi's Sarcoma
  Lymphoma
  Metastases

Ischemic
  Scars/Fibrosis

Miscellaneous
  Trauma (including factitial)
  Burns
  Pressure Sores
  Neuropathic Ulcers
  Bites (spiders, scorpions, snakes)
  Sweet's Syndrome
  Ulcerative Lichen Planus
  Bullous Diseases (epidermolysis bullosa)
  Idiopathic

ulceration with recurrent bleeding, rolled borders, or a fungating appearance can indicate malignancy, and such lesions should always be biopsied.

The single most important diagnostic consideration is to rule out arterial insufficiency. Intact pulses militate against an arterial etiology. Unlike venous ulcers, arterial ulcers tend to be punched out and covered with a hard black eschar. Debridement of the eschar reveals a surprising depth, often involving underlying structures of the leg. Complicating the situation is the fact that about 20% of patients with venous ulcers have concomitant arterial insufficiency.[1] Inappropriate leg compression in a patient with arterial insufficiency may cause extensive infarction requiring arterial reconstruction or bypass. Doppler examination can indicate the presence of arterial disease (see Chapter 2). With the patient supine, systolic pressures are taken at the brachial and posterior tibial arteries. The brachial:tibial ratio should be at least 0.8. If it is 0.7 or below, pulse volume recordings or angiodynographic studies should be done. These studies should also be done in cases where the arteries are non-compressible (e.g., diabetes).

A thorough medical check must be done to rule out aggravating conditions such as cardiac decompensation. Laboratory examinations should include hemoglobin and urine glucose.[15] If the legs show a mottled pattern with atrophy, which indicates atrophy blanche, one should biopsy the ulcer's edge to confirm microthrombi and fibrin deposition in the mid-dermal blood vessels.[16] Plasma cryofibrinogen levels and serum cryoglobulins may be checked if warranted. A VDRL (Venereal Disease Research Laboratory) test and an anticardiolipin antibody can exclude anti-phospholipid syndrome. Generally speaking, however, an extensive and expensive laboratory workup is not necessary, and studies should be done based on clinical evaluation.

MANAGEMENT

In venous leg ulcers, calf pump dysfunction and increased venous pressure are the problems. Leg elevation and compression are the main solutions.[17] Because it is virtually impossible to enforce leg elevation outside a hospital setting, professionals have focused tremendous energy on compression. A bewildering array of elastic and inelastic compression bandages are available. These are used in combination with layers of gauze, thus creating the multi-layer compression bandage, which maximizes uniform compression and encourages re-epithelialization. Usually these are fastened on the outside with an elastic wrap. Given constant stretch, the compression under such a bandage is proportional to the number of layers.[18] Gradually, the number of layers can be increased to patient tolerance. Custom-fitted compression stockings, with 30 to 40 mmHg compression, may be beneficial in controlling edema and skin breakdown.

Often it is an Unna Boot that is placed over the ulcer itself. The Unna Boot, an inelastic bandage impregnated with zinc oxide, provides physical support to improve the function of the calf muscle pump. It needs to be changed only once or twice weekly, an important consideration in patient compliance. Zinc oxide is slowly solubilized, and may correct local zinc deficiency. In addition it may directly enhance re-epithelization and decrease inflammation and bacterial growth.[18] The Unna Boot, however, does not adapt to decreased edema and may induce allergic contact dermatitis. As many as 4% of the leg ulcer patients demonstrate patch test sensitivity to the former.[19] Even so, the Unna Boot, gauze, and elastic wrap compression bandage remain in common use. Brand names of Unna Boots and elastic wraps may be found in Table 7-2.

The development of occlusive dressings is based on principles of wound healing. In an initial inflammatory phase, macrophages digest microorganisms and nonviable tissue.[20] Epithelial cells at the ulcer's edge, and sometimes at islands within the ulcer, proliferate and begin to migrate to cover the gap. When new blood vessels, macrophages, fibroblasts, and loose connective tissue proliferate, the wound is said to be forming granulation tissue or "granulating." Numerous cytokines, including growth factors, prostaglandins, interleukins, and colony stimulating factors improve granulation tissue, tensile strength, and re-epithelialization.[21] Developers of topical treatments and occlusive dressings have acted to enhance what our bodies have provided. Hydrocolloid dressings such as DuoDERM appear to decrease trauma to granulation tissue during dressing changes, and they decrease the risk of both contamination and pain.[22] Calcium alginate dressings appear particularly easy to use and quite capable of absorbing copious amounts of exudates.[23] According to Mian and associates[24] lyophilized type I collagen is more helpful than hydrocolloid dressings in venous leg ulcers. They posit that the collagen recruits platelets and macrophages that produce growth factors that activate the wound healing cascade. Cony and associates[25] observed superior re-epithelialization with dressings of cultured keratinocytes adhering to a collagen film. Yet another

Table 7-2. List of Different Brands of Leg Compression Bandages

Types of Bandages	Company
Inelastic	
Dome-Paste	Miles
DuoDERM Adhesive Compression Bandage	ConvaTec
Gelocast Unna Boot	Beiersdorf Inc.
Medicopaste Unna Boot	WTS
Unna-Flex	Glenwood Inc.
Unna-Flex	ConvaTec
Unna-Pak	Glenwood Inc.
Viscopaste PB7	Smith & Nephew
Unna Boot Bandage	ABCO
Elastic	
Coban	3M
Elastoplast	Beiersdorf Inc.
Medi'rip	Conco
Setopress	Acme United Corp.
Versalon	Kendall

dressing features topical prostaglandin E-2 in hydrocolloid granules.[26] Although occlusive dressings in combination with compression appear promising, they are still underutilized, perhaps because of fear of causing infections.[27]

Numerous reports have cited pentoxifylline (Trental) as a valuable adjunct to venous leg ulcer therapy.[28-31] Although these studies report improved healing, one study found that Doppler continuous wave ultrasound studies were not improved over controls. One beneficial program is 200 mg intravenously daily and 400 mg orally three times daily for 7 days, followed by 400 mg orally three times daily for another 60 days. Local inflammation in venous ulcers causes accumulation of neutrophils in capillaries and interstitial fluid. Pentoxifylline probably works by decreasing the plasma fibrinogen level and enhancing neutrophil motility.

A relatively new treatment modality is the use of a sequential compression pump. Whether or not pumps increase oxygen tension is being debated.[32,33] Although expensive, these pumps are quite helpful for elderly or inactive patients with calf pump inadequacy. The sequential compression pumps are usually used for 1 hour daily at a pressure less than diastolic, and a ratio of 90 seconds on to 30 seconds off.

BACTERIAL COLONIZATION: A TREATMENT TRAP

Sterilizing a leg ulcer is virtually impossible because it is inhabited by a variety of bacteria. Some of these bacteria, including *Group A Strep, Group G Strep*,[34] and *Pseudomonas*, are responsible for pyodermas and sepsis. *Staph aureus* and *Pseudomonas* may be associated with delayed graft healing.[35] Still, the role of bacterial colonization is not clear. The type of flora present does not necessarily correlate with the presence or absence of clinical signs of infection. Adding systemic antibiotics to compressive bandaging has not been reported to produce healing rates faster than compressive bandaging alone.[36] Use of systemic antibiotics may favor colonization by resistant strains.[37] Overt cellulitis or pyoderma, of course, demand culture and antibiotic treatment. Since increased pain and elevated C-reactive proteins may also be associated with occult infection, antibacterial therapy is probably also warranted here.[38] However, routine use of systemic antibiotics, simply to cover colonization, seems unwise.

Even more unwise is the use of topical antibiotics in leg ulcers. They probably do little to alter bacterial counts, and they interfere with epithelial migration. Silver nitrate compresses (0.25%), which dry exudates and precipitate bacterial proteins, are probably more effective than topical antibiotics. Allergic sensitization is a major problem in leg ulcers. Not only are local eruptions common, but widespread "id" reactions can occur. Neomycin, a potent antibiotic sensitizer, induces sensitivity when applied to ulcers in 30% of patients.[39] Other topical sensitizers in leg ulcers include EDTA, lanolin, nitrofurazone, parabens, and vitamin E cream. Topical antibiotics should probably not be used, and any topical treatment of leg ulcers should be considered with extreme caution.

SURGICAL MANAGEMENT

Venous leg ulcers are usually managed medically rather than surgically. When ulcers are large, nonhealing, or painful, skin grafting may help restore barrier function.[40] Split-thickness grafts require less revascularization than full-thickness grafts and therefore have a greater chance of survival. Recently there has been much interest in allografts of cultured keratinocytes which can be frozen and stored in skin banks.[41] Cultured epithelial allografts do not permanently survive on the ulcer, and giving immunosuppressive drugs to sustain them is not justified.[42,43] Beele and associates[44] noted that allografts appear to enhance granulation and re-epithelialization starting from the periphery of the ulcer. Possibly these cultured keratinocytes release cytokines that stimulate multiplication and migration of the host's own keratinocytes. Cultured epidermal grafts, a simple outpatient procedure, may represent a painless, noninvasive adjunct to medical treatment of venous leg ulcers.[45,46]

The value of surgery on the veins themselves has been debated. Ligation of the communicating veins and saphenous vein stripping have been reported to accomplish healing in only 25% of the cases.[47] When valvuloplasty was also done, the healing rate increased to 87%. Adjunctive use of an elastic stocking and sequential compression reduces postoperative edema and improves the long-term prognosis. Surgical correction of venous incompetence prevents reflux and restores the normal vasodilator response to exercise.[48] With tissue oxygenation thus maintained, the ulcers heal at the maximum rate. It would appear that communicating vein ligation, saphenous vein stripping, and valvuloplasty offer an aggressive alternative in refractory venous ulcers.

ARTERIAL ULCERS

Arterial ulcers, also known as ischemic ulcers or infarcts, are caused by arterial insufficiency. These generally occur in patients over 50 years of age but are occasionally seen in younger patients with diabetes mellitus and hyperlipidemia.

ETIOLOGY
Arterial insufficiency commonly results from main vessel occlusion and less commonly from small vessel occlusion. Interference with the arterial supply can be extramural, as in impingement by scar tissue; mural, as in vasculitis or arteriosclerosis; or intramural, as in thrombosis. The cutaneous blood supply is not adequate to meet the demands of local tissue metabolism and results in skin breakdown. Although arterial ulcers are more common in males, smoking and dietary factors increase their incidence in females.[49] With increasing longevity of the population, arterial ulcers are becoming more common. Peripheral vascular disease accounts for about 10% of leg ulcers, but ischemia is also a complicating factor in many venous ulcers.

The anatomy of the leg predisposes it to arterial ulcers. Although there are no less than five collateral vessels present about the knee joint, collateral circulation in the popliteal artery system is inadequate. Sudden occlusion here is frequently associated with infarction of the leg.[50]

CLINICAL FEATURES
Several features distinguish arterial ulceration from venous ulceration (Table 7-3). While venous ulcers are most common in the medial malleolar area, arterial ulcers frequently involve the pretibial area or dorsum of the toes or feet. Arterial ulcers tend to be more painful than venous ulcers. While leg elevation lessens the pain of venous ulcers, it aggravates the pain of ischemic ulcers because gravity assists arterial flow. For this reason, rising and walking abates the pain of arterial ulcers. Intermittent claudication occurs on walking and is relieved promptly by rest. Cold, windy weather shortens claudication distance whereas warm weather allows the patient to walk farther.

Arterial ischemic ulcers are generally irregular in shape (Figure 7-3). The edges of the ulcers are smooth and well defined. The base of the ulcer is usually obscured by pale yellow purulent exudate and yellow or greenish necrotic debris, often with islands of gangrenous skin. Usually very little or no granulation tissue is present. The ulcers are usually deep and tendons are often visible. Edema is present around wound margins, and a variable amount of

Table 7-3. **Clinical Differentiation of Arterial, Venous, and Neuropathic Ulcers**

	Arterial Ulcers	Venous Ulcers	Neuropathic Ulcers
Location	Lower one third of leg, toe, feet, interdigital spaces	Typically just proximal to medial malleolus of ankle	Plantar surface of foot beneath metatarsal head
Pedal Pulses	Diminished or absent	Usually present	Diminished or absent
Appearance	Irregular shape Edges smooth, well defined Minimal to no granulation Usually deep	Irregular shape Good granulation Usually shallow Marked edema Intact skin dark, fibrotic	Punched out shape Good granulation Callus around ulcer Intact skin shiny Lack of sensations
Pain	Severe pain Increased with ambulation Decreased with rest	Minimal to moderate pain Increased with ambulation Decreased with elevation	No pain

tenderness is present around the ulcer. The skin around the ulcer is dry and cracked. Hyperpigmentation, usually marked in skin around a venous ulcer, is minimal in ischemic ulcers. The skin is also usually cold around and distal to the ulcer. Patients may present with marked edema of the extremity because they tend to keep the extremity in a dependent position almost all the time. Patients usually have a weak or absent pulse around and distal to the ulcer. None of the above features are, however, diagnostic. Doppler studies and angiography are frequently helpful in differentiating arterial from venous ulcerations. These studies can significantly impact on the management of venous ulcers with an ischemic component.

MANAGEMENT

In treating arterial leg ulcers, the management team should follow the dictum: "First, do no harm." Particularly, avoid compression bandages, since they restrict the blood flow, and avoid sensitizing topical medications. Local treatment of ischemic ulcers is the most important aspect of care. Pressure must be removed from the area of skin breakdown. Bedrest, with the head of the bed elevated to 5 to 7 degrees, produces an increase in oxygen tension and skin temperature in the ischemic leg. Leg elevation reduces blood flow to the leg and should be avoided. During walking, a non–weight-bearing position to avoid excessive muscular activity of the leg might

help. Further, vigorous exercises of the extremity should also be avoided. Conservative debridement and hydrotherapy treatments can aid in cleaning and encouraging re-epithelialization. Hydrocolloid dressings provide a moist environment that may be beneficial for ischemic ulcers.

The pharmacopoeia has limited application in ischemic leg ulcers. Because of its actions in increasing erythrocyte flexibility, increasing fibrinolysis, and decreasing platelet aggregation, pentoxifylline is a valuable adjunct to treatment of ischemic ulcers. The prostacyclin analog iloprost has been reported to be markedly superior to aspirin for healing and abating ischemic pain.[51] Norgren and associates,[52] on the other hand, found iloprost to offer no advantage over placebo in recalcitrant arterial ulcers. Propionyl-1-carnitine appears to increase flow velocity in arterial ulcers and enhance healing.

Despite the efficacy of many medical treatment modalities, arterial ulcers frequently need surgery. Bypass grafts using the saphenous vein and percutaneous transluminal angioplasty have saved many limbs. Endarterectomy, however, may be as beneficial as bypass and may also be better than angioplasty while saving the saphenous vein for use if endarterectomy fails and bypass is needed.[53] If arterial surgery is not feasible, epidermal spinal electrical stimulation may increase blood flow, decrease pain, and promote healing.[54]

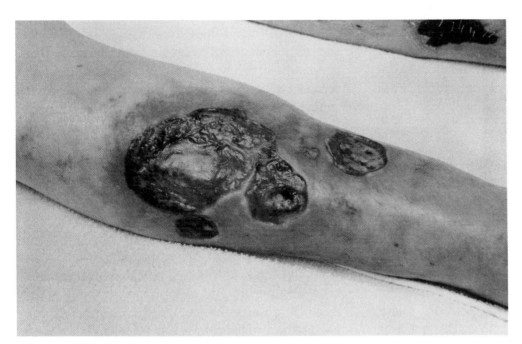

Figure 7-3. Arterial ulcer of the leg. *Photo courtesy of Smith & Nephew.*

DIABETIC ULCERS

Diabetic ulcers of the lower extremities account for more than half of the lower extremity amputations done in the United States. Not only are they responsible for much suffering and disability, their treatment costs half a billion dollars a year.[55] Treating diabetic ulcers requires patience and a thorough understanding of the principles of wound healing.

ETIOLOGY

Most diabetic ulcers are based on a combination of ischemia and neuropathy. For any given ulcer, however, one etiology or the other usually predominates. Primary ischemic ulcers are relatively rare, but peripheral neuropathy places the diabetic foot at extreme risk. Motor neuropathy leads to degeneration of small foot muscles. Altering of foot bone relationships leads to hammer toes, pes caves, and abnormal pressure points over the first and fifth metatarsal heads. As the foot becomes progressively deformed, pressure from ill-fitting shoes and stress from walking lead to ischemia and ulceration. Insensitive to early signs of inflammation, the patient with diabetic neuropathy continues to walk on the pressure points resulting in increased damage. Tissue injury causes a hyperkeratosis, and autonomic dysfunction causes cessation of sweating with subsequent scaling and fissuring. Autonomic neuropathy causes loss of perspiration resulting in fissuring of skin which acts as nidus for ulceration. Ulcer formation is initiated by skin cracks and fissures, repeated minor trauma, careless pedicure, or fungal infection. These ulcers are usually preceded by erythema, blisters, and calluses, and wound healing is impaired. Although the mechanisms of faulty healing are not well understood, Pecoraro and associates[56] concluded that peri-wound oxygen perfusion is the critical determinant in diabetic ulcer healing. A peri-ulcer PO_2 less than 20 mmHg is associated with a poor prognosis for healing.

CLINICAL FEATURES

The typical neuropathic foot ulcers occur on the plantar surface of the foot in areas of maximum pressure such as heel, toes, and metatarsal heads (Figure 7-4). The ulcers are usually deep and infected. The ischemic limb is cool, with a dusky rubor on dependency and pallor on elevation.[57] The skin is shiny and atrophic. Posterior tibial and dorsalis pedis pulses may be absent, but a strong popliteal pulse can be found. Usually the ulcer itself is painless, but the patient may complain of burning pain and paresthesia in the extremities. Pain, which is worst in the supine position, is reduced by dependency and exertion. In the neuropathic ulcer, touch, pressure, and proprioception are lost. Forty-one percent of these patients are unaware of sensory loss.[58]

DIAGNOSIS

It is very important to evaluate for both neuropathy and ischemia. Sensations are assessed by lightly applying a cotton swab to the toe pads, metatarsal area, instep, and heel. With the foot rested on the opposite knee, the patient should be able to localize the area of touch. A nylon filament can be applied to the plantar surface, and the patient should be able to tell when touched. While the normal person can detect 1 or 2 g of pressure, many diabetics are unable to detect 10 g, the point at which the filament bends.[59] If pulses are not palpable or if there are signs of ischemia, Doppler studies and, if indicated, arteriography should be done. Tibial and peroneal artery occlusion are more common in diabetics than in the general population.

MANAGEMENT

Prevention is the first line of defense against diabetic ulcers. A foot care program is imperative; its routine use would probably save over half the limbs amputated in diabetics.[60] All diabetics should check their feet daily for erythema, edema, and callosities, which can indicate new pressure points. A podiatrist should also be part of the management team. Running shoes with custom orthotic inserts can distribute pressure over the whole surface of the sole, and thus prevent localized pressure and consequent ulceration.[61] For the severe, irregular deformity of a Charcot's foot, a soft, molded custom shoe often decreases some of the abnormal stresses against the foot. Vigilance should be maintained for detection of new pressure sites and refitting or modifications to the shoe done as needed because such feet are constantly changing shape.

The importance of skin care in maintaining the epidermal barrier cannot be overemphasized. If hyperkeratosis is severe, or there is cracking of the epidermis, keratolytics such as urea or lactic acid (Lachydrin) can soften the surface and eliminate superficial fissuring. In severe hyperkeratosis these preparations can be occluded (loosely) with plastic wrap or a baggie for several hours. Washing with salicylic acid soap and a Buf-Puf will further the removal of excess keratin. Petrolatum fully penetrates the stratum corneum and provides an impermeable barrier.[62] A further advantage of petrolatum is that it is neither irritating nor allergenic. Fungal infections usually worsen hyperkeratosis, and if present, should be vigorously treated. Terbinafine hydrochloride (Lamisil) applied twice daily for a month is highly effective, as are econazole nitrate (Spectazole), oxiconazole nitrate (Oxistat), sulconazole nitrate (Exelderm), and ciclopirox olamine (Loprox). According to the author's experience, the last four need to be applied for at least 8 weeks. If the fungus proves refractory, systemic griseofulvin, ketoconazole, or itraconazole should be used if liver function permits.

Once an ulcer develops, management should be geared toward improving perfusion and relieving localized pressure. Hyperkeratosis and necrosis should be thoroughly mechanically debrided. The resulting clean base provides a start for granulation and re-epithelialization. Wet-to-dry dressings and enzymatic debridements are usually far from sufficient. Patients should be cautioned that any weight bearing on an ulcer can do great harm. Going barefoot should be strictly proscribed. Total contact casting or healing shoes with Plastazote inserts can be very helpful in protecting the foot, distributing pressure, and allowing mobility.[57] See Chapter 10 for treatment of diabetic ulcers with total contact casting.

Certain topical modalities should be avoided. Wet-to-dry saline dressings impede epithelial migration, and iodine and peroxide can damage fibroblasts. As always, topical sanitizers such as neomycin should be strictly avoided. Occlusive dressings are of limited use because they prevent day-to-day visualization of the ulcer. Further, the maceration they cause can lead to extension of the ulcer underneath the dressing.

Topical, activated, platelet supernatant, CT-

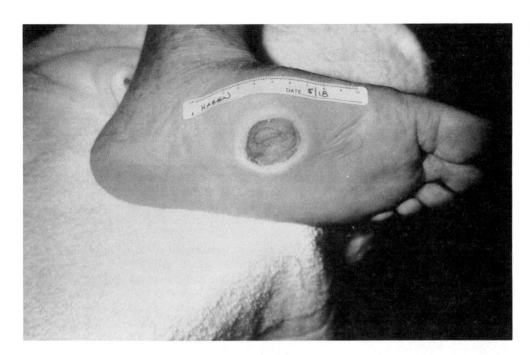

Figure 7-4. Diabetic foot ulcer. *Photo courtesy of Smith & Nephew.*

102, prepared from homologous platelets, contains numerous growth factors that appear to significantly accelerate wound healing including diabetic ulcers.[63,64] While it is logical that they would be effective, this modality is still experimental and requires further evaluation.

TWO SPECIAL SITUATIONS

LIVEDOID VASCULITIS

A hyalinizing vasculopathy, livedoid vasculitis shows both a venous and an arterial component. Microthrombi and deposition of fibrin in the mid-dermal blood vessels leads to epidermal infarction, ulcers, and stellate scars.[65] Decreased fibrinolysis and the presence of tissue plasminogen activator (tPA) causes a hypercoagulant state. Having given 10 mg of recombinant tPA intravenously over 4 hours every day for 14 days, Klein and Pittelkow noted dramatic improvement in five of six patients. A combination of the anti-platelet drugs ticlopidine hydrochloride, dipyridamole, and aspirin may also cause major improvement in 30 days.[65] Sulfasalazine, 1 g orally three times daily, may be beneficial.[66] As might be expected, pentoxifylline, with its effects on platelet aggregation, fibrinolysis, neutrophil motility, prostacyclin synthesis, and erythrocyte flexibility is probably also beneficial in the treatment of livedoid vasculitis.[67]

SICKLE CELL ULCERS

Sickle cell anemia occurs because of inheritance of an abnormal hemoglobin, hemoglobin S. Occurring mostly in areas where malaria is endemic, the abnormal hemoglobin may confer some resistance to malaria. In patients homozygous for hemoglobin S, the abnormal hemoglobin polymerizes in the erythrocytes which lose their flexibility. Blood flow is impeded through the microcirculation resulting in some very refractory leg ulcers. The goal is specific therapy to inhibit polymerization of hemoglobin S. This is a goal that has not yet been achieved.[68]

Many treatment approaches have been tried. Pentoxifylline may be useful because of its ability to decrease blood viscosity and enhance erythrocyte flexibility.[69] In a study, el-Momen gave a patient 600 to 800 IU/kg of recombinant human erythropoietin subcutaneously weekly, and the patient responded with complete resolution of the ulcer and pain.[70] Khouri and Upjohn[71] achieved healing of a refractory leg ulcer with a free latissimus dorsi transfer. Before they proceeded, however, they did exchange transfusions to bring the concentration of hemoglobin S down below 30%. In this way they appeared to reduce the sickling in the microcirculation. Until a way to interfere with sickling in the blood vessels is found, however, the management of sickle cell ulcers is going to remain a management challenge.

CONCLUSION

Management of ulcers of the lower extremities requires a team approach by professionals who approach the problem from varying, and sometimes conflicting, points of view. For the team to work effectively, each member must understand what the others are doing. If everyone on the team communicates, the resulting organized approach provides gratifying results for the team, and more importantly for the patient as well.

REFERENCES

1. Falanga V. Venous ulceration. *J Dermatol Surg Oncol.* 1993;19:764-771.
2. Callam MJ, Ruckley CV, Harper DR, Dale JJ. Chronic ulceration of the leg: extent of the problem and provision of care. *BMJ.* 1985;290:1855-1856.
3. Young JR. Differential diagnosis of leg ulcers. *Cardiovasc Clin.* 1983;13:171-193.
4. Anning JT. *Leg Ulcers: Their Cause and Treatment.* London: Churchill Livingston; 1954.
5. Demis DJ, chief ed. *Clinical Dermatology.* 20th rev. Philadelphia, PA: JB Lippincott Co; 1993.
6. Rook A, Wilkinson DS, Ebling FJG, Champion RH, Burton JL, eds. *Textbook of Dermatology.* 4th ed. Oxford, London: Blackwell Scientific Publications; 1986.
7. Stacey MC, Burnand KG, Pattison M, Thomas ML, Layer GT. Changes in the apparently normal limb in unilateral venous ulceration. *Br J Surg.* 1987;74:936-939.
8. Claudy AL, Mirshahi M, Soria C, Soria J. Detection of undegraded fibrin and tumor necrosis factor: alpha in venous leg ulcers. *J Am Acad Dermatol.* 1991;25:623-627.
9. Falanga V, Eaglstein WH. The "trap" hypothesis of venous ulceration. *Lancet.* 1993;341:1006-1008.
10. Wise F. Purpura annularis telangiectoides (Majocchi) and progressive pigmentary dermatosis (Schamberg). *J Invest Dermatol.* 1942;5:153-166.
11. Fishman HC. Pigmented purpuric lichenoid dermatosis of gougerot-blum. *Cutis.* 1982;29:260-261.
12. Milligan A, Graham-Brown RA, Burns DA, Anderson I. Prolidase deficiency: a case report and literature review. *Br J Dermatol.* 1989;121:405-409.
13. Schiff TA, Goldman R, Sanchez M, et al: Primary lymphocutaneous nocariosis caused by an unusual species of nocardia: nocardia transvalensis. *J Am Acad Dermatol.* 1993;28(2 Pt 2):336-340.
14. Colemont LJ, Harrier HD, Shoemaker WC. Vasopressin related bullous diseases of the legs. *J Clin Gastroenterol.* 1991;13:91-93.
15. Eriksson G. Local treatment of venous leg ulcers. *Acta Chir Scand.* 1988;544(suppl):47-52.
16. Klein KL, Pittelkow MR. Tissue plasminogen activator for treatment of livedoid vasculitis. *Mayo Clin Proc.* 1992;67:923-933.
17. Riordan CA. The management of venous ulcers of the legs. *Australas J Dermatol.* 1991;32:111-116.
18. Agren MS. Studies on zinc in wound healing. *Acta Derm Venereol (Stockh).* 1990;154:1-36.
19. Brandrup F, Menne T, Agren MS, Stromberg HE, Holst R, Frisen M. A randomized trial of two occlusive dressings in the treatment of leg ulcers. *Acta Derma Venereol (Stockh).* 1990;70:231-235.
20. Clark RF. Basis of cutaneous wound repair. *J Dermatol Surg Oncol.* 1993;19:693-706.
21. Falanga V. Growth factors and wound healing. *J Dermatol Surg Oncol.* 1993;19:711-714.
22. Annoni F, Rosina M, Chiurazzi D, Cava M. The effects of a hydrocolloid dressing on bacterial growth and the healing process of leg ulcers. *Int Angiol.* 1989;8:224-228.
23. McMullen D. Clinical experience with a calcuim alginate dressing. *Dermatol Nurs.* 1991;3:216-219.
24. Mian E, Mian M, Beghe F. Lyophilized type I collagen and chronic leg ulcers. *Int J Tissue React.* 1991;13:257-269.
25. Cony M, Donatien P, Beylot C, et al. Treatment of leg ulcers with an allogenic cultured—keratinocyte-collagen dressing. *Clin Exp Dermatol.* 1990;15:410-414.
26. Eriksson G, Torngren M, Aly A, Johansson C. Topical prostaglandin E-2 in the treatment of chronic leg ulcers: a pilot study. *Br J Dermatol.* 1988;118:531-536.
27. Eaglstein WH. Occlusive dressings. *J Dermatol Surg Oncol.* 1993;19:716-720.
28. Barbarino C. Pentoxifylline in the treatment of venous leg ulcers. *Curr Med Res Opin.* 1992;12:547-551.
29. Angelides NS, von-der-Ake CW, Themistocleus P. Comparison of skin and muscle biopsies before and after pentoxifylline treatment in patients with leg ulcers due to deep venous incompetence. *Int Angiol.* 1991;10:72-76.
30. Colgan MP, Dormandy JA, Jones PW, Schraibman IG, Shanik DG, Young RA. Oxpentifylline treatment of venous ulcers of the leg. *BMJ.* 1990;300:972-975.
31. Ward A, Clissold SP. Pentoxifylline: a review of its pharmacodynamic and pharmacokinetic properties, and its therapeutic efficiency. *Drugs.* 1987;34:50-97.
32. Nemeth AJ, Falanga V, Alstadt SP, Eaglstein WH. Ulcerated edematous limbs: effect of edema removal on transcutaneous oxygen measurements. *J Am Acad Dermatol.*

1989;20(2 Pt 1):191-197.

33. Kolari PJ, Pekanmaki K, Pohjola RT. Transcutaneous oxygen tension in patients with post-thrombotic leg ulcers: treatment with intermittent pneumatic compression. *Cardiovasc Res*. 1988;22:138-141.

34. Nohlgard C, Bjorklind A, Hammar H. Group G streptococcal infections on a dermatological ward. *Acta Derm Venereol (Stockh)*. 1992;72:128-130.

35. Gilliland EL, Nathwani N, Dore CJ, Lewis JD. Bacterial colonization of leg ulcers and its effect on the success rate of skin grafting. *Ann Royal Coll Surg Eng*. 1988;70:105-108.

36. Alinovi A, Bassissi P, Pini M. Systemic administration of antibiotics in the management of venous ulcers. *J Am Acad Dermatol*. 1986;15:186-191.

37. Valtonen V, Karppinen L, Kariniemi AL. A comparative study of ciprofloxacin and conventional therapy in the treatment of patients with chronic lower leg ulcers infected with pseudomonas aeruginosa or other gram-negative rods. *Scand J Inf Dis*. 1989;60(suppl):79-83.

38. Goodfield MJ. C-reactive protein levels in venous ulceration: an indication of infection? *J Am Acad Dermatol*. 1988;18(5 Pt 1):1048-1052.

39. Fisher A. *Contact Dermatitis*. 3rd ed. Philadelphia, PA: Lea and Febiger; 1986.

40. Kirsner RS, Falanga V. Techniques of split-thickness grafting for lower extremity ulcerations. *J Dermatol Surg Oncol*. 1993;19:779-783.

41. DeLuca M, Albanese M, Cancedda R, et al. Treatment of leg ulcers with cryopreserved allogeneic cultured epithelium. *Arch Dermatol*. 1992;128:633-638.

42. Phillips TJ, Gilchrist BA. Clinical applications of cultured epithelium. *Epithelial Cell Biol*. 1992;1:39-46.

43. Fabre JW. Epidermal allografts. *Immun Lett*. 1991;29:161-165.

44. Beele H, Naeyaert JM, Goeteyn M, De-Mil M, Kint A. Repeated cultured epidermal allografts in the treatment of chronic leg ulcers of various origins. *Dermatologica*. 1991;183:31-35.

45. Phillips TJ, Bigby M, Bercovtich L. Cultured allografts as an adjunct to the medical treatment of problematic leg ulcers. *Arch Dermatol*. 1991;127:799-801.

46. Marcusson JA, Lindgren C, Berghard A, Toftgard R. Allogeneic cultured keratinocytes in the treatment of leg ulcers: a pilot study. *Acta Derm Venereol (Stockh)*. 1992;72:61-64.

47. Sottiurai VS. Comparison of surgical modalities in the treatment of recurrent venous ulcer. *Inter Angiol*. 1990;9:231-235.

48. Sarkany I, Dodd HJ, Gaylarde PM. Surgical correction of venous incompetence restores normal skin blood flow and abolishes skin hypoxia during exercise. *Arch Dermatol*. 1989;125:223-226.

49. Woods BO. Clinical evaluation of the peripheral vasculature. *Cardiol Clin*. 1991;9:413-427.

50. Hollinshead H, Rosse C. *Textbook of Anatomy*. 4th ed. Philadelphia, PA: Harper and Row; 1985.

51. Fiessinger JN, Schafer M. Trial of iloprost versus aspirin treatment for critical limb ischemia of thromboangiitis obliterans. *Lancet*. 1990;335:555-557.

52. Norgren L, Alwmark A, Angqvist KA, et al. A stable prostacyclin analog (iloprost) in the treatment of ischaemic ulcers of the lower limb. *Euro J Vasc Surg*. 1990;4:463-467.

53. van der Heijden FH, Eikelboom BC, van Reedt-Dortland RW, et al. Endarterectomy of the superficial femoral artery: a procedure worth reconsidering. *Euro J Vasc Surg*. 1992;6:651-658.

54. Jivegard L, Augustinsson LE, Carlsson CA, Holm J. Long-term results by epidural spinal electrical stimulation (ESES) in patients with inoperable severe lower limb ischemia. *Euro J Vasc Surg*. 1987;1:345-349.

55. *Diabetes Surveillance, 1980-1987*. US Department of Health and Human Services: The Division of Diabetes Translation. 1990:23-25.

56. Pecoraro RE, Ahroni JH, Boyko EJ, Stensel VL. Chronology and determinants of tissue repair in diabetic lower extremity ulcers. *Diabetes*. 1991;40:1305-1313.

57. Miller OF. Essentials of pressure ulcer treatment. *J Dermatol Surg Oncol*. 1993;19:759-763.

58. Holewski JJ, Moss KM, Stess RM, et al. Prevalence of foot pathology and lower extremity complications in a diabetic outpatient clinic. *J Rehab Res Dev*. 1989;26:35-44.

59. Duffy JC, Patout CA. Management of the insensitive foot in diabetes: lessons learned from Hansen's disease. *Milit Med*. 1990;575:155-159.

60. Bild DE, Selby JV, Sinnock P, Browner WS, Braveman P, Showstack JA. Lower extremity amputation in people with diabetes: epidemiology and prevention. *Diabetes Care*. 1989;12:24-31.

61. Soulier SM. The use of running shoes in the prevention of plantar diabetic ulcers. *J Am Podiatr Med Assoc*. 1986;76:395-400.

62. Ghadially R, Halkier-Sorenson L, Elias PM. Effects of petrolatum on stratum corneum structure and function. *J Am Acad Dermatol*. 1992;26:387-396.

63. Steed DL, Goslen JB, Holloway GA, Malone JM, Bunt TJ, Webster MW. Randomized prospective double-blind trial in healing chronic diabetic foot ulcers: CT-102 activated platelet supernatant, topical versus placebo. *Diabetic Care*. 1992;15:1598-1604.

64. Knighton DR, Ciresi K, Fiegel VD, Schumerth S, Butler E, Cerna F. Stimulation of repair in chronic, nonhealing cutaneous ulcers using platelet-derived wound healing formula. *Surg Gynecol Obstet*. 1990;170:56-60.

65. Yamamoto M, Danno K, Shio H, Imamura S. Antithrombotic treatment in livedo vasculitis. *J Am Acad Dermatol*. 1988;18(1 Pt 1):57-62.

66. Gupta AK, Goldfarb MT, Voorhees JJ. The use of sulfasalazine in atrophie blanche. *Int J Dermatol*. 1990;9:663-665.

67. Ely H, Bard JW. Therapy of livedo vasculitis with pentoxifylline. *Cutis*. 1988.42:448-53.

68. Steingart R. Management of patients with sickle cell disease. *Med Clin North Am*. 1992;76:669-682.

69. Frost ML, Treadwell P. Treatment of sickle cell leg ulcers with pentoxifylline. *Int J Dermatol.* 1990;29:375-376.

70. al-Momen AK. Recombinant human erythropoietin induced rapid healing of a chronic leg ulcer in a patient with sickle cell disease. *Acta Haematol.* 1991;86:46-48.

71. Khoury RK, Upton J. Bilateral lower limb salvage with free flaps in a patient with sickle cell ulcers. *Ann Plast Surg.* 1991;27:574-576.

Chapter 8

Wound Debridement and Hydrotherapy

Robin Ryan Marquez, MS, PT

Wound healing is either delayed or prevented in the presence of devitalized tissue in the wound bed. Wound cleansing and preparation is the most important step for reducing the risk of wound infection. It is, therefore, essential that all contaminants and nonviable tissues be removed prior to wound closure. Otherwise, the risks of infection and of a cosmetically poor scar are greatly increased. In wound management, this step is most time consuming and tedious. Neither good suturing technique nor the use of prophylactic antibiotics can replace meticulous cleaning, irrigation, and debridement. The purpose of this chapter is to provide the reader with guidelines for various types of wound debridement, indications for hydrotherapy and wound irrigation, and alternative options for the conservative management of wounds. A table containing recommended concentration of commonly used whirlpool additives is also provided.

ROLE OF DEBRIDEMENT

Debridement is the removal of necrotic and extraneous tissue from a wound. This is particularly important when attempting to minimize the risk of

infection. The presence of nonviable tissue is associated with an increased number of bacteria.[1] The removal of necrotic tissue significantly decreases the number of bacteria and allows the patient's own defense system to be more effective in combating infection.[1] Application of topical antimicrobial agents is most successful when used following debridement since they are unable to penetrate the avascular necrotic tissue.[2]

Wounds with necrotic tissue exhibit delayed healing and are unable to complete the normal phases of wound healing including re-epithelialization and wound contraction. Both of these phases are critical for the normal sequence of wound healing.[3] Studies have shown that the presence of eschar or scab in a dry wound results in slower re-epithelialization of the wound bed compared with faster epithelization in the presence of moist wound environment.[4]

The wound bed is very delicate and must be handled carefully. In clean wounds with healthy granulation, tissue debridement is not indicated. The presence of an eschar over a bone or a tendon often does not require debridement unless there is an associated cellulitis present. Clinicians should be particularly careful when working with eschar-covered wounds with arterial insufficiency. It is recommended that prior to revascularization, arterial wounds with eschar be maintained in a dry state. Following revascularization to the involved area, eschar can be debrided slowly from the surrounding tissue.

Prior to proceeding with cleansing and irrigation of a laceration or wound, several issues must be considered. These include hand washing, personnel precautions, and pain control. A simple, brief hand washing should be performed before the procedure is performed and after finishing up with a patient. Because the process of preparing and cleansing a wound brings wound care personnel into contact with blood and other secretions, it is recommended that appropriate gloves and eyewear be worn at all times. Water-resistant gowns are also recommended but they are not always practical. The most infectious agents that are of concern in these settings are the hepatitis B and the human immunodeficiency virus (HIV).

Wound cleansing and debridement often can be uncomfortable, if not outright painful, for the patient. Most patients require pain medications and/or topical anesthetics prior to treatment. Not only will the patient be more comfortable, but the cleaning can be more vigorous and possibly more effective.

TYPES OF DEBRIDEMENT

There are two types of debridement (Table 8-1): selective and non-selective. Selective debridement removes only nonviable tissue from a wound, whereas non-selective debridement indiscriminately removes both viable and nonviable tissue from a wound.

SELECTIVE DEBRIDEMENT

Selective debridement may be performed in one of three ways:
(1) sharp/surgical debridement
(2) enzymatic debridement
(3) autolytic debridement
Sharp/surgical debridement is the most effective, aggressive, and fastest means of removing large amounts of devitalized tissue. However, there are certain associated risks such as sepsis and bleeding. Healthy tissue may also be disrupted, and the pain associated with this type of debridement often requires anesthesia. Many patients are not candidates for surgical debridement secondary to associated risk factors and complications of undergoing general anesthesia. Surgical debridement should be used cautiously on patients with low platelet counts or those taking anticoagulants. Enzymatic debridement includes application of topical agents or enzymes. It is a conservative alternative to selectively debride necrotic tissue or eschar since these enzymes only digest devitalized tissue and do not harm healthy tissue. Autolytic debridement is another safe and conservative means of removing nonviable tissue from a wound bed. Certain occlusive dressings facilitate the body's own autolytic process resulting in the self-digestion of necrotic tissue and eschar liquification by enzymes naturally present in the wound fluid. However, autolytic debridement is not recommended when clinical infection is present.

NON-SELECTIVE DEBRIDEMENT

Non-selective forms of debridement are considered mechanical debridement. It may include any one or a combination of the following: dry-to-dry, wet-to-dry, wet-to-wet gauze dressings; Dakin's solution; hydrogen peroxide application; whirlpool jet agitation; and/or high-powered wound irrigation/lavage. A non-selective form of debridement is recommended for wounds containing extensive necrotic tissue and debris that may be promoting an infectious process. Debridement of necrotic tissue must be performed to allow the healing process of granulation development and fibroblastic deposition of collagen upon which epidermal cells can migrate and close the wound.[5] As granulation tissue becomes more prevalent a more selective method of debridement will be required to decrease damage to healthy granulation tissue. Various forms of gauze dressings should be used cautiously because, upon removal, not only the necrotic tissue but also the delicate epithelium and granulation tissue cling to the dressing. The same care should be taken when

Table 8-1. Types of Debridement

Type of Debridement	Method of Debridement	Indications for Use
Surgical/Sharp	Surgical excision	Wounds with large amounts of necrotic tissue
	Scalpel, scissors, forceps	Indicated for diabetic patients or when infection threatens the patient's life
Mechanical	Hydrotherapy	Softens hard eschar prior to conservative sharp debridement
	Irrigation (high-power or syringe)	For wounds with undermining of soft tissue or sinus tracts
	Hydrogen peroxide	Wounds with large amounts of necrotic tissue
	Wound scrubbing	Assists with removal of superficial loose debris and minimizes bacterial growth around the wound periphery
	Wet-to-dry dressings	Useful to debride wounds with moderate amounts of exudate and necrotic tissue
Enzymatic/Chemical	Topical application of enzymes (i.e., Travese, Elase, Collagenese)	Used with Stages III and IV wounds with large amounts of necrotic tissue
		Used to penetrate hard eschar after cross-hatching with a scalpel
		Discontinue after removal of devitalized tissue to avoid damage

Autolytic	Semi-occlusive/occlusive dressings
	  Transparent films
	  Hydrocolloids
	  Hydrogels
	  Calcium alginates
		Used with Stages III and IV wounds with light to moderate exudate

		Will assist with rehydration and liquidation of necrotic debris and eschar
		Cannot be used when clinical infection is present

performing vigorous wound cleansing by whirlpool or high-powered irrigation on necrotic wounds because the mechanical action created by the turbulence can wash away healthy tissue along with necrotic tissue. Hydrogen peroxide should not be used with granulating wounds since it has been found to cause blisters of new tissue as well as oxidization of wound debris and healthy tissue protein.[6] Hydrogen peroxide has also proven to cause trauma to new granulation tissue when used with deep tunneling wounds.[7]

Sharp/Surgical Debridement

In spite of efforts to cleanse and irrigate the wound, gross contaminants can still remain adherent to the injured tissues. If this occurs, sharp debridement should be carried out prior to closure of the wound. Removal of imbedded or adherent debris can be accomplished with tissue scissors or by scalpel excision (Figure 8-1).

Basic Instruments

Minor wound debridement can be accomplished with the following set of instruments: dissection scissors, iris (tissue) scissors, tissue forceps, scalpel handle, and the appropriate scalpel blades. There are also numerous disposable instrument sets that meet the needs of many minor wound care problems.

Scissors There are three basic types of scissors that are useful in minor wound care: iris or tissue scissors, dissection scissors, and bandage scissors

Figure 8-1. Technique to debride deep dermis and subcutaneous fat.

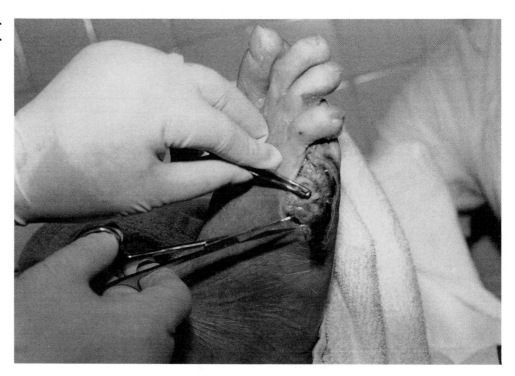

(Figure 8-2). The 4-inch iris scissors, both curved and straight, are predominantly used to assist in wound debridement and revision. These scissors are very sharp and are appropriate in situations that require very fine control. For heavier tissue revision, as might be necessary for wound undermining, blunt dissection scissors are recommended. Bandage scissors with a single blunt-tip are most useful for cutting sutures, adhesive tape, sponges, and other dressing materials. Because of their size and bulk, these scissors are very durable and practical.

Forceps When forceps are applied to the skin or other tissues, inadvertent damage to viable cells can occur if an improper technique is used. The currently recommended forceps are 4 $^3/_4$-inch Adson with small teeth (Figure 8-3). Teeth decrease the need to apply excessive force to grasp and secure tissue. Forceps without teeth are to be discouraged because the flat surface of their jaws tend to crush tissue more easily (Figure 8-4). Figure 8-5 demonstrates the correct and incorrect way to hold forceps manually.

Scalpel and Blades There are three primary blades used for wound debridement (Figure 8-6).

The #10 blade is used in minor wound care for the removal of thick callous tissue and is helpful for larger excisions during wound revision. Very commonly used and quite versatile is the #15 blade. It is small and well suited for precise debridement and wound revision. The #11 blade is configured ideally for incision and drainage of superficial abscesses.

Tissue Debridement and Techniques

Devitalized tissue can be recognized by its shredded, ischemic, blue, black, or brown appearance. Occasionally, these appearances can be misleading and true demarcation between viable and devitalized tissue cannot be made for several days. Therefore, one overriding principle of wound debridement is to spare as much tissue as possible. Further excision and debridement of the wound can be made at later intervals.

Technique for Simple Debris Excision

Most debridement can be carried out by simple excision of debris-laden tissue, using tissue forceps and iris scissors (Figure 8-7). Subcutaneous adipose tissue under the dermis can be freely excised without any concern for cosmetic results. Soiled,

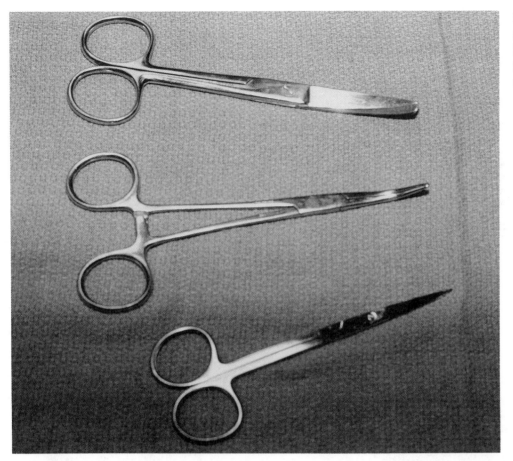

Figure 8-2. Three types of scissors useful for wound care: iris scissors (bottom), dissection scissors (middle), and bandage scissors (top).

Figure 8-3. Two types of Adson forceps: with teeth (left) and without teeth (right).

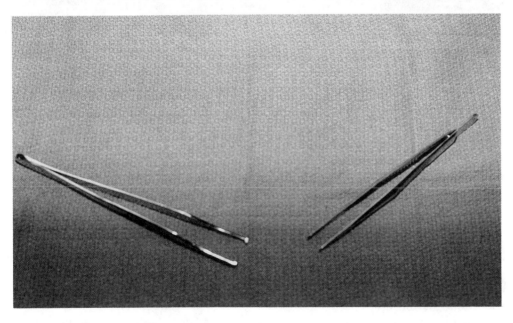

devitalized fatty tissue is a fertile substrate for the growth of bacteria with subsequent development of infection.[8]

Tendon, bone, nerves, and vascular structures should be avoided during the debridement procedure. These structures should not be uncovered by

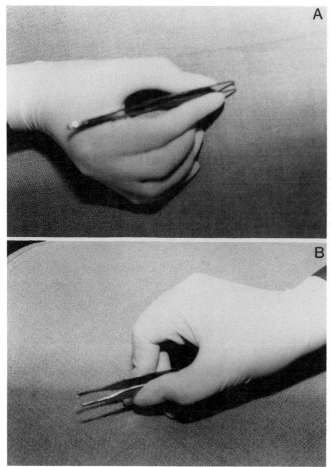

Figure 8-4. The correct and incorrect way to grasp tissue with forceps. (A) The correct way to grasp the tissue by the subcutaneous tissue. (B) The incorrect way to grasp tissue is by crushing the dermis and epidermis between the jaws of the forceps.

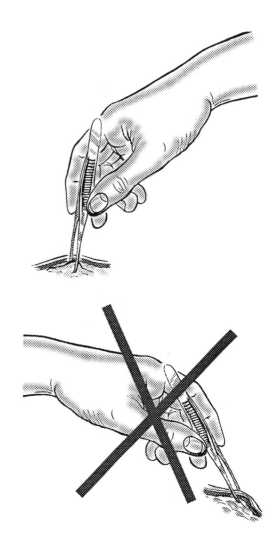

Figure 8-5. The correct (top) and incorrect (bottom) way to hold forceps to avoid tissue trauma.

debriding nonviable tissue until the physician is notified. All vital structures usually will be deep to subcutaneous tissue. If debridement reveals a fistula tract that goes into another tissue plane, the debridement should be stopped. A general guideline is that if the patient complains of pain, even after pain medication, the debridement should be stopped. Nonviable tissue is dead and removal should be painless. Viable tissue removal will often cause pain.

Bleeding is an undesirable problem when debriding. The removal of nonviable tissue should not produce bleeding. Wounds should not be debrided so deeply as to cause profuse bleeding. In addition to the problem of adequate wound visualization with active bleeding, hematomas can cause an in-crease in the rate of infection and delay the healing process.[9] If bleeding is encountered, the debridement should be stopped and a pressure with non-adherent dressing should be applied. If possible, the involved extremity should be elevated. Silver nitrate sticks have also been proven to be helpful in cauterizing superficial capillary bleeding.

Technique for Excision of Damaged Dermis

More care has to be taken in debriding and excising the epidermis and dermis. The best principle is to trim as little skin as possible. Wound margins should only be trimmed to the point in which viable tissue is first exposed.

Wounds covered with thick eschar should be debrided in stages. First, the eschar should be allowed to soften. The utilization of occlusive dressings will allow the eschar to rehydrate. The use of chemical enzymatic debriding agents in conjunction with an occlusive dressing accelerates this process. In order to obtain best results, it is recommended to use a scalpel to score or cross-hatch the eschar to allow for better penetration of the enzymes. Figure 8-8 demonstrates technique for cross-hatching eschar.

Enzymatic Debridement

The enzymatic method of debridement is one option that offers a safe, conservative, selective approach to the removal of gross necrotic tissue. This form of debridement requires the application of an enzyme capable of breaking down fibrin, denatured collage, and elastin.[10] A prescription from a physician must be obtained to use enzymatic debridement and should specify which enzymatic preparation is to be used. It is not recommended that enzymatic agents be used on dry eschar since enzymes are not easily activated. Enzymes will debride most efficiently in a moist environment. Occlusive dressings will allow rehydration of eschar and prevent the enzymatic preparation from drying out. When enzymatic debridement is used for a totally dry eschar crosshatching the eschar with a scalpel is recommended to allow for greater penetration of the enzymes. Chemical disinfectants such as sodium hypochlorite and benzoyl peroxide are still used, but these agents have been shown to be cytotoxic. Their use is generally discouraged by most wound healing experts. For more information on specific enzymatic debriding agents, please refer to Chapter 4.

Autolytic Debridement

Autolytic debridement is a selective technique that allows the body to lyse or break down necrotic tissue by using the body's own enzymes and moisture to rehydrate, soften and liquefy hard eschar and slough. Autolytic debridement, without exogenous

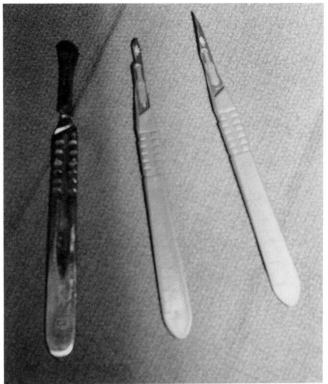

Figure 8-6. Scalpel handle and #11 (left), #10 (middle), and #15 (right) scalpel blades.

enzymes, may take place in chronic wounds in 7 to 10 days under semi-occlusive and occlusive dressings but is not observed under gauze dressings.[11]

Transparent films, hydrocolloids, and calcium alginates may all be used to enhance autolytic debridement. Generally, these dressings are changed on a daily or every other day schedule during the debridement phase. Wounds are cleaned at each dressing change with normal saline. Transparent films and occlusive wafer dressings are usually ineffective for the purpose of promoting autolysis in malnourished individuals. They are contraindicated in immunosuppressed patients and must be used with care on patients with potential or known anaerobic infections, especially diabetic patients.[12] Totally occlusive hydrocolloid dressings may create an environment supportive of anaerobic organisms. Calcium alginate dressings may be used in sloughy and infected wounds, but they are contraindicated in dry wounds. Hydrogels generally hasten the autolytic process by quickly rehydrating necrotic tissue. Gels can be held in place by transparent films and/or gauze.

Figure 8-7. Sharp debridement of necrotic debris using forceps and iris scissors.

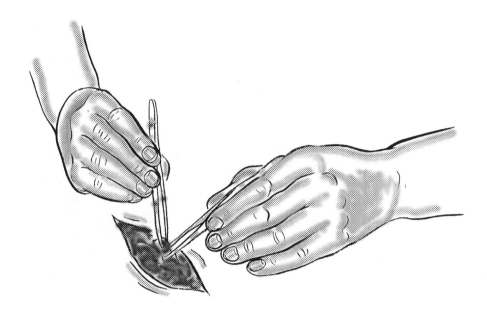

Mechanical Debridement

Another method to accomplish debridement is mechanical. This is achieved with any of the following techniques: wound cleansing via scrubbing, damp-to-dry gauze dressings, hydrotherapy, and irrigation. Mechanical debridement is non-selective and removes both viable and nonviable tissue from the wound bed.

Technique for Scrubbing the Wound Periphery

The actual technique for scrubbing the wound periphery is illustrated in Figure 8-9. It is important for the clinician to be gentle with debridement and start at the wound itself. The motion should be circular, with gradually larger circles away from the wound. At no time should the sponge or gauze be brought from the periphery back towards the wound because this maneuver will carry unwanted organisms from unsterile skin areas back to the area of the cleansed wound site. Scrubbing continues until the skin is visibly free of contaminates and dried blood. There is no specific time for scrubbing, but it should last at least 2 to 3 minutes.

DAMP-TO-DRY DRESSINGS

Mechanical debridement of wounds can be performed with damp-to-dry dressings. The gauze is dampened with normal saline and then completely opened to a single layer and lightly packed into the wound bed. In order for this technique to be effective, the gauze must be completely dry in the wound bed (approximately 6 hours) before it is removed. As the gauze dries, it entraps necrotic debris and wound exudate within the fibers. The tightness of the weave and the absorbency and adherency of the gauze will determine the extent of mechanical debridement. This method is painful and indiscriminately removes granulation tissue as well as necrotic debris.

HYDROTHERAPY

INDICATIONS FOR USE

Wound soaking is a common practice and patients are often referred to physical therapy for hydrotherapy services. Hydrotherapy is believed to loosen debris, break up blood coagulum, remove toxic resi-

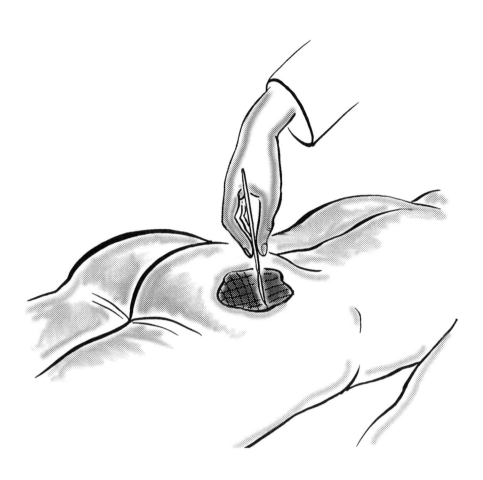

Figure 8-8. Cross-hatching of eschar with a scalpel.

due from various topical agents, and produce a moist environment for wound healing. Wound soaking and use of water agitation is helpful in loosening, softening, and removing gross contaminants but it is not a substitute for mechanical skin cleansing and wound irrigation. In addition, various antimicrobial agents may be added to the water of a whirlpool to kill bacteria present in infected wound.[13,14]

In full-thickness dermal ulcers with necrotic debris or eschar, hydrotherapy is indicated to facilitate softening and separation of eschar and necrotic tissue. Whirlpool is most effective when used in conjunction with interim wound dressings. Whirlpool can be performed daily or twice a day with wet-to-dry gauze dressings to assist with the debridement of wounds covered with a yellow fibrous debris or gelatinous surface exudate. The mechanical action of the water turbulence and

removal of the wet-to-dry dressing will help to debride surface debris and exudate.

Clean wounds with healthy red granulation tissue and migrating epidermal cells should not be subjected to even minimal water agitation which mechanically damages fragile endothelial and epithelial cells. Clean wounds are not indicated for hydrotherapy, but should be managed with appropriate non-adherent, protective dressing.

WHIRLPOOL ADDITIVES

There are several antibacterial agents which may be added to whirlpool water to help reduce wound infection. It is important to remember that all open wounds contain microflora, but this does not necessarily mean the wound is infected. Therefore, the clinician must give careful consideration when weighing the benefits of using such agents

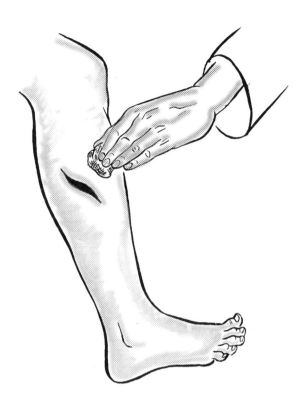

Figure 8-9. Note the spiral technique of scrubbing a wound periphery by beginning at the center and moving away to the periphery without crossing back over the actual wound area.

to prevent infection versus the suppression of tissue repair secondary to cytotoxic effects. If a wound is clean, with healthy red granulation tissue and minimum serious drainage, it is advised not to use a whirlpool additive. If whirlpool additives are to be used, it is critical that the recommended concentration be used to prevent cytotoxicity of wound tissue.

The most frequently used whirlpool additives are povidone-iodine (Betadine), sodium hypochlorite (household bleach), chloramine-T (Chlorazene), chlorhexidene gluconate (Hibiclens), and Tide laundry detergent (without perfume). See Table 8-2 for dilutions and dosages for whirlpool additives and indications for their use.

Povidone-Iodine (Betadine)

Povidone-iodine, or Betadine, is probably one

of the most frequently misused antiseptics in the clinical setting. It is routinely used as a presurgical scrub and is effective for this purpose because of its ability to destroy viruses, yeasts, bacteria, and fungi. However, iodine toxicity has occurred in patients receiving dressing changes or irrigation with full-strength povidone-iodine dressings in wound beds. It is important to remember that povidone-iodine was never approved by the FDA for use in open wounds.

Lineaweaver and associates[15] found that topical application of povidone-iodine diluted to a 0.001% concentration is bactericidal to staphylococcus aureus, yet is noncytotoxic to cultured human fibroblasts. The results of this study argue against the use of povidone-iodine at concentrations greater than 0.001% and should caution the clinician against using povidone-iodine and other topical agents for prolonged periods of time.

Kucan and associates[16] reported that the application of 10% povidone-iodine to chronic human pressure sores every 6 hours was no more effective than saline washes in reducing bacteria counts. Additional research studies have reported povidone-iodine to be ineffective in wound colonized with greater than five organisms per gram of tissue.[17,18]

The clinician should be cautioned that sufficient evidence exists which indicates tissue cytotoxicity and diminished antimicrobial effectiveness when povidone-iodine is used topically in concentrations greater than 0.001%. In addition, clinicians must be aware of the possible long-term effects of topical povidone-iodine solutions that may occur through system absorption of iodine with repeated use.[19] One can only speculate that new wound tissue subjected to submersion and irrigation with this agent will be equally affected, even if it is used at the recommended concentrations. However, further research is indicated to assess the cytotoxic effect of povidone-iodine as a whirlpool additive.

Sodium Hypochlorite (Household Bleach)

The addition of sodium hypochlorite (in a 0.5% solution) to the whirlpool water results in the release of free chlorine which acts as an effective antimicrobial

Table 8-2. **Dilution and Dosage for Whirlpool Additives**

Whirlpool Agent	Indications for Use	Recommended Dilution and Dosage
Chlorhexidine Gluconate (Hibiclens)	Superficial clean wounds with granulation tissue and minimal to moderate amount of seropurulent drainage	Hubbard tank (425 gal) = 4 oz* High-boy whirlpool (95 gal) = 2 oz Low-boy whirlpool (80 gal) = 2 oz Hand whirlpool = 1 oz
Sodium Hypochlorite (household bleach) 5.25%	Infected wounds with foul odor, copious amount of exudate, and/or necrotic debris	1:240 dilution Hubbard Tank (425 gal) = 1 gal, 48 oz* High-boy whirlpool (95 gal) = 25 oz Low-boy whirlpool (80 gal) = 21 oz Hand whirlpool (30 gal) = 7 oz
Chloramine-T (Chlorazene) 12.20% free chlorine	Infected wounds with foul odor, copious amount of exudate, and/or necrotic debris	1:5000 dilution (200-300 ppm)** 282 to 423 gal = 320 g 77 to 116 gal = 88 g 44 to 66 gal = 50 g 33 to 50 gal = 20 g 18 to 26 gal = 20 g
Tide	Wounds with a high concentration of adipose tissue*	Hubbard tank (425 gal) = 4 oz* High-boy whirlpool (95 gal) = 2 oz Low-boy whirlpool (80 gal) = 2 oz Hand whirlpool (30 gal) = 1/2 oz

*Based on author's clinical experience
**Based on manufacturer's recommendations

agent to control sepsis. Although the antimicrobial effectiveness of this chlorine-liberating compound has been demonstrated, such compounds may be cytotoxic. Lineaweaver and associates[15] found 0.5% sodium hypochlorite to be cytotoxic to cultured human fibroblasts and adversely affected wound healing in an animal model. This study also showed that a 0.005% solution is bactericidal in vitro but is noncytotoxic to fibroblasts.

Chloramine-T (Chlorazene)

This is a powder substance which contains the chlorine molecule linked to a hydrogen-nitrogen bond forming an amine, known as chloramine-T. This germicidal whirlpool agent is recommended to be used in concentration of 200 to 300 parts per million (a 1:5000 dilution). Chlorazene is reported to be less irritating and cytotoxic than sodium hypochlorite. The molecular structure of the substance allows for a slower release of free chlorine into the water, and this, therefore, increases the bactericidal effects for a longer period of time. This is the only additive that should be added to the water prior to wound submersion.

Chlorhexidene Gluconate (Hibiclens)

Chlorhexidene gluconate, or Hibiclens, is routinely used as a presurgical scrub on intact skin. When used as a whirlpool additive it produces a strong antiseptic activity and a persistent antimicrobial and bactericidal effect against a wide range of microorganisms. It is similar to povidone-iodine in action, and is reported to cause cytotoxic effects to cultured human fibroblast cells but to a lesser degree.[15] Research indicates that prolonged topical use of chlorhexidene gluconate results in decreased mobility of macrophages and neutrophils to the affected area. It is recommended that wounds which involve more than the superficial layers of the skin should not be routinely treated with this agent.

Tide

Although there is no research published to date on the use of Tide laundry detergent as a whirlpool additive, it has proven to be clinically effective in treating wounds with high concentrations of adipose tissue. Tide detergent contains a high concentration of phosphorus which acts as a fat emulsifier to accelerate the liquification of adipose tissue. This is particularly helpful in wounds located on the upper thigh, abdomen, or buttocks. Like any additive, Tide should not be used for prolonged periods. Its use should be limited to the point until the necessary adipose tissue has been eliminated.

It should be noted that antimicrobial agents should be added once adequate temperature and water level have been achieved, and just before the patient enters the tank due to the short kill time of many agents. The only exception is Chlorazene which, because of its molecular structure, is able to provide a slower release of free chlorine. Therefore, manufacturers recommend that Chlorazene be added to the water 5 minutes prior to patient submersion. The treatment time should also be limited to 15 minutes versus the typical 20 minutes due to the short antimicrobial kill time of many agents.

IRRIGATION/WOUND LAVAGE

Wound irrigation is probably the most effective way to remove debris and contaminants in partially healed wounds or those without hard eschar. Irrigation is also the single most effective method of reducing bacterial counts on wound surfaces or in sinus tracts.[20]

In comparing methods of irrigation for highly contaminated wounds, high-pressure streams of saline are clearly superior to low pressure streams such as those that might be obtained with a bulb-type syringe.[20,21] Regardless of the technique, irrigation must be accomplished gently to avoid damage to the healing tissue. For "clean" wounds with low levels of contamination, some authorities recommend reducing the force of the stream to minimize any potential for unnecessary tissue trauma from the irrigation itself.[22]

For the purpose of infection control, universal precautions should be observed when performing wound irrigation/lavage. Protective eyeware, face shield, gloves, and water-resistant gowns should always be worn.

SYRINGE IRRIGATION

When performing syringe irrigation, the flow should be directed at right angles to the wound and the fluid allowed to drain by gravity. A basin to collect irrigant should be placed under the involved area. This requires careful positioning of the patient, either in bed or in a chair.

Indications for Use

Syringe irrigation can be used for both clean and small infected wounds. When irrigating a clean wound base use a 35 cc syringe with normal saline. The clinician should make sure to use enough irrigant to cleanse the base thoroughly. At least one syringe full should be used. For infected wounds, normal saline delivered via a 50 cc syringe with a 19 gauge needle will provide enough pressure to effectively remove wound debris and dressing residue without irritating new granulation tissue.[23] One must be careful not to prick the wound base with the needle. The wound base should be irrigated thoroughly so as to completely cover the wound base. The number of full syringes depends on the size of the wound and the amount of necrotic debris present.

HIGH-PRESSURE IRRIGATION/LAVAGE

Indications for Use

High-pressure irrigation/lavage is recommended for large or multiple wounds with necrotic tissue. This form of debridement applies a stream or spray under a controlled pressure to mechanically debride the wound, thereby removing more adherent material that would be unaffected by conventional techniques (Figure 8-10). Normal saline is used most often as the irrigant solution, but in cases

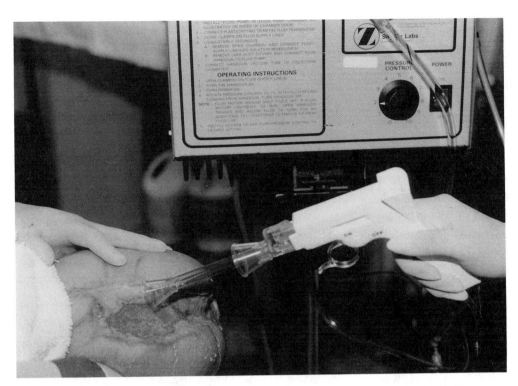

Figure 8-10. Pulsavac Lavage Debridement System by Snyder Labs, a subsidiary of Zimmer, 200 West, Ohio Ave, Dover, Ohio.

of severe infection antimicrobial solutions may be used to irrigate the wound.

This technique has the advantage of cleaning the wound in a shorter period of time compared with hydrotherapy and the wound tissue is also not traumatized during transfers. This treatment is easily portable and has the option of using a return suction feature (to collect excess fluids) which makes it ideal for treating those patients at bedside who are too critically ill to be transported and require constant monitoring, or those patients who are ventilator dependent. It is also recommended for the elderly individual with extremity contractures and thin skin over bony prominences resulting in multiple breakdown areas.

FOLLOW-UP

It is essential that any changes in the wound or wound treatment be re-evaluated by the clinician. The appearance of a wound often changes from one day to the next. Any new or unusual changes in the wound should be reported to the physician. Any changes in the method of debridement or dressing regime should be done in collaboration with the physician. The purpose of any form of debridement is to remove devitalized tissue and should be carefully monitored to make sure normal tissue is not damaged. It is helpful to re-evaluate the wound after changing dressing products or types of dressings to determine the effect of the dressing. Since each wound is individual, frequent wound evaluations should be performed at regular intervals or whenever there is a change in the wound bed or dressing management.

CONCLUSION

An overview has been presented for the management of wounds requiring debridement. Sharp debridement is a quick method of removing nonviable tissue which can impede wound healing and increase the risk of infection. The clinician must demonstrate the education and technical skill to practice sharp debridement in a collaborative role with the primary care physician. Enzymatic debridement is a conservative, pain-free method in which topical enzymes are used to digest necrotic debris. The type of enzymes used should be specific to the type of devitalized tissue present in the wound. Autolytic debridement relies on the body's own defense mechanisms to assist with the lysis of necrotic tissue. The use of semi-occlusive and occlusive dressings enables the body to use its own enzymes to rehydrate eschar or slough within the wound. Mechanical debridement can be performed via a variety of techniques, all of which apply a mechanical force on the wound surface to assist with the desiccation and separation of necrotic debris or dressing residual and decrease bacterial growth. The necessary guidelines for wound debridement should be followed and frequent wound evaluations performed if wound status changes or the treatment regime is altered.

REFERENCES

1. Halpin-Landry JE. How do you score? Test your skills in pressure-ulcer management. In: Krasner D. *Chronic Wound Care: A Clinical Source Book for Health Professionals.* King of Prussia, PA: Health Management Publications; 1990:194-205.

2. Zink M, Rousseau P, Holloway GA. Lower extremity ulcers. In: Bryant RA. *Acute and Chronic Wounds.* St. Louis, MO: CV Mosby; 1992:164-212.

3. Hunt TK, Heppenstall RB, Pines E, Rovee D. *Soft and Hard Tissue Repair: Biological and Clinical Aspects.* New York, NY: Praeger Publishers; 1984.

4. Winter GD. Formation of scab and the rate of epithelialization in superficial wounds in the skin of the domestic pig. *Nature.* 1962;193:293-294.

5. Feedar JA, Kloth LC. Conservative management of chronic wounds. In: Feedar JA, Kloth LC. *Wound Healing: Alternatives in Management.* Philadelphia, PA: FA Davis Co; 1990:135-172.

6. Bassen M, Shalev O, Dudai M. Near fatal oxygen embolism due to wound irrigation with hydrogen peroxide. *Post Grad Med J.* 1982;58:448-450.

7. Gruber RP, Vistnes L, Pardae R. The effect of commonly used antiseptics on wound healing. *J Plast Reconstr Surg.* 1975;55:472-476.

8. Haury B, Rodeheaver GT, Vensco J, Edgerton M, Edlinch R. Debridement: an essential component of wound care. *Am J Surg.* 1978;135:238-242.

9. Altemeier W. Principals in the management of traumatic wounds and infection control. *Bull NY Acad Med.* 1979;55:123-138.

10. Levin ME. The diabetic foot: pathophysiology, evaluation and treatment. In: Levin ME, O'Neal LW. *The Diabetic Foot.* St. Louis, MO: CV Mosby Co; 1988:1-50.

11. Mertz PM. Intervention: dressing effects on wound healing. In: Eaglstein WH. *New Directions in Wound Healing: Wound Care Manual.* Princeton, NJ: ER Squibb & Sons, Inc; 1990:83-96.

12. Alvarez O, Rozint J, Wiseman D. Moist environment for healing: matching the dressing to the wound. *Wounds.* 1989;1:35-51.

13. Simonetti A, Miller R, Gristina J. Efficacy of povidone-iodine in the disinfection of whirlpool baths and hubbard tanks. *Phys Ther.* 1972;52:1277-1282.

14. Steve L, Goodhart P, Alexander J. Hydrotherapy burn treatment: used of chloramine-T against resistant microorganisms. *Arch Phys Med Rehabil.* 1979;60:301-303.

15. Lineaweaver W, Richard H, Soucy D, et al. Topical antimicrobial toxicity. *Arch Surg.* 1985;120:267-270.

16. Kucan JO, Robson MC, Heggers JP, Ko F. Comparison of silver sulfadiazine, povidone-iodine and physiologic salin in the treatment of chronic pressure ulcers. *J Am Geriatr Soc.* 1981;29:232-235.

17. Robson MC, Schaerf RH, Krizek TJ. Evaluation of topical povidone-iodine ointment in experimental burn wound sepsis. *Plast Reconstr Surg.* 1974;54:328-334.

18. Tommey RC, Norberg HP, Guernsey JM. The use of povidine-iodine in the treatment of burns: a literature review. *J Okla State Med Assoc.* 1980;73:406-408.

19. Aronoff TG, Friedman S, Doedens D, Lavelle K. Increased serum iodide concentration from iodine absorption through wounds treated topically with povidone-iodine. *Am J Med Sci.* 1980;279:173-176.

20. Peterson LW. Prophylaxis of wound infection. *Arch Surg.* 1945;50:177-183.

21. Stevenson TR, Thacker JG, Rodeheaver GT. Cleansing the traumatic wound by high pressure syringe irrigation. *J Am College Emerg Phys.* 1976;5:17-21.

22. Edlich RF, Rodeheaver GT, Morgan RF, Berman DE, Thacker JG. Principals of emergency wound management. *Am Emerg Med.* 1988;17:1284-1302.

23. Rogness H. High pressure wound irrigation. *J Enterostomal Ther.* 1985;12:27-28.

Chapter 9

Wound Dressings

Jan Cuzzell, MA, RN, and Diane Krasner, MS, RN, CETN

Treating and dressing a variety of wounds present enormous challenges to the clinician. Wound dressing selection is complex, and decisions often need to be modified based on changes in the patient's condition. For example, exacerbation of chronic disease or changes in wound status such as localized infection require re-evaluation of the care plan. Timely adjustments of the topical treatment protocol can mean the difference between a wound that heals and one that rapidly deteriorates.

The red-yellow-black color classification system takes much of the guesswork out of the assessment process[1-3] and provides practical guidelines for dressing selection. Familiarity with many dressing materials now available will help the clinician match the right dressing to the wound, patient, and setting.[4] Furthermore, by individualizing dressing protocols, patient outcomes will be optimized. The purposes of this chapter are to describe wound dressings by generic category, to present a systematic approach to wound assessment and dressing selection that clinicians can use in all settings, and to provide a list of dressing manufacturers.

TRADITIONAL SURGICAL DRESSING

CONTACT LAYER

This is the first layer of the dressing which is placed either directly over the wound or after the application of a topical medication. The contact layer usually consists of a non-adherent dressing material such as an ointment-impregnated or fine mesh gauze. This non-adherent layer prevents new epithelium from sticking to the dressing and from being inadvertently removed when the dressing is changed. The contact layer also wicks or draws exudate away from the wound.

INTERMEDIATE OR ABSORBENT LAYER

This is the second layer of the dressing which generally consists of gauze sponges placed on top of the contact layer. It absorbs the exudate and blood extruded from the wound. This layer also protects the wound from external trauma. The combination of both the contact and intermediate layers is known as the primary dressing. Many dressings combine both layers in a single dressing.

OUTER LAYER

The outer or third layer of the dressing consists of absorbent cotton pads placed over the primary dressing. This layer is secured by either adhesive tape or other dressing retainers. It provides additional protection by acting as a splint to immobilize the wound until healing is underway. Most commercially available dressings are available as separate dressing components.

DRESSINGS BY GENERIC CATEGORY

Over 2,000 dressing materials are available

commercially. It is rather impossible for a clinician to remember trade names, actions, indications, and contraindications of all products. In order to make it convenient for the clinician, dressings should be organized by generic categories. Eight commonly used dressing categories, including properties, indications, and contraindications are described below. Table 9-1 presents a list of generic dressing categories and their manufacturers.

GAUZE DRESSINGS

Gauze dressings are manufactured from yarn or thread. There are many types of gauze dressings such as cotton mesh gauze, non-woven gauze, and impregnated gauze. They are highly permeable to air. These dressings readily absorb exudate and the porosity allows for rapid moisture evaporation. Indications for use include initial treatment of wounds with necrotic tissue when debridement is needed or when other, more occlusive dressings are contraindicated. Gauze can be used for wet-to-wet, wet-to-moist, or wet-to-dry debridement. Wounds with undermining or tunneling can be loosely packed with cotton mesh roll gauze or gauze packing strips to prevent exudate accumulation and to prevent premature closure of the wounds. Cotton mesh gauze with large interstices is often used for debridement, while non-woven gauze is primarily used for absorption. Although gauze dressings are readily available and are cost-effective, they have several disadvantages. Gauze is permeable to bacteria, thus potentially increasing the opportunity for wound infection. These dressings stick to the wound bed and may damage newly formed granulation tissue and epidermis when removed from the wound surface. Further, gauze fibers can become enmeshed in dried serous wound exudate which can cause increased pain during dressing changes. Both woven and non-woven gauze tends to shed lint and fibers which can act as foreign material and lead to prolonged inflammation and infection. Gauze dressings do not absorb excessive amount of exudate, therefore, frequent dressing changes are necessary or maceration may result. Gauze dressings should be used with caution and after careful assessment of the wound.

NON-ADHERENT DRESSINGS

Non-adherent dressings limit the risk of the dressing sticking to the base of the wound. Available as either impregnated, e.g., Vaseline®, or non-impregnated, e.g., Telfa®, these dressings are useful for skin tears, donor sites, and skin grafts. They are also useful when the intact skin around the wound is highly friable and tears easily. These dressings only absorb minimal amounts of exudate. They do not stick to the wound bed and are not painful when removed. Non-adherent wound dressings usually require a secondary dressing to cover them. Impregnated, non-adherent dressings containing antimicrobial agents may be cytotoxic to fibroblasts.[5]

HYDROCOLLOID DRESSINGS

Hydrocolloid dressings are made up of gelatin, pectin, and/or carboxymethylcellulose (CMC) in a polyisobutylene adhesive base. Impermeable to water, oxygen, and bacteria, these dressings are effective in absorbing minimal to moderate amounts of exudates. The occlusive properties are useful in autolysing minimal to moderate amounts of necrotic tissue. Hydrocolloids are highly conformable, adhere well in the presence of moisture, and are used in both acute and chronic, partial- or full-thickness, granulating and epithelializing wounds. They are particularly well suited for high friction areas. As hydrocolloids interact with wound fluids, they leave residues in the wound bed or on the margins which are difficult to remove. Since these dressings are impermeable to oxygen, they are not recommended for dressing wounds with anaerobic infections.

SEMI-PERMEABLE FILMS

Film dressings are manufactured from transparent polyurethane membranes with water-resistant adhesives. They are highly elastic, conform easily to body contours, provide optimal visual wound monitoring, and are cost-effective. These dressings are semi-permeable to moisture vapor and oxygen, but occlusive to bacterial invasion. Indications include superficial wounds and burns, postoperative wounds, and donor sites. They are also used for retention of primary dressings. Because films are

Table 9-1. **Wound Care Products by Generic Category**

Product	Manufacturer
Alginate Dressing	
Algiderm	Viaderm Pharmaceuticals
ALGOSTERIL	Johnson & Johnson Medical
Curasorb	Kendall
Kaltostat	Calgon Vestal
Sorbsan	Dow B. Hickam
Biosynthetic Dressings	
Biobrane II	Dow B. Hickam
Silon	BioMed Sciences
Cleansers	
a. Saline	Multiple
b. Hydrogen peroxide	Multiple
c. Skin cleansers	
Eucerin Cleanser	Beiersdorf
Peri-Wash	Sween
Triple Care	Smith & Nephew United
d. Wound cleansers	
Biolex	Bard
Cara-Klenz	Carrington
Clinical-Care	Care-Tech Labs
Constant-Clens	Sherwood Medical
Dermal Wound Cleanser	Smith & Nephew United
Micro-Klenz	Carrington
Puri-Clens	Sween
Royl-Derm	Acme United
SAF-Clens	Calgon Vestal
Shur Clens	Calgon Vestal
Ultra-Klenz	Carrington
Composite Dressings	
Airstrip	Smith & Nephew United
Alldress	Scott Health Care
BAND-AID	Johnson & Johnson Medical
Covaderm	DeRoyal
Coverlet	Beiersdorf
CURAD Bandages	Kendall
Curity Cover	Kendall
Cutifilm Plus*	Beiersdorf
ETE	Scott Health Care
Exu-Dry	Frastec
LyoFoam A,C	Acme United
Metalline	Selomas
Microdon	3M
NU-DERM	Johnson & Johnson Medical
Odor-Absorbent Dressing	Hollister
PolyDerm WBC	Laivan
POLYMEM	Ferris Manufacturing Corp.
Primapore	Smith & Nephew United
Release	Johnson & Johnson Medical
Sofsorb	DeRoyal
STERI-PAD	Johnson & Johnson Medical
SURGIPAD Combine Dressings	Johnson & Johnson Medical
TELFA	Kendall

Table 9-1. **Wound Care Products by Generic Category (Continued)**

Product	Manufacturer
TELFA Island Dressing	Kendall
TENDERSORB Wet-Pruf Abdominal Pad	Kendall
Topper Dressing Sponge	Johnson & Johnson Medical
Transorb	Brady Medical
Ventex	Kendall
Viasorb	Sherwood Medical
Enzymes/Debridings Agents	
Elase	Fugisawa
Elase and Chloromycetin	Fugisawa
Panafil Ointment	Rystan
Panafil White Ointment	Rystan
Santyl	Knoll Pharmaceuticals
Travase	Flint
Foam Dressings	
Allevyn	Smith & Nephew United
Cutinova	Beiersdorf
EpiGard	Ormed
Epi-Lock	Calgon Vestal
Lyofoam	Acme United
MitraFlex	Calgon Vestal
Flexzan	Dow B. Hickam
Gauze Dressings	
a. Woven	Multiple
b. Non-woven	
EXCILON	Kendall
NU GAUZE General Use Sponges	Johnson & Johnson
SOF-WICK	Johnson & Johnson
VERSALON	Kendall
c. Packing	
Kerlix	Kendall
NU-BREDE	Johnson & Johnson Medical
NU-GAUZE Packing Strips	Johnson & Johnson Medical
d. Conforming/Wrapping	
Conform	Kendall
Elastomull	Beiersdorf
Kerlix Lite	Kendall
Kling	Johnson & Johnson Medical
SOF-KLING	Johnson & Johnson Medical
SOF-BAND	Johnson & Johnson Medical
e. Debriding	
NU-BREDE	Johnson & Johnson Medical
f. Impregnated Gauze Dressings	
Adaptic	Johnson & Johnson Medical
Aquaphor	Beiersdorf
Carrington Hydrogel Wound Dressing Saturated Pad	Carrington
Curity Oil Emulsion	Kendall
Curity Packing Strips (iodoform)	Kendall
Curity Packing Strips (plain)	Kendall
Curity Petrolatum Gauze	Kendall
Curity Wet Dressing (saline)	Kendall

Table 9-1. **Wound Care Products by Generic Category (Continued)**

Product	Manufacturer
Curity Wet Dressing (water)	Kendall
Dermagran Wet Dressings (saline)	Dermasciences
Dermagran Wet Dressings (zinc-saline)	Dermasciences
Kendall Xeroform	Kendall

Hydrocolloid Dressings
Actiderm	ConvaTec
Comfeel	Coloplast
Cutinova	Beiersdorf
DuoDERM	ConvaTec
Hydrapad	Baxter
Intact	Bard
Orahesive	
RepliCare	Smith & Nephew United
Restore	Hollister
Sween-A-Peel	Sween
3M Tegasorb	3M
ULTEC	Sherwood Medical

Hydrogel Dressings
Aquasorb	DeRoyal
Biolex Wound Gel	Bard
Carrington Gel Wound Dressing	Carrington
ClearSite	New Dimensions in Medicine (NDM)
Dermagran Wound Dressing	Dermasciences
Elasto-Gel	Southwest Technologies Inc.
Geliperm Wet/Granulate	Fougera
Hypergel	Scott Health Care
Inerpan	Sherwood Medical
IntraSite Gel	Smith & Nephew United
Normlgel	Scott Health Care
Nu-Gel	Johnson & Johnson Medical
Royl-Derm	Acme United
Second Skin	Spenco
Spand-Gel	Medi-Tech
Vigilon	Bard

Paste, Powders, Beads, Contact Layers
Bard Absorption Dressing/EasyPak	Bard
Comfeel Paste	Coloplast
Comfeel Powder	Coloplast
Chronicure	ABS Life Sciences
Debrisan	Johnson & Johnson Medical
Dermanet Wound Contact Layer	DeRoyal
DuoDERM Granules	ConvaTec
DuoDERM Paste	ConvaTec
Geletin-Pectin Powder (generic)	Multiple
HolliHesive Paste	Hollister
HydraGran	Baxter
Karaya Paste	Hollister
Karaya Powder (generic)	Multiple
Multidex Hydrophilic Powder	Lange Medical Products
N-TERFACE	Winfield Laboratories
Premium Paste	Hollister

Table 9-1. **Wound Care Products by Generic Category (Continued)**

Product	Manufacturer
Premium Powder	Hollister
ReliCare Paste	Smith & Nephew United
ReliCare Powder	Smith & Nephew United
Tegapore	3M
Skin Sealants	
AllKare	ConvaTec
Barri-Care Barrier Film	Care-Tech Laboratories
Incontinence Protective Barrier Film	Bard
Nu-Gard	Nu-Hope
Prep-Site	Acme United
Protective Barrier Film	Bard
Skin Gel	Hollister
Skin Prep	Smith & Nephew United
Skin Shield	Mentor
Sween Prep	Sween
Transparent Film Dressings	
Acu-Derm	Acme United
Bioclusive	Johnson & Johnson Medical
BlisterFilm	Sherwood Medical
Ensure-It	Deseret
Opraflex	Professional Medical
OpSite	Smith & Nephew United
Polyskin	Kendall
Tegaderm	3M
Transorb	DeRoyal
Wound Pouches	
Wound Drainage Collector	Hollister
Wound Manager	ConvaTec

minimally absorbent, they trap moisture and facilitate autolytic debridement. However, moisture accumulation can cause maceration in wounds with moderate to heavy exudate. In addition, they can be difficult to apply without wrinkles or channeling, and do not hold well in high friction areas. Furthermore, these dressings are adhesive and can tear healthy skin in the elderly.

SEMI-PERMEABLE HYDROGELS

Semi-permeable hydrogel dressings contain approximately 96% water or glycerin. These products are three-dimensional hydrophilic polymers manufactured from gelatin or polysaccharides. Transparent, highly conformable, moisture-retentive, and permeable to oxygen, hydrogels are available in

either sheet or gel form. Indications include acute and chronic, partial- and full-thickness wounds with minimal to moderate amounts of exudate. Because of high water content, they promote autolytic debridement and are effective in the removal of eschar and sloughy tissue. Hydrogel sheets are good to use for ultrasound treatment. A cover dressing should be used over gel forms. These dressings should be avoided for wounds with moderate to heavy exudate.

SEMI-PERMEABLE FOAMS

Foam dressings are polyurethane non-adhesive, hydrophilic dressings. They are hydrophilic at the wound contact surface and hydrophobic on the outer side. Capable of absorbing moderate

Table 9-1. **Wound Care Products by Generic Category (Continued)**

Product	Manufacturer
Not Otherwise Classified (NOC)	
Adhesives	
Adhesive Skin Closures	
Adhesive Removers	
Antimicrobials, Antiseptics, and Antibiotics	
Bandages	
Barrier Ointments	
Collagen	
Compression Wraps	
Dressing Covers	
Growth Factors	
Health Care Personnel Handrinse	
Leg Ulcer Wraps	
Lubricating/Stimulating Sprays	
Moisturizers	
Ointments	
Sterile Fields	
Surgical Tapes	
Chloresium Ointment/Solution	Rystan
Circulon System	ConvaTec
Comprilan	Beiersdorf
Dermagran Ointment	Dermasciences
Dermagran Moisturizing Spray	Dermasciences
Dome Paste	Miles
Gelocast	Beiersdorf
Granulex	Dow B. Hickam
Hydron Wound Dressing	Bioderm Sciences
Hypafix	Smith & Nephew United
Medifil	BioCore
Mefix	Scott Health Care
Odor Absorbent Dressing	Hollister
Optipore Sponge	Calgon Vestal
Proderm	Dow B. Hickam
SkinTemp	BioCore
Steri-Drape Irrigation Pouch	3M
Steri-Strip Skin Closures	3M
Unna-Flex	ConvaTec
Unna Pack	Glenwood

While every attempt has been made to be as inclusive as possible in the development of this listing, the multiplicity of products and the rapid pace of new product development may mean that certain products were inadvertently omitted. Frequent revision of this listing will be necessary in order to maintain its currency. No endorsement of any product is intended. With each category, products must be individually evaluated. All products within a category do not necessarily perform equally.

©Diane Krasner 1993

amounts of exudate, foams are permeable to both moisture vapor and oxygen. Extremely conformable, foam sheets can be easily customized to fit a particular wound. They are also available in the form of cavity fillers which are composed of chips of polyurethane foam encapsulated in a layer of thin, perforated polymeric film. Like other semi-permeable materials, foams are moisture retentive and promote autolytic debridement. Indications include partial- and full-thickness draining wounds, deeper wounds with cavities, and skin protection around tracheostomy sites. These dressings may dehydrate the wound bed of granular, non-draining wounds.

EXUDATE ABSORBING DRESSINGS

A variety of products such as powders, pastes, beads, and hypertonic saline gauze fall under this dressing category. The calcium alginate dressings are also included here. These hydrophilic products absorb several times their weight in exudate. They are used to fill highly exudating, deep wounds that have uneven wound beds. Permeable to oxygen, they help control bacterial proliferation, provide cleansing, and reduce odor. They also conform easily to body contours and easily irrigate out of wounds. Use of these products with dry or minimally exudating wounds is not recommended. They also require a secondary dressing to cover them.

BIOLOGIC DRESSINGS

Biologic dressings are derived from human or animal sources and are usually indicated for large wounds such as massive burns. Their use is limited with chronic wounds, but they have been used to treat leg ulcers. A cutaneous autograft is a skin graft taken from one part of the body and transplanted to another part of the same person. This is the ideal permanent wound coverage, but usually difficult to accomplish in massive wounds because of lack of available donor sites. A cutaneous allograft is a skin graft taken from a human cadaver or live donor and transplanted to another person. Unlike autografts, allografts only provide temporary wound coverage. A xenograft is a skin graft taken from an animal and transplanted to a human (e.g., pig skin). Xenografts are sometimes used as a "test" graft prior to applying autograft or allograft. Good xenograft adherence increases the likelihood of autograft/allograft "take." Disadvantages of the biologic dressings include limited availability, high cost, possible disease transmission, and graft rejection.

OVERVIEW OF WOUND CLOSURE TECHNIQUES

When a person experiences skin or tissue trauma, a complex series of cellular, biochemical, and physiological processes are initiated.[6] These processes, which include granulation, wound contraction, and re-epithelialization, are aimed at restoring tissue integrity and re-establishing the body's protective barrier. The result is a healed wound. Frequently, healing occurs at different rates in different individuals and the events of tissue repair overlap. The challenge to the clinician is to identify treatment protocols that facilitate the different healing events as they occur until wound closure is complete.[7]

Primary intention healing occurs when the edges of a wound are reapproximated at the time of wounding and held together with sutures, staples, or adhesive skin closures. Examples include surgical incisions and clean lacerations. The wound space is small and very little granulation tissue is required for healing because healthy tissue planes are held in such close proximity. As a result, epidermal continuity is restored rapidly, wound contraction is negligible, and the end result is usually a relatively thin scar with minimal deformity.

Secondary intention healing occurs when the wound edges are not reapproximated and a large wound space is left to fill in with granulation tissue. Examples include dehisced surgical wounds and many chronic wounds such as pressure ulcers, leg ulcers, and diabetic ulcers. Infected surgical wounds are often left open to allow for drainage and prevent deep infection. Compared with primarily closed wounds, wounds that heal by secondary intention require much more granulation tissue to be deposited to fill the wound space. Wound contraction is a significant mechanism for healing and considerable epithelial cell migration is required to resurface the wound. The result is a much longer healing time with a larger scar and more deformity.

Third intention healing, also known as delayed primary healing, is a closure technique that is used for wounds with a high potential for infection. Surgical wounds may be considered clean-contaminated or contaminated as a result of breaks in surgical technique or the entering of nonsterile body cavities. To prevent postoperative wound infections, many surgeons elect not to close the incision at the time of surgery. Instead, wound edges are held open with gauze or other packing material. After several days (usually 3 to 5), when edema and drainage diminish and infection is less likely, the wound is closed primarily.

Prolonged healing produces a chronic wound. Usually one or more impairments to tissue repair exist when a chronic wound is present. Common impairments include malnutrition, poor tissue oxygenation, wound infection, and chronic disease. Iatrogenic causes, such as steroids or cytotoxic agents, can also delay healing.[8] Assessment for these factors and finding ways to optimize the local wound environment are important tasks in the ongoing evaluation of the wound healing process.

Taking into consideration the type of wound closure and the existing impairments to tissue repair, the challenge for the clinician is to identify treatment protocols and dressing materials that will optimize the wound healing process, be readily available and user-friendly for the patient and caregiver, and minimize complications. If the patient is an inpatient, different options may be available than in an outpatient setting, where caregiver and reimbursement constraints may significantly impact treatment choices. A systematic approach to wound dressing selection can be extremely efficacious. When choosing a category of dressing, begin by considering the type of wound and the wound closure technique.

DRESSINGS FOR WOUNDS CLOSED BY PRIMARY INTENTION

The functions of dressings that are placed over sutures, staples, or adhesive skin closures include: protection from additional trauma with movement or friction, prevention of exogenous microbial con-

tamination, and partial immobilization of the wound site. Many clinicians choose to use all three layers of sterile cotton-gauze material for wound coverage in the immediate postoperative period.[9,10] Blood and serous drainage tends to ooze from incision lines during the first 24 hours after surgery. If left at the wound site, these fluids provide an excellent medium for bacterial proliferation and can potentiate low-grade infection in the form of stitch abscesses. Therefore, surgical wounds should be dressed with an absorbent dressing such as gauze. This type of surgical dressing is usually left in place for a minimum of 48 hours which, in healthy patients, is sufficient time for epidermal resurfacing to occur and the barrier function of the skin to be restored.[10] If blood or wound drainage saturates the gauze layer and seeps through the outer layer, a phenomenon known as "strike-through," the dressing should be changed immediately. A moist outer layer destroys the barrier capacity of the dressing, permitting microbes from the environment to enter and migrate rapidly to the unhealed wound surface and increasing the risk of wound infection.

If strike-through is observed on the dressing of a primarily closed wound, the clinician should immediately reinforce the dressing with additional absorbent cotton pads and notify the nurse or surgeon. If the surgeon requests that the dressing be changed, the old dressing can be removed and a new dressing applied using a sterile or no-touch dressing technique.[11] Moist dressings should be removed down to the contact layer, leaving the contact layer in place whenever possible. Dry sterile gauze sponges and absorbent cotton pads can then be applied and the dressing edges sealed securely with tape or surgical netting. This provides additional support against mechanical stresses. A dressing change is also indicated if a dressing becomes moist or contaminated from exogenous sources such as urine, feces, or other body fluids.

After 48 hours, dressing change frequency for primarily closed wounds is dictated by the condition of the wound, the patient, and by clinician preference. If the skin edges are well approximated and the suture line is dry, the incision may be left open to air. If, on the other hand, the patient is immunocompromised, incontinent, or at high risk for wound infection or dehiscence, continuing the dressing would be reasonably prudent practice.

Daily dressing changes, using a sterile or no-touch technique, may be needed for an extended period of time (even after staples, sutures, or adhesive skin closures are removed) to prevent friction damage or maceration. Continuous and careful assessment of the wound should be made for signs of clinical infection—edema, erythema, exudate, local tenderness—each time the dressing is changed. If any crusting or dried exudate around the sutures or staples is observed, this should be gently removed with a cotton-tipped swab moistened with sterile saline or 3% hydrogen peroxide. If an antimicrobial ointment or cream is prescribed, it should be applied in a very thin layer to both the incision and the suture sites to minimize maceration of the tissue.

Occlusive or semi-occlusive synthetic dressings can be used in lieu of gauze for the dressing of primarily closed wounds. In vitro studies have demonstrated that epidermal resurfacing is up to 40% faster under occlusive dressings than under conventional gauze dressings.[12,13] Furthermore, decreased inflammation and pain, as well as improved cosmetic outcomes, have been reported when occlusive dressings are utilized.[14-16] The effect of a decreased inflammatory response on the strength of scar tissue over time has not been well researched with respect to occlusion. Additionally, the potential for increased bacterial infection under occlusion is another controversial issue, particularly if patients are immunocompromised.[17,18] Metaanalysis of occlusive dressings indicates that wound infection rates are higher with conventional gauze dressings than with occlusive dressings.[19] Until there are further studies to support the use of occlusive dressings for the treatment of large surgical wounds, they should be used with caution, especially in patients who are at high-risk for infection.

DRESSINGS FOR WOUNDS HEALING BY SECONDARY INTENTION

Open wounds exhibit observable changes as they progress through the three phases of the wound healing process: inflammatory phase, fibroblastic phase, and remodeling phase (see Chapter 1). Regardless of the etiology of the wound, its appearance can help guide the clinician in selecting a treatment plan that will optimize healing. Generally, four factors will guide dressing selection: the color of the wound, the amount of drainage, the wound depth, and the condition of the surrounding skin.

Wound Color

In wounds healing by secondary intention, wound color is often a reflection of the balance between new tissue and necrotic tissue. Healing chronic wounds with minimal to no necrotic tissue appear red or pink, because the wound space is filled with granulation tissue and new epithelium. In contrast, wounds with soft devitalized tissue or fibrous exudate often appear yellow or cream-colored, and may be complicated by infection. Finally, tissue necrosis causes denaturation and increased collagen fibers in the wounded area. The result is the formation of a thick, leathery eschar in the wound space that is black, brown, or tan in color. Wound color complements other assessments of wound condition and can also guide treatment selection.

Red Wounds

Examples of red wounds include donor sites, clean granulating or dehisced wounds, and chronic wounds immediately following thorough sharp debridement. The goal of red wound management is to provide a moist wound environment that minimizes damage to newly forming tissue. Red wounds should be gently cleansed with an isotonic solution to remove any exudate or adherent debris from the wound surface. Except in the case of deep tunneling soft tissue cavities that collect drainage, hydrotherapy is rarely indicated for cleansing of red wounds. In fact, the mechanical action of the agitators can cause tissue trauma if cleansing is too vigorous. Likewise, rubbing the wound surface with gauze should be avoided, because this may injure fragile cells. Once cleansing is complete, select a dressing material that will keep the wound moist and not adhere to the newly forming granulation tissue or epithelium. Ideal dressings for red wounds include non-adherent and impregnated gauzes, transparent films, hydrocolloids, and hydrogels. Wet-to-dry gauze dressings in red wounds should be avoided because of the potential for tissue trauma when they are removed. Bleeding during cleansing or when a dressing is removed is an indication that cell injury has occurred and that healing tissue is being disrupted.

If a wound has recently been excised or incised, initially the surface may appear more yellow than red due to exposed subcutaneous fat. Close inspection may reveal tiny capillaries that will eventually cover the wound surface with new vascular tissue through the process of angiogenesis. The absence of devitalized tissue in a red wound does not preclude the occurrence of wound infection.

Yellow Wounds

Yellow wounds containing soft devitalized tissue (slough) or fibrous exudate provide an optimal environment for rapid bacterial growth. Whether or not the wound becomes infected depends on several factors including wound size, local tissue perfusion, and the immune status of the patient. Consequently, whether local or systemic signs of infection are present will influence the selection of the dressing. If the yellow wound displays no signs of infection, the cleansing and dressing procedures should be aimed at actively removing exudate and debris. Hydrotherapy is an excellent choice for the mechanical cleansing of yellow wounds. If hydrotherapy is contraindicated or unavailable, a 35 cc syringe with an 18 gauge venous access catheter (angiocath) and an isotonic saline solution can be used to thoroughly irrigate the wound surface. This provides a safe pressure of approximately 15 psi at the wound surface.[5] Any undermined areas at the wound margins or any sinus tracts or pockets should be cleansed thoroughly.

A dressing technique should be selected that debrides soft necrotic tissue and actively absorbs exudate. For example, a wet-to-damp saline gauze dressing can be used to non-selectively debride necrotic tissue. An occlusive/adhesive dressing (such as a transparent film, hydrocolloid, or hydrogel) can be used to promote autolysis of the necrotic tissue.[7] In autolysis, the occlusive environment promotes the action of naturally occurring cellular enzymes that act to liquefy the avascular tissue and increase wound drainage. Exudate absorbers, such as copolymer starches, foams, or alginates, can be used if exudate is copious. Use of enzymatic debriding agents as an alternative therapy may be useful only if the yellow tissue is thick and relatively dry.

For clinically infected yellow wounds, use of an aggressive cleansing procedure similar to that described above is indicated. However, irrigation of the wound with a noncytotoxic antimicrobial solution is sometimes preferred over saline.[5] Systemic antibiotics and use of a topical antimicrobial agent should be considered until the infection is under control, especially if the patient is immunocompromised. Occlusive dressings should be used only with extreme caution if the wound is infected, since an occlusive environment may exacerbate infection.

Black Wounds

Black wounds are frequently encountered by clinicians, especially those in outpatient and long-term care settings with a large chronic wound population. Examples of black wounds that are commonly seen include full-thickness leg and foot ulcers, Stages III and IV pressure ulcers, gangrene, and deep burns. Occasionally, traumatic wounds contain significant amounts of black necrotic tissue, also known as eschar. The necrotic tissue provides an excellent medium for bacterial growth and proliferation and prolongs the inflammatory phase of the healing process. Additionally, eschar provides a physical obstacle to tissue repair by interfering with wound contraction and epidermal migration. For these reasons, the goal of treatment for black wounds is usually to remove the devitalized tissue as quickly as possible. In selected patients where tissue perfusion is compromised or immunosuppression significant enough to prevent aggressive intervention, a decision may be made to manage the wound conservatively. In such cases, the eschar is left intact, kept dry, and monitored carefully.

Sharp/surgical debridement is one method of selectively debriding black tissue. It is an effective and efficient intervention, especially in large infected wounds with associated bacteremia. Large wounds usually require surgical or laser debridement in a surgicenter, a specially equipped treatment room, or an operating room. However, surgical or laser debridement may be contraindicated for patients with coagulopathies and immunosuppression. If the amount of necrotic tissue is limited, debridement can be performed by a trained professional with minimal blood loss or pain to the patient.

Alternative methods for treating black wounds are often selected when sharp debridement is contraindicated, or when no one is available to perform the procedure. These methods include enzymatic, autolytic, and mechanical forms of debridement. Most enzymatic debriding agents are selective, but are labor intensive and only minimally effective in deep wounds with subcutaneous tissue involvement.[20] Autolysis of eschar can be accomplished with the use of occlusive or moisture-retentive dressings. These dressings promote softening and melt-out of the eschar by stimulating local bacterial proliferation, enzymatic activity, and lysis of collagen, an extremely selective process.[17,21,22] As with yellow wounds, autolysis should be used with caution in infected wounds and in immunosuppressed patients.

Most wounds in the "real world" are not, of course, uniform in color. Wound healing is a complex and dynamic process, and wounds usually present as a combination of colors depending on the amounts of necrotic tissue at different depths of injury, the existing systemic and local impairments to healing, and current and past therapies. When using color to guide interventions, the treatment should be selected that will address the most severe situation first: black before yellow before red. For example, the goal of treatment for a granulating leg ulcer with yellow debris is to remove the debris while protecting any exposed granulation tissue. Therefore, the correct

intervention is to select a dressing that actively removes debris without adhering to healthy, healing tissue.

DRAINAGE, DEPTH, AND SURROUNDING SKIN

When selecting a dressing, it is also important to consider the viscosity and amount of wound drainage, wound depth, and the condition of the surrounding skin. For example, watery wound drainage is easily wicked away from the wound surface by the gauzes, alginates, or exudate absorbers, while viscous drainage is not. Copious amounts of liquid drainage can also be managed using wound pouches. It is important to manage excess drainage because too moist an environment can cause maceration of the wound margins, promote bacterial and yeast colonization, and impair wound healing. Likewise, too dry an environment can lead to desiccation of granulation tissue and a deeper wound. Ideally, a dressing material should be selected that maintains a slightly moist wound environment.[23]

While superficial wounds can be easily managed with films, foams, or hydrocolloids, wounds with cavities need "fillers." Fillers remain in contact with the wound surface, obliterating dead space where drainage tends to pool, thus contributing to abscess formation. Filler dressings include gauze, packing foams, alginates, and exudate absorbers (starches, pastes, beads, and powders).

Finally, the skin needs to be inspected around the wound for intactness and fragility. Repeated dressing changes should be avoided with adhesive materials that can strip the epidermis or can cause skin tears, especially in the very young and the elderly. If the skin is at risk for breakdown or is already broken, use of adhesive materials should be avoided or discontinued and non-adhesive/non-adherent dressing materials should be chosen whenever possible.[24] If taping is unavoidable, tape with a non-aggressive adhesive. A transparent film dressing, elastic netting, or Montgomery straps may also be used to secure the dressing. In addition, protecting intact, peri-wound skin with a skin sealant before applying an adhesive dressing or tape will help minimize adhesive stripping. When adhesive stripping is unavoidable, hydrocolloid or gelatin-pectin wafers can be cut into strips and used to "window-pane" a wound, providing an alternative surface for anchoring the dressing.

Familiarity with the numerous types of dressing materials available today increases the chances for selecting the optimal dressing for a particular wound (see Table 9-1). Knowing the performance criteria for each dressing type, as outlined by Turner,[23] can help to maximize use of dressing materials (Table 9-2). Matching the appropriate dressing to the patient, wound, and setting requires critical thinking. Awareness of currently accepted standards for wound care is important. Clinicians are encouraged to base their wound care practices on the principles embodied in the AHCPR *Clinical Practice Guidelines* on pressure ulcers.[25,26]

CONCLUSION

Selecting wound dressings is challenging because of advances in available dressing options and the dynamic status of each wound. Proper dressing selection requires accurate wound assessment and careful identification of the stage of healing. Repeated assessment of wound progress and timely changes in the dressing regimen are essential. Because of the many factors that can impair wound healing, a multidisciplinary, holistic approach to patient care is required. A systematic method for wound assessment, like the one presented here, allows the clinician to consider appropriate interventions and help minimize the complications associated with open wounds.

REFERENCES

1. Cuzzell J. The new RYB color code. *Am J Nurs.* 1988;10:1342-1346.

Table 9-2. Performance Criteria for Wound Management Products

To remove excess exudate and toxic components
To maintain a high humidity at wound/dressing interface
To allow gaseous exchange
To provide thermal insulation
To afford protection from secondary infection
To be free from particulate or toxic contaminants
To allow removal without trauma at dressing change

Adapted with permission from Turner.[23]

2. Stotts NA. Seeing red and yellow and black: the three color concept of wound care. *Nursing 90.* 1990;2:59-61.
3. Moriarty MB. How color can clarify wound care. *RN.* 1988;51(9):49-54.
4. Krasner D. Resolving the dressing dilemma: selecting wound dressings by category. *Ostomy Wound Manage.* 1990;35:62-70.
5. Rodeheaver G. Controversies in topical wound management: wound cleansing and wound disinfection. In: Krasner D. *Chronic Wound Care: A Clinical Source Book for Healthcare Professionals.* King of Prussia, PA: Health Management Publications; 1990:282-289.
6. Cohen IK, Diegelmann RF, Linblad WJ. *Wound Healing: Biochemical and Clinical Aspects.* Philadelphia, PA: WB Saunders; 1992.
7. Alvarez O, Rozint J, Meehan M. Principles of moist wound healing: indications for chronic wounds. In: Krasner D. *Chronic Wound Care: A Clinical Source Book for Healthcare Professionals.* King of Prussia, PA: Health Management Publications; 1990:266-281.
8. Stotts N. Impaired wound healing. In: Carrieri-Kohlman V, Lindsey AM, West CM. *Pathophysiological Phenomena in Nursing.* 2nd ed. Philadelphia, PA: WB Saunders; 1993:443-469.
9. Peacock EE. *Wound Repair.* 3rd ed. Philadelphia, PA: WB Saunders; 1984.
10. Ponder RB, Krasner D. Gauzes and related dressings. *Ostomy Wound Manage.* 1993;39:48-60.
11. Krasner D, Kennedy KL. Using the no-touch technique for pressure ulcer dressing changes. *Nursing 94.* 1994;April.
12. Winter GD. Formation of the scab and the rate of epithelialization of superficial wounds in the skin of the young domestic pig. *Nature.* 1962;193:293-294.
13. Alvarez OM, Mertz DM, Eaglstein WH. The effect of occlusive dressings on collagen synthesis and reepithelialization in superficial wounds. *J Surg Res.* 1983;35:142-148.

14. Linsky CB, Rovee DT, Dow T. Effect of occlusive dressings on wound inflammation and scar tissue. In: Dineen P, Hildick-Smith G. *The Surgical Wound.* Philadelphia, PA: Lea & Febiger; 1981:191-206.

15. Eaglstein WH, Mertz PM, Falanga V. Occlusive dressings. *Am Fam Phys.* 1987;35:211-216.

16. Barnett A, Berkowitz RL, Mills R, Vistnes LM. Comparison of synthetic adhesive moisture vapor permeable and fine mesh gauze dressings for split thickness skin graft donor sites. *Am J Surg.* 1983;145:379-381.

17. Aly R, Shirley C, Cunico B, Maibach HI. Effect of prolonged occlusion on microbial flora, pH, carbon dioxide, and transepidermal water loss on human skin. *J Invest Dermatol.* 1978;71:378-381.

18. Shelanski MV, Nicholson SE, Shelanski JB, Constantine BE. The influence of moisture vapor transmission rates of polymer dressings on the rate of wound healing and bacterial proliferation on wound surfaces. *Wounds.* 1989;2:115-121.

19. Hutchinson JJ. Prevalence of wound infection under occlusive dressings: a collective survey of reported research. *Wounds.* 1989;2:123-133.

20. Silverstein P, Maxwell P, Duckett L. Enzymatic debridement. In: Boswick JA. *The Art and Science of Burn Care.* Rockville, MD: Aspen Publishers, Inc; 1987:75-81.

21. Mertz PM, Eaglstein WH. The effect of semi-occlusive dressings on the microbial population in superficial wounds. *Arch Surg.* 1984;119:287-289.

22. Katz S, McGinley K, Leyden LL. Semi-permeable occlusive dressings: effects on growth of pathogenic bacteria and reepithelialization of superficial wounds. *Arch Dermatol.* 1986;122:58-62.

23. Turner TD. The development of wound management products. In: Krasner D. *Chronic Wound Care: A Clinical Source Book for Healthcare Professionals.* King of Prussia, PA: Health Management Publications; 1990:31-46.

24. Doughty DB. Principles of wound healing and wound management. In: Bryant RA. *Acute and Chronic Wounds: Nursing Management.* St. Louis, MO: CV Mosby; 1992:31-68.

25. Panel for the Prediction and Prevention of Pressure Ulcers in Adults. *Pressure Ulcers in Adults: Prediction and Prevention. Clinical Practice Guideline, No. 3.* AHCPR Publication No. 92-0047. Rockville, MD: Agency for Health Care Policy and Research, Public Health Service, US Department of Health and Human Services, May 1992.

26. Bergstrom N, Bennett MA, Carlson CE, et al. *Treatment of Pressure Ulcers. Clinical Practice Guidelines, No. 14.* AHCPR Publication No. 95-0642. Rockville, MD: Agency for Health Care Policy and Research, Public Health Service, US Dept of Health and Human Services, December 1994.

Chapter 10

Total Contact Casting for Wound Management

David R. Sinacore, PhD, PT, and Michael J. Mueller, PhD, PT

Total contact casting (TCC) is an effective therapy for healing chronic neuropathic plantar ulcers in individuals with diabetes mellitus. The use of TCC and other pressure relieving methods[1] in the clinical management of neuropathic wounds has gained considerable acceptance over the past 30 years, largely through the seminal efforts of Brand and colleagues at the Gillis W. Long National Hansen's Disease Center in Carville, Louisiana. Brand has theorized that most plantar ulcers originate from a history of repetitive trauma in the presence of insensitivity of the feet (i.e., sensory neuropathy).[2]

Despite Brand's efforts, the use of TCC and its management principles have remained limited to few clinical settings in the United States. There are several reasons for the limited use of TCC. Foremost, there is a reluctance on the part of many medical practitioners to appreciate the role that sensory neuropathy plays in pathogenesis of diabetic foot ulcers. Secondly, even today, traditional medical opinion presumes that the majority of diabetic foot ulcers are due to vascular insufficiency, and are therefore not amenable to pressure-relieving or protective methods of management. Lastly, TCC was adapted from treatment of neuropathic ulcers in

Hansen's disease (leprosy) which originated in third-world, tropical countries. While its use may be widespread in other countries, the simple principles of TCC have not been readily adapted to other diseases where sensory neuropathy is prevalent as with diabetes mellitus, spina bifida, or chronic alcoholism.[3] Perhaps, the methods of TCC are not "high tech" enough for the practice of modern-day medicine in this country, or possibly the medical-legal risks associated with TCC in the diabetic patient are considered "too high" for the general medical practitioner. Whatever the reasons, TCC has not gained complete acceptance in the management of diabetic plantar ulcers in the United States. This is unfortunate, especially in light of the numerous favorable reports using TCC.[3-12]

The purpose of this chapter is to describe TCC in the management of neuropathic, plantar ulcers. Some of the criteria used to classify the ulcer are briefly described. The importance of classifying ulcers is emphasized since only neuropathic ulcers are appropriate for treatment with TCC or other pressure-relieving methods.[13] The most common pathways leading to ulcer generation are briefly described, including the theories supporting the effectiveness of the casting method. The application of the cast is described including necessary wound debridement and dressings inside the cast. Finally, the effectiveness of TCC, as demonstrated by clinical studies is discussed, as are factors which may complicate its clinical usefulness. Future research questions are posed concerning the use of TCC to aid in the prevention of subsequent ulceration, infection, and amputation.

CLASSIFICATION OF ULCERS

We, among others,[14-17] have found it useful to classify ulcers by the predominating factor of its suspected etiology. Ulcers in the individual with diabetes mellitus can be classified as predominantly vascular or neuropathic. In some cases there may be signs and symptoms of both types of ulcers; these ulcers can be classified as mixed.

The classification of wounds into vascular or neuropathic is not strict or absolute, nor is it based on a single test or criterion. Rather, the classification of wounds is based on several factors including: the wound's appearance, the typical location/site of occurrence, symptoms of pain associated with the wound, and the results of other special tests such as Doppler pressures, ankle/arm indices, and arteriography (Table 10-1). At times, the results of these special tests are either not available or were not performed prior to the initial visit. When this occurs, a careful medical history followed by a thorough physical examination should be used to classify wounds in order to decide which treatment approach is most beneficial.

Classifying wounds helps the clinician select the appropriate therapeutic strategies which address the primary, underlying etiology. Typically, there is no single etiology, but a predominant factor, which if identified, should maximize therapeutic intervention. In all wounds, it may be necessary to delay therapeutic interventions in order to ascertain whether an underlying infection is present. The clinician must always be mindful of the possibility of an underlying infection in the diabetic foot. If uncertain, it may be wise to delay

intervention just long enough to rule out the presence of underlying infection by various clinical methods such as cultures, x-rays, leukocyte scans, or bone biopsies.[18]

In some cases where no predominant etiology is obvious, and no infection is present, it may be prudent to institute a therapeutic intervention, then closely monitor the ulcer for evidence of healing (i.e., progression through the stages of wound repair described in Chapter 1) or development of complications. If the ulcer is not progressing through the stages of wound repair as anticipated, or develops acute complications which could delay wound healing or threaten the limb, the therapy should be altered immediately.

ULCERS WITH PREDOMINANTLY NEUROPATHIC ETIOLOGY

Neuropathic ulcers are most common on the plantar surfaces of the feet. In general, neuropathic ulcers demonstrate signs and symptoms which are distinct from a vascular etiology. Neuropathic ulcers are typically round or ovoid in appearance (Figure 10-1). They most often occur in the presence of warm feet with readily palpable pulses.[4] Local signs of inflammation in the surrounding tissues are almost always present, including redness, swelling, and elevated local skin temperatures. The hallmark of these ulcers is markedly diminished or absent pain sensation. Typically neuropathic ulcers are surrounded by rims of callus buildup which is indicative of the excessive plantar pressures. With local tissue debridement, these ulcers readily bleed. The most common sites of ulceration are the metatarsal heads,[1,3] though the precise location of the ulcer correlates with the foot type, presence of foot deformity, and location of excessive pressure.[19] Neuropathic, plantar ulcers have been called diabetic ulcers, mal perforans ulcers, or pedal ulcers. Although these names are all descriptive, they fail to capture the underlying causative agent, namely the sensory neuropathy which results in the loss of protective sensation. In a foot with diminished or absent sensation of pain, even minor repetitive trauma can lead to tissue damage resulting in ulceration.[20]

Table 10-1. Summary of Signs, Symptoms, and Special Tests Used to Determine the Predominant Etiology of Arterial, Venous, and Neuropathic Ulcers

Primary Etiology	Signs	Symptoms	Special Tests
Arterial Ulceration	Often located on toes, interdigital spaces, or malleoli	Pain at wound site	Ankle/arm index <0.70
	Minimal granulation tissue, border of wound is rough	Increased pain with ambulation	Positive arteriogram
	Diminished or absent peripheral pulses	Decreased pain with rest	
Venous Ulceration	Located on leg, proximal to medial malleolus	Usually minimal pain	Usually none required
	Leg often edematous		May perform Doppler ultrasound
	Edges of wound slope to a central crater		
	Thick, dark, hard skin around wound		
Neuropathic Ulceration	Usually on plantar surface of foot beneath metatarsal heads	Lack of pain/temperature sensation	Ankle/arm index ⩾1.0
	Punched out appearance	Debridement is painless, bleeds easily	Unable to sense 5.07 Semmes-Weinstein monofilament
	Rim of callus surrounds entire or portion of ulcer		Diminished NCV or vibratory sense
	Usually good peripheral pulses		
	Usually good granulation tissue		

Adapted from Mueller MJ. Wound care in the elderly patient with diabetes. In: Protas EJ, ed. *Twenty-First Century Healing: Twenty-First Century Geriatric Care.* Professional Health Educators, Inc: 1993.

ULCERS WITH MIXED ETIOLOGY

Macrovascular disease and neuropathy (i.e., sensory, motor, and autonomic) characterize the diabetic foot, therefore, circulatory impairments often accompany impaired or absent protective sensation. In fact, Pecoraro and associates[21] identified 55% of the diabetic subjects who had cutaneous ulceration which eventually resulted in a major lower extremity amputation, had evidence of significantly impaired arterial circulation and sensory neuropathy. As a rule, neuropathic ulcers, which are accompanied by severe compromise of the vascular supply to the foot, do not heal as quickly or as readily. Failure of ulcer healing in an ischemic foot carries a poor prognosis. Defective ulcer healing appears to be a major factor contributing to limb loss.[22]

ASSESSMENT

ASSESSMENT OF INSENSITIVITY OF THE FEET

As part of the ulcer assessment, the clinician should thoroughly explore the causes of the ulcers. Often patients will be unaware and unable to recall any single precipitating event. Typically, patients will report the development of a minor blister or reddening of the skin which later devel-

Figure 10-1. Typical neuropathic ulcer on the plantar surface of the foot in an individuals with long standing type II diabetes mellitus.

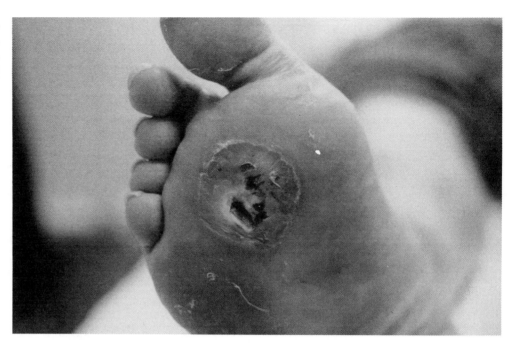

ops into a large ulcer. Such a history should alert the clinician to the prospect of diminished sensation and a neuropathic component. The confirmation and assessment of sensory neuropathy can be accomplished by any number of ways. Some of the more commonly recommended methods include vibration assessment or temperature assessment.[1] We[3] and others[23,24] use a series of Semmes-Weinstein monofilament probes at multiple sites on the plantar and dorsal surfaces of the feet to assess light pressure (touch). The Semmes-Weinstein monofilament probes have been shown to be an easily administered, reliable method to discriminate between groups of patients at risk for ulceration.[23] The inability to sense the 5.07 monofilament probe at the majority of preselected sites on the foot indicates a decrease in "protective sensation" and the presence of a significant sensory neuropathy. Based on his clinical experience, Levin[16] suggests the severity of the neuropathy progresses stereotypically in the chronic diabetic, initially losing vibratory sensation, then deep tendon reflexes, and finally, protective sensation of light touch or pressure. Such stereotypical signs may be used to judge the severity and progression of the diabetic neuropathy.

DURATION OF ULCER PRESENCE

In most cases, neuropathic ulcers have been present (open) for several weeks or months. In large part, this may be due to neglect, since the ulcer may go unnoticed for variable periods of time. Often, patients unsuccessfully attempt to manage their own foot ulcers using home dressings or healing agents. The longer the ulcer is present, the greater the possibility of an underlying infection. Ambulating on an open wound can cause an otherwise localized infection to spread into surrounding tissues, leading to cellulitis, osteomyelitis, or widespread sepsis.[25] By the time patients seek medical attention for their nonhealing foot ulcers, the possibility of a severe, deep infection is quite high.[26,27]

ULCER ASSESSMENT

Any excessive callus buildup is indicative of high pressures on the plantar aspect of the foot. Callus buildup must be evaluated for the presence of an underlying ulcer. Excessive callus buildup should be trimmed or pared down and probed for a potentially ulcerated area below. It is not unusual to find evidence of a blister with coagulated blood beneath a plantar callus.

Every ulcer must be thoroughly evaluated for

any evidence of sinuses or penetrating tracks. If the ulcer is deeper than it is wide, the ulcer must be opened so that the width is equal to its depth to ensure adequate drainage and healing of the wound's inner layers and prevent premature superficial healing. The ulcer should be cleaned and all necrotic tissue debrided. The surrounding callus should be trimmed to reduce pressure at the margins of the ulcer (see Chapter 8 for more information).

The ulcer size and depth are measured by a millimeter ruler or depth gauge. The perimeter of the ulcer (size) also may be traced onto sterile clear acetate (exposed x-ray film) using an indelible ink marker. Alternatively, the clinician can quantitate the wound size by estimating the circumference using a wound grid. This tracing should later be placed in the patient's record for subsequent comparison measurements. The depth of the ulcer can be measured using a depth gauge inserted at the deepest part of the wound to the ulcer surface. These are reliable and useful methods of quantifying the size and depth of the ulcer[28] because they give the patient visual feedback regarding the effectiveness of therapeutic intervention. This method is also helpful in convincing the reluctant patient to continue with a given therapeutic intervention if healing is slow.

ASSESSMENT FOR PRESENCE OF AN ACTIVE INFECTION

The presence of an active, deep infection is a serious complication in the diabetic foot.[25] If an active infection is present, TCC should not be used. While the depth of the ulcer is not a strict contraindication to using TCC in general, the deeper the ulcer involving tendons or ligaments being exposed, the greater the likelihood of infection. In one recent study, osteomyelitis was present in the majority of ulcers involving deep structures such as bone, tendon, or joint capsule.[27]

If an active infection is suspected, it is wise to delay TCC. A period of strict immobilization by complete bedrest along with antibiotic therapy may often be required prior to instituting TCC. Some

vascular surgeons advocate aggressive, surgical wound debridement and revascularization to promote wound healing depending on the status of the circulation.[26] Once the acute infection has subsided, a carefully molded TCC may be applied.

MECHANISM OF NEUROPATHIC ULCER GENERATION

Mechanical factors appear to play a significant role in the etiology of neuropathic ulcers. The primary mechanical factors which contribute to skin breakdown appear to be magnitude of force, duration of force, and repetition of force. Force on a biological tissue is measured according to its area of application, namely the resultant pressure. Clinically, the three attributes of force or pressure can combine to contribute to skin breakdown by three different scenarios:

(1) low pressures exerted for long durations resulting in tissue ischemia
(2) high pressures for short durations resulting in acute trauma and skin breakdown
(3) repeated bouts of moderate pressure resulting in injury similar to cumulative trauma[20,29]

Low pressures for extended periods of time can cause ischemia and skin breakdown. In his classic experiment, Kosiak[30] applied varying amounts of pressure for varying amounts of time to the anesthetized skin of dogs. He found an inverse time-pressure relationship. Microscopic pathological changes were noted in tissues subjected to as little as 60 mmHg (8 KPa or 1.16 psi) for only 1 hour. Ulceration occurred with pressures as low as 20 KPa (2.9 psi) for times of approximately 11 hours. Ulceration did not typically occur until 3 days after the application of pressure. This type of ulceration can occur in patients with insensitivity who develop ulcers after wearing tight shoes or positioning their heels on a bed for many hours. Figure 10-2 depicts two heel ulcers which occurred in a 49-year-old male with chronic, type II diabetes mellitus after wearing a new pair of shoes for several hours. This individual had the complete loss of "protective

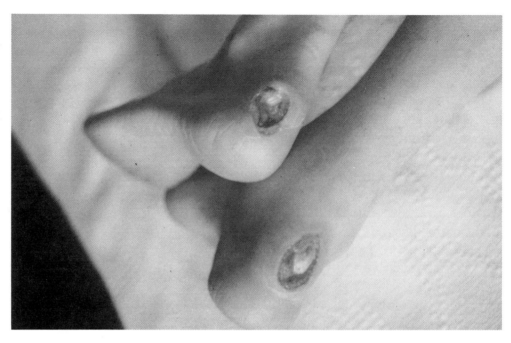

Figure 10-2. Bilateral neuropathic ulcers in a 49-year-old male with 10-year history of type II diabetes mellitus. He has lost protective sensation and unknowingly developed severe heel ulcers after wearing a new pair of shoes for several hours.

sensation" due to sensory neuropathy. In general, appropriate treatment for these patients must include thorough education regarding their sensory neuropathy, in addition to obtaining proper protective footwear and instruction in proper positioning programs.

The second mechanism of injury is high pressure for a short duration. The ultimate tensile strength of skin on the sole of the foot is approximately 0.95 kg/mm². [31] This means that a single bout of trauma would require 0.95 kg/mm² or 1300 pounds per square inch (8.97 megapascal) of pressure to cause a break in the skin. Such injuries could occur only if large amounts of force are concentrated over a small area. Such a situation would arise if a person stepped on a tack or a sharp piece of glass. We have had many patients with plantar wounds who were unaware that they stepped on a nail or tack. This type of injury is best prevented by the constant use of protective footwear that is inspected before wearing.

Brand was the first to postulate that plantar wounds on the insensitive feet of patients with diabetes mellitus or Hansen's disease can be caused by repeated bouts of moderate pressure (in the range of 20 to 70 psi). [29] As supporting evidence, he anesthetized the footpads of rats and subjected

them to 10,000 repetitions of 20 psi/day for several days. Although a single bout at 20 psi will not even cause discomfort, 10,000 repetitions/day caused noticeable inflammation after 3 days and skin breakdown in 7 days. [20]

This mechanism of injury appears to be responsible for the common metatarsal head ulcer seen in the diabetic. High peak pressures under prominent metatarsal heads are repeated hundreds of times a day during the course of a patient's normal ambulation. Limited joint mobility in the feet of patients with diabetes appears to further contribute to high plantar pressures. [32,33] This high pressure would cause pain in a foot with intact sensation, but patients with peripheral neuropathy continue to ambulate until a wound develops. Our experience indicates these wounds respond favorably to TCC. [3,9]

THEORY SUPPORTING EFFECTIVENESS OF TCC

There are several characteristics of TCC which may allow neuropathic wounds to heal. The primary mechanism is thought to be that the total contact cast significantly increases the surface area for weight-bearing forces, thereby reducing peak pressures at the ulcer site. Rather than bearing most of the forces at the prominent metatarsal heads, the total contact nature of the cast allows the entire longitudinal arch and portions of the calf to bear weight. In one study, pressures were reduced 84% at the third metatarsal head and 75% at the first metatarsal head when subjects walked in a total contact cast compared to regular shoes.[34] The reduction of peak pressures by an increase in weight-bearing surface area is thought to contribute to wound healing.

A secondary benefit of TCC is that it seems to reduce edema in the casted region. Although there is limited data to support this contention, we observe that most casts become loose within the first week after initial application. The loosening of the cast appears to be due to a reduction in edema or a redistribution of tissue fluids. Unless significant edema remains, subsequent casts typically remain snug. The TCC provides a rigid protection against increasing edema and some investigators have speculated that along with the plantar flexor muscles, casting acts like a pump to reduce edema actively.[35] Another benefit of TCC is that it helps prevent and localize infection to the tissues surrounding the ulcer. In our controlled clinical trial, none of the patients receiving TCC developed a deep infection while 26% of the patients using traditional footwear and daily dressing changes required hospitalization.[9] TCC not only appears to protect the wound from outside contaminants, but helps prevent the spread of local infection.

A related characteristic of the TCC that may contribute to healing is that it immobilizes the foot, ankle, and injured tissues. Immobilization may help to protect the tissues, reduce trauma, and allow the body to mount an effective response of healing. Finally, the TCC may be beneficial to wound healing because it interferes with the patient's mobility. Although decreased ability to walk may be viewed as a disadvantage of casting, decreased ambulation results in decreased forces on the plantar foot and appears to contribute to healing. Patients typically are unable to walk as readily as they did prior to casting. We instruct patients to reduce their walking and weight-bearing activities to one third their usual daily amount. In addition to being somewhat awkward, the TCC acts as an effective reminder to reduce ambulation. From a mobility perspective, TCC may be considered a compromise between bed rest and unrestricted ambulation.

TOTAL CONTACT CAST APPLICATION

WOUND CARE PRIOR TO CASTING

As a rule, no special dressings or antibiotic ointments are needed to promote ulcer healing. We routinely apply a thin dressing in order to collect any drainage from the ulcer throughout the casting period. We apply a small, thin, wet-to-dry dressing using saline-soaked, fine mesh gauze placed over the ulcer, then cover with a dry, thin Telfa pad or gauze dressing. This dressing is secured with paper tape. It is important that any dressing be kept as thin and small as possible to avoid excessive pressures from the dressing on the ulcer inside the cast. If the ulcer is deep, a loosely packed, wide mesh gauze may be used to fill the ulcer to the surface, followed by a thin Telfa dressing. We have found some topical antiseptics can cause the ulcer bed to dry out prematurely and may delay some wound healing, therefore, it is unnecessary to apply a topical antiseptic on the ulcer.

It is common in diabetic patients with chronic plantar ulcers to have excessive edema at the foot and lower extremity. It may be necessary to elevate the edematous foot and leg before casting to reduce the swelling. Using a sequential compression pump for 30 to 60 minutes is effective in transiently reducing moderate to extensive foot and leg edema.

To apply a total contact walking cast, place the patient in the prone position with the ipsilateral knee and ankle flexed to 90 degrees (the plantar surface of the ulcerated foot should be parallel to the floor). This position prevents further edema, takes the stretch off the gastrocnemius muscle, and allows the extremity to be held up easily while the inner layers of the cast are forming, thus preventing dents or other high-pressure areas in the cast.

A small amount of cotton padding is placed loosely between adjacent toes to absorb any moisture and prevent maceration and rubbing of the toes. A 3- or 4-inch wide, closely fitting cotton stockinette is rolled over the foot and leg up to just below the knee. The toe end of the stockinette should be sewn closed or can be folded into the toe sulcus and taped closed. The stockinette is pulled tight so it is wrinkle free. Wrinkles, occurring at the dorsum of the ankle, are cut with the edges overlapped then taped with paper tape to prevent a seam (an area of high pressure) when applying the total contact layers of plaster.

Next, a layer of $1/2$-inch adhesive-backed foam (Sifoam) or felt is applied to cover and protect all the toes. This foam layer should be placed over the closed stockinette and extended dorsally from the metatarsophalangeal area around the toes to the toe sulcus on the plantar surface. The edges of the foam should be trimmed medially and laterally and beveled to minimize pressure. The toes in the total contact cast are enclosed in plaster to protect the insensitive foot and prevent damage to the toes from striking objects or from objects being lodged in the cast.

The leg should now be supported by an assistant and the foot and ankle held stable in the neutral position (90 degrees at the ankle), with the toes passively dorsiflexed only slightly. Many diabetic patients are unable to achieve the neutral or 90 degree position of the ankle joint secondary to joint or muscle limitations. Attempts to achieve this position passively may result in abnormal pronation and a prominent talus or navicular bone on the medial aspect of the foot. Bony prominences in the abnormally pronated foot may cause areas of high pressure in the cast, so excessive pressure to achieve the neutral position is not recommended. A small amount of equinus can easily be accommodated in the cast by building up the posterior portion of the sole of the cast with plaster to level the weight-bearing surface.

Next, two circular pieces (approximately 2 inches in diameter) of $1/4$-inch adhesive-backed felt are placed over the malleoli on the stockinette. The felt pieces should be beveled along the edges to reduce the pressure along the felt-to-plaster interface. Another felt pad, 18 to 20 inches long and 2 inches wide, is beveled along the edges and placed along the anterior aspect of the leg and dorsum of the foot from just below the tibial tuberosity distal to the metatarsal heads. This felt pad protects the prominent tibial crest and facilitates cast removal. Felt pads prevent the cast from rubbing on bony prominences. Occasionally, additional bony prominences such as the styloid process of the fifth metatarsal, achilles tendon insertion on to the calcaneus, or the talonavicular area may be padded, depending on the foot type. No other padding is generally required.

One to two layers of an extra fast-setting, creamy plaster bandage (Gypsona®II) are wrapped loosely around the lower leg and foot from the proximal to the distal direction. The plaster bandage should commence below the previously marked fibular head (approximately 1 to 1.5 inches below) and continue distally to beyond the metatarsal heads. Care must be taken to avoid any gaps in the plaster or wrinkles in the stockinette. The plaster bandage should be rolled quickly and without tension. The bandage is then rubbed continuously to conform to the shape of the foot and leg until it has firmly set. The plaster is molded and contoured around bony prominences and felt padding. Particular attention should be given to molding the plaster to the contours of the sole of the foot. This thin layer of plaster is the most critical part of the total contact cast. The patient should be instructed not to move the foot or leg during the application of these initial layers of plaster. After this "eggshell" layer has been applied, the assistant supporting the leg and foot should not move the foot or apply excessive pressure to the plaster, because this could distort or dent it and cause potential areas of high pressure. The inner layer should be allowed to set fully before any more plaster is applied.

Once the inner layer of plaster has set (approximately 4 to 5 minutes), additional layers should be added for reinforcement and strength. Plaster splints (five splints in thickness), approximately 30 inches long, are applied anteriorly to posteriorly from the dorsal surface of the toes around on the plantar aspect of the foot and up to the posterior aspect of the leg. A second set of splints is wrapped in a medial to lateral direction around the calcaneus and up the proximal side of the leg. These splints reinforce the plantar and posterior portions of the cast.

To complete the cast, a rubber walking heel is incorporated on the plantar surface of the cast. A 1/4-inch plywood board is used between the walking heel and the cast to minimize the danger of cracks in the sole of the cast from pressure on the heel. The 1/4-inch plywood board should be cut smaller than the length of the foot. It should extend from the heel to the toe sulcus and be slightly narrower than the foot's width. The area between the contoured sole of the foot and the board should be filled with a plaster roll to level the plantar surface.

The placement of the walking heel is critical. The walking heel is placed on the board just behind the midline of the foot. Placing the heel too far forward on the foot will cause the patient to have difficulty with balance and may cause excessive movement of the foot and leg in the cast. Placing the heel too far posteriorly will cause the patient to roll forward onto the toe of the cast and may contact the ground, breaking the toe region of the cast. The walking heel is attached to the cast, and the toes are fully enclosed by an additional one or two rolls of plaster. Every attempt should be made to keep the anterior portion of the cast thin to facilitate removal. We use a fiberglass tape to attach the heel and complete the outer layers. This material is lightweight, durable, quick setting, and water resistant. However, fiberglass roll is not molded as easily to the extremity. We recommend the use of this material, particularly with patients who may need to bear weight soon after application.

The completed cast should now be allowed to dry thoroughly (Figure 10-3). As an added precaution, the patient is instructed not to bear weight for at least 24 hours after application to allow the inner layers to harden. Before dismissing the patient, the cast should be checked for proper fit and the patient instructed in proper cast care and precautions.

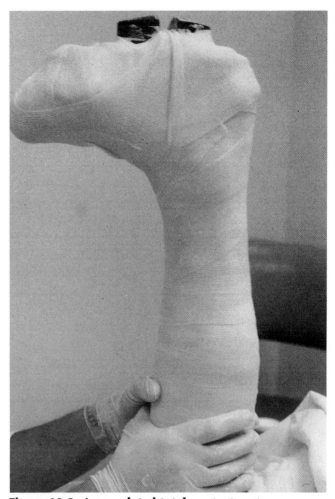

Figure 10-3. A completed total contact cast.

STUDIES SUPPORTING USE OF TCC

The effectiveness of TCC has been documented in several clinical reports over the past decade.[3-12] A review of 259 neuropathic ulcers in 235 subjects with diabetes mellitus demonstrates that 73% to 100% of the ulcers healed (Table 10-2). Healing times have consistently averaged 37 to 44 days from the initial date of casting. The healing times are quite remarkable considering the average length of time the ulcers were present prior to TCC was nearly 7 months. It should be noted that these healing times do not differ markedly in non-diabetic individuals without evidence of peripheral vascular disease or severe ischemic changes.[36] It is generally believed that diabetics

Table 10-2. **Summary of Studies Using Total Contact Casting for Neuropathic Plantar Ulcers in Individuals With Diabetes Mellitus***

Study/Year	Number of Patients	Number of Ulcers	Number of Days Ulcer Present Prior to Casting	Healed (%)	Number of Days Until Ulcer Healed
Pollard et al, 1983	6	8	--	100	38
Helm et al, 1984	22	24	267	73	38
Boulton et al, 1986	7	8	224	100	43
Sinacore et al, 1987	30	33	438	82	44
Walker et al, 1987	51	55	303	--	37
Diamond et al, 1987	1	1	300	100	39
Nawoczenski et al, 1989	1	1	26	100	43
Mueller et al, 1989	21	21	155	90	42
Laing et al, 1992	36	43	507	77	44
Myerson et al, 1992	60	65	156	89	38

*Includes insulin-dependent (IDDM or type I) and non-insulin dependent (NIDDM or type II) diabetes mellitus

with ankle-arm indices less than or equal to 0.45 and distal lower extremity pressures less than 70 mmHg are unlikely to heal using TCC. We have found that some individuals with chronic diabetes, demonstrating evidence of severe peripheral vascular disease, are able to heal in a similar time using TCC.[3] Though healing rates were similar, clinicians should be aware that diabetics with evidence of vascular compromise may be prone to developing more severe types of complications as a result of casting. We[3] and others[7] have observed more severe complications in diabetics with average Doppler index below 0.61 (range 0.38 to 0.81).

COMPLICATING FACTORS IN THE USE OF TCC

TCC is not without its risks and complications. One study reported that as many as 43% of diabetic subjects who received TCC developed complications.[4] The most well-known complications are superficial abrasions and fungal infections. Abrasions can be caused by improper application of the cast, excessive movement of the foot or leg inside a loosely fitting cast, and damage to or breakage of the cast from moisture or trauma. Despite our warnings not to alter or tamper with the casts, we have had patients chisel windows in their casts, thereby causing underlying tissues to herniate through these windows resulting in severe abrasions in areas surrounding the windows. As a rule, abrasions occur over or around bony prominences in 27% of the patients treated by TCC.[3,37] Most often, these abrasions heal readily and do not delay subsequent cast applications or ulcer healing. In our experience, some patients treated by TCC develop local, fungal infections, usually on the digits. Diabetics appear to be susceptible to fungal foot infections more than non-diabetics.[18] The type of offending fungus varies, but typically they respond to broad-spectrum, topical, anti-fungal agents. In one study, we have observed 15% of the diabetic subjects treated by TCC develop fungal infections. Generally, these fungal infections were minor and did not prevent further casting.[9]

Clinicians, particularly physical therapists, may be concerned that 6 weeks or longer of TCC may cause immobilized foot and ankle joints to become stiff, resulting in additional limited joint mobility. Limited joint mobility caused by chronic diabetes may be exacerbated by TCC and contribute further to the high peak plantar pressures we are attempting to reduce. In a study by Diamond and associates[38] ankle and foot joint mobility did not significantly change after 6 weeks of TCC compared to the non-casted extremity, therefore, TCC does not place the foot with the recently healed ulcer at risk for further limited joint mobility.

Though minor complications occur with TCC, we believe the benefits far outweigh the complications reported. Most of the complications can be minimized with careful application and close patient follow-up at frequent intervals over a casting period. The skills required to learn the safe application of TCC is well worth the investment.

ULCER RECURRENCE

It has been estimated that 15% of all diabetics will develop at least one foot ulcer during their lifetime.[39] The natural history of single or recurrent foot ulcer development, over a number of years of having diabetes mellitus, is uncertain, but it appears to be quite high. Diabetic foot complications account for approximately 20% of all diabetic hospital admissions.[40] Most diabetics over the age of 65 require at least one hospitalization per year for

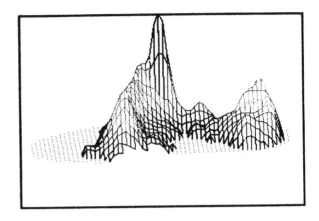

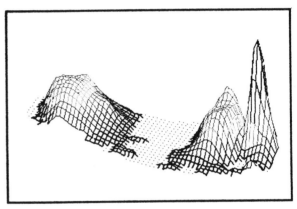

Figure 10-4. A three-dimensional F-scan tracing of the peak plantar surface pressures during the stance phase of gait in an individual with diabetes mellitus.

foot-related complications.[41]

Neuropathic plantar ulcers recur frequently. A few longitudinal studies of the recurrence rates indicate that re-ulceration within the first 6 months after initial healing are high, prompting some to consider healing successful only after 6 months of skin closure.[41,42] Using this criteria, Aplequist and associates[43] report an ulcer recurrence rate of 34%, 61%, and 70% after 1, 3, and 5 years, respectively during follow-up observation. Follow-up at 2 years after initial ulcer healing indicates the recurrence rates vary between 20% to 35%.[37,44] The recurrence rates for ulcers in subjects having sensory neuropathy with or without diabetes mellitus appears to be similar.[36]

Most ulcers recur within the first 6 months following initial ulcer healing, typically within the 3 or 4 weeks. As Brand has pointed out, this is a particularly vulnerable period for re-ulceration.[2] The recently healed ulcer is not fully mature and not yet able to withstand the vertical and shear stresses placed on it. Brand recommends extreme caution, with limited weight-bearing activities during this period, to allow complete wound consolidation and connective tissue remodeling.[2] The successful outcome using TCC, like other forms of therapeutic intervention, depends on the definition of healing. We have defined wound healing as the complete closure of the ulcer with intact skin (complete epithelialization), without evidence of drainage or sinus formation.[3,9] We routinely calculate the time it takes (in days) for the ulcer to completely heal from the time of initial casting. As indicated earlier, other investigators define successful wound healing for up to 6 months after initial ulcer closure.[42,43] This definition obscures the recidivism rates after initial healing as well as the risk of re-ulceration early after TCC removal. Two groups of investigators have observed ulcer recurrence rates between 35% and 57% within the first month after TCC.[37,44] In general, we have observed that reducing the recidivism rate largely depends on: the ability of definitive, prescriptive footwear to relieve excessive pressures on the plantar aspects of the feet; the patient's understanding of their sensory neuropathy and the role of excessive pressure on insensitive feet; and the patient's compliance with limiting weight-bearing activities for a period of 3 to 6 weeks following initial healing.

Immediately upon healing, we prescribe patients who have a loss of protective sensation with custom-made footwear. Generally, the custom-made footwear consists of extra-depth shoes with rigid, rocker-bottom soles and total contact plasti-zote inserts.[45] We closely monitor in-shoe plantar pressures using commercially-available, pressure sensing devices (F-scan®) (Figure 10-4). In addition, we instruct patients in a "wearing/break-in" schedule for their custom-made footwear over several days. We routinely require individuals to use assistive devices when ambulating for several weeks following initial ulcer healing. In addition, we have found that instructing patients with recently healed, forefoot ulcers to walk using a gait pattern, which discourages active push-off late in the stance phase

of gait and can further reduce peak plantar pressures in the forefoot.[46] We believe all of these factors are critical and can help protect against ulcer recurrence. Failure to achieve complete ulcer healing with TCC has been reported in several studies. Laing and associates[7] reported a failure rate of 22% in 36 diabetic patients treated by TCC, while Helm and associates[6] estimated 27% of the initial subjects casted failed to heal. We initially observed a failure rate of 18%,[3] and later, in a controlled follow-up study, we reported that 10% of the ulcers failed to heal.[9] The majority of reported failure rates include those patients who tried a therapeutic course of TCC, but refused subsequent casts despite evidence of ulcer healing.[3] When examining failure rates, it is necessary to distinguish those patients for whom TCC was an appropriate form of therapy and may have healed neuropathic ulcers from those patients who may have had underlying (vascular) pathology where TCC may not have been a suitable form of therapy. Some of the failure rates using TCC include individual subjects who did not heal due to undiagnosed deep tissue infection, while others include subjects who failed to comply with proper follow-up procedures. Thorough descriptions of the reasons for failure should be reported for the clinician to judge who is or is not a good candidate for TCC.

PREDICTING SUCCESSFUL OUTCOMES WITH TCC

Many clinicians are interested in predicting the likelihood of healing a foot ulcer. Historically, ankle/arm indices and Doppler arterial pressures in the tibial, pedal, and toe vessels have been used to predict a successful healing outcome.[16] Though used, ankle/arm indices and segmental Doppler pressures are notoriously poor predictors of both the ability to heal an ulcer and the level at which healing is likely when a limb-salvaging amputation is considered. Not surprising, ankle/arm indices and segmental Doppler pressures are generally poor prognostic indicators of successful outcome (i.e., complete healing) using TCC.[3] At present there is no published data that allow the clinician to judge when TCC will likely be successful in healing plantar ulcerations. More recently, the use of transcutaneous oxygen pressures (TcPO$_2$) have improved the prediction accuracy of wound closure and wound failure.[47] In general, peri-wound TcPO$_2$, less than 20 mmHg, were highly predictive of early wound healing failure. TcPO$_2$ measurements made adjacent to wound margins reflect local skin oxygenation and underscore the important role cutaneous circulation (as opposed to deep arterial circulation) has in predicting a successful healing outcome. Future research using peri-wound TcPO$_2$ tensions may help to predict not only the potential for ulcer healing using TCC, but perhaps also those individuals who may or may not be suitable for TCC.

WOUND HEALING FAILURE AND AMPUTATION

The consequences of failing to achieve complete wound healing can be dramatic. The amputation rate due to wound healing failure has been reported to vary from 17% to 44%.[48,49] In a review of 31 studies, the primary criteria for diabetic amputations were gangrene, infection, and nonhealing ulcers (65%).[50] Failure to recognize and manage the underlying sensory neuropathy may, in part, be responsible for the high amputation rates following unsuccessful wound healing (unpublished observations). Unfortunately, the survival rate of non-amputated, contralateral limbs of a diabetics is also poor. Less than 50% of the contralateral (non-amputated) limbs survive more than 5 years after one major amputation. Clearly, the threat of another subsequent major amputation is large, so the underlying sensory neuropathy must be addressed.

AUTONOMIC NEUROPATHY

The presence and severity of the autonomic neuropathy in the diabetic foot should never be underestimated. As Brand pointed out, based on his many years of practice and experience treating neuropathic ulcerations, he rarely knew "a foot which sweats normally to develop an ulcer."[29] Such astute observations underscore the importance of evaluating the presence of autonomic neuropathy.

In patients with chronic diabetes mellitus, it is rare that autonomic neuropathy would occur in the absence of clinically significant sensory or motor neuropathy. However, it is unknown to what extent autonomic neuropathy alone can either cause an ulcer or delay wound healing. A recent study by Gilmore and associates[51] demonstrated that multiple measures of peripheral autonomic neuropathy were worse in the feet of diabetics with a history of unilateral ulceration compared to the non-ulcerated (contralateral) foot. Furthermore, peripheral sympathetic neuropathy was more severe than what was found in feet of diabetics without a previous history of ulceration.[51] In the same study, Gilmore and associates suggest that peripheral autonomic neuropathy may be a major contributing factor to the development of diabetic foot ulcerations, and may help explain the occurrence of foot ulceration in some diabetics with intact circulation and minimal evidence of somatic neuropathy.[51]

With regards to TCC, the presence and severity of peripheral autonomic neuropathy may be partly responsible for the wound healing failures observed with this method. In general, the presence and increasing severity of peripheral autonomic neuropathy carries a poor prognosis, being associated with a significantly higher morbidity and mortality.[52] Future research should address the role peripheral autonomic (sympathetic) impairments may have in the generation and management of diabetic foot ulcerations.

ADVANTAGES/DISADVANTAGES OF TCC

TCC has the major advantage of being an extremely cost-effective therapy for healing chronic neuropathic ulcers. In general, applications of total contact casts cost very little when compared to in-hospital stays including daily wound care by a professional nursing staff. The actual direct costs for diabetic (neuropathic) foot ulcers in the United States is not known.[53] Smith and associates[41] performed a 2-year prospective study of 429 ambulatory patients with diabetes mellitus who were classified as either high, medium, or low risk for hospitalizations. They reported that 58% of the high-risk diabetics averaged 1.47 hospitalizations per patient over the 2 years and averaged 14.6 hospital days per patient compared to 8.6 days for medium-risk and 5.3 days for low-risk diabetics. We conservatively estimate the average hospital room costs for an in-hospital stay of 5.3 days to be $2,252. These estimates are conservative in that they do not reflect the costs of procedures, medications, or physician's costs. By contrast, we estimate the current outpatient costs of TCC, including six to eight cast changes and ulcer debridement over a typical 8-week duration, averages $810 to $1,050. These costs are far less than the costs associated with one annual stay in the hospital. It appears TCC is not only an extremely effective therapy but also an extremely cost-effective therapy for healing chronic neuropathic ulcers.

A major advantage of TCC is that it allows the patient to remain ambulatory throughout the healing period. Though TCC allows individuals to maintain an ambulatory status, we require the use of assistive devices such as canes, crutches, or walkers to reduce plantar pressures and restrict individuals' walking velocities. The patients, in addition to remaining ambulatory, are often able to maintain their employment status, so no loss of wages (indirect costs) is incurred. Another advantage of TCC is that it requires very little participation by the patient or family members to perform daily wound care. This makes it an ideal therapy for patients unable to participate in their own wound care.

The major disadvantages of TCC are the difficulties reported by patients such as clumsiness and awkwardness. Most individuals have difficulty with ambulation, reporting unsteadiness and instability. Like traditional plaster casts, most people complain of general discomforts while sleeping and difficulty with activities of daily living such as bathing. With wounds that drain profusely, there may be unpleasant odors that are socially embarrassing, and therefore, require more frequent cast changes. It is not uncommon for individuals to complain of transient itching and burning inside the cast, particularly those with painful diabetic neuropathy.

We believe the advantages far outweigh any disadvantages of TCC, however, consideration must be given to the reluctant patient or the individual who would be unsafe with TCC. In these cases, alternative forms of therapy must be explored and utilized.

CONCLUSION

Research indicates that TCC currently is the most effective therapy for healing neuropathic ulcers. This chapter outlines proper methods to be used with TCC. Given proper application of the cast, chances for complications are minimized. Careful follow-up, after complete healing of the wound, is necessary to minimize the risks for re-ulceration. Successful treatment of neuropathic ulcers with TCC should result in a lower incidence of infection, hospitalization, and lower extremity amputation in this group of patients with chronic disease.

REFERENCES

1. Boulton AJM, Veves A, Young MJ. Etiopathogenesis and management of abnormal foot pressures. In: Levin ME, O'Neal LW, Bowker JH. *The Diabetic Foot.* 5th ed. St. Louis, MO: CV Mosby; 1993:233-246.
2. Brand PW. The insensitive foot (including leprosy). In: Jahass MH. *Disorders of the Foot.* Philadelphia, PA: WB Saunders; 1982:1266-1286.
3. Sinacore DR, Mueller MJ, Diamond JE, Blair VP III, Drury D, Rose SJ. Diabetic neuropathic ulcers treated by total contact casting: a clinical report. *Phys Ther.* 1987;67:1543-1549.
4. Boulton AJM, Bowker JH, Gadia M, et al. Use of plaster casts in the management of diabetic neuropathic foot ulcers. *Diabetes Care.* 1986;9:149-152.
5. Diamond JE, Sinacore DR, Mueller MJ. Molded-double rocker plaster shoe for healing a diabetic plantar ulcer: a case report. *Phys Ther.* 1987;67:1550-1552.
6. Helm PA, Walker SC. Total contact casting in diabetic patients with neuropathic foot ulcerations. *Arch Phys Med Rehabil.* 1984;65:691-693.
7. Laing PW, Cogley DJ, Klenerman L. Neuropathic foot ulceration treated by total contact casts. *J Bone Joint Surg.* 1992;74B:133-136.
8. Myerson M, Papa J, Eaton K, Wilson K. The total contact cast for management of neuropathic plantar ulceration of the foot. *J Bone Joint Surg.* 1992;74A:261-269.
9. Mueller MJ, Diamond JE, Sinacore DR, et al. Total contact casting in treatment of diabetic plantar ulcers: a controlled clinical trial. *Diabetes Care.* 1989;12:384-388.

10. Nawoczenski DA, Birke JA, Graham SL, Koziatek E. The neuropathic foot—a management scheme: a case report. *Phys Ther.* 1989;69:287-291.

11. Pollard JP, LeQuesne LP. Method of healing diabetic forefoot ulcers. *BMJ.* 1983;286:436-437.

12. Walker SC, Helm PA. Total contact casting and chronic diabetic neuropathic foot ulcerations: healing rates by wound location. *Arch Phys Med Rehabil.* 1987;68:217-221.

13. Sinacore DR, Mueller MJ. Total contact casting in the treatment of neuropathic ulcers. In: Levin ME, O'Neal LW, Bowker JH. *The Diabetic Foot.* 5th ed. St Louis, MO: CV Mosby; 1993:283-304.

14. Apelqvist J, Castenfors J, Larsson J, Stenstrom A, Agardh CD. Wound classification is more important than site of ulceration in the outcome of diabetic foot ulcers. *Diabetic Med.* 1989;6:526-530.

15. McCulloch JM, Kloth LC. Evaluation of patients with open wounds. In: Kloth LC, McCulloch JM, Feedar JA. *Wound Healing: Alternatives in Management.* Philadelphia, PA: FA Davis Co; 1990:99-118.

16. Levin ME. Pathogenesis and management of diabetic foot lesions. In: Levin ME, O'Neal LW, Bowker JH. *The Diabetic Foot.* 5th Ed. St. Louis, MO: CV Mosby; 1993:17-60.

17. Edmonds M, Foster AVM. Diabetic Foot Clinic. In: Levin ME, O'Neal LW, Bowker JH. *The Diabetic Foot.* 5th ed. St. Louis, MO: CV Mosby; 1993:587-603.

18. Little JR, Kobayashi GS, Bailey TC. Infection of the diabetic foot. In: Levin ME, O'Neal LW, Bowker JH. *The Diabetic Foot.* 5th ed. St. Louis, MO: CV Mosby; 1993:181-198.

19. Mueller MJ, Minor SD, Diamond JE, Blair VP. Relationship between foot deformity and location of ulcer in patients with diabetes mellitus. *Phys Ther.* 1990;70:356-362.

20. Brand PW. Management of the insensitive limb. *Phys Ther.* 1979;59:8-12.

21. Pecoraro RE, Reiber GE, Burgess EM. Pathways to diabetic limb amputation: basis for prevention. *Diabetes Care.* 1990;13:513-521.

22. Pecoraro RE. The nonhealing diabetic ulcer: a major cause for limb loss. *Prog Clin Biol Res.* 1991;365:27-43.

23. Holewski JJ, Stress RM, Graf PM, Grunfeld C. Aesthesiometry: quantification of cutaneous pressure sensation in diabetic peripheral neuropathy. *J Rehabil Res Dev.* 1988;25:1-10.

24. Birke JA, Sims DS. Plantar sensory threshold in the insensitive foot. *Lepr Rev.* 1986;57:261-267.

25. Klamer TW, Towne JB, Bandyk DF, Bonner MJ. The influence of sepsis and ischemia on the natural history of the diabetic foot. *Am Surg.* 1987;53:490-494.

26. Tannenbaum GA, Pomposelli FB Jr, Marcaccio EJ, et al. Safety of vein-bypass grafting to the dorsal pedal artery in diabetic patients with foot infection. *J Vasc Surg.* 1992;15:982-988.

27. Newman LG, Waller J, Palestro CJ, et al. Unsuspected osteomyelitis in diabetic foot ulcers: diagnosis and monitoring by leukocyte scanning with indium in 111 oxyquinoline. *JAMA.* 1991;266:1246-1251.

28. Diamond JE, Mueller MJ, Delitto A, Sinacore DR. Reliability of a diabetic foot evaluation. *Phys Ther.* 1989;69:797-802.

29. Brand PW. The diabetic foot. In: Ellenberg M, Rifkin H. *Diabetes Mellitus, Theory and Practice.* 3rd ed. New York, NY: Medical Exam Publishing Co; 1983;829-849.

30. Kosiak M. Etiology and pathology of ischemic ulcers. *Arch Phys Med Rehabil.* 1958;40:62-69.

31. Yamaguchi T. Study on the strength of human skin. *J Kyoto Pref Med.* 1960;67:347-379.

32. Mueller MJ, Diamond JE, Delitto A, Sinacore DR. Insensitivity, limited joint mobility and plantar ulcers in patients with diabetes mellitus. *Phys Ther.* 1989;69:453-462.

33. Fernando DJS, Masson EA, Veves A, Boulton AJM. Relationship of limited joint mobility to abnormal foot pressures and diabetic foot ulceration. *Diabetes Care.* 1991;14:8-11.

34. Birke JA, Sims DS, Buford WL. Walking casts: effect on plantar pressures. *J Rehabil Res Dev.* 1985;22:18-25.

35. Mooney V, Wagner FW. Neurocirculatory disorders of the foot. *Clin Orthop Related Res.* 1977;122:53-61.

36. Søderberg G. Follow-up of application of plaster-of-paris casts for non-infected plantar ulcers in field conditions. *Lepr Rev.* 1970;41:184-190.

37. Helm PA, Walker SC, Pullium GF. Recurrence of neuropathic ulceration following healing in a total contact cast. *Arch Phys Med Rehabil.* 1991;72:976-970.

38. Diamond JE, Mueller MJ, Delitto A. Effect of total contact cast immobilization of subtalar and talocrural joint motion in patients with diabetes mellitus. *Phys Ther.* 1993;73:310-315.

39. Palumbo PJ, Melton LJ, Harris MI, Hamman RF. Peripheral vascular disease and diabetes. In: *Diabetes in America.* Washington, DC: US Government Printing Office; 1985. XVI-XV20 DHHS NIH publ. no. 85-1468.

40. *Report of the National Diabetes Advisory Board.* Bethesda, MD: US Government Printing Office; 1980. NIH publ. no. 81-2284.

41. Smith DM, Weinberger M, Katz BP. A controlled trial to increase office visits and reduce hospitalizations. *J Gen Intern Med.* 1987;2:232-238.

42. Apelqvist J, Larsson J, Agardh CD. Long-term prognosis for diabetic patients with foot ulcers. *J Intern Med.* 1993;233:485-491.

43. Apelqvist J, Larsson J, Agardh CD. The importance of peripheral pulses, peripheral edema, and local pain for the outcome of diabetic foot ulcers. *Diabetic Med.* 1990;7:590-594.

44. Diamond JE, Mueller MJ, Delitto A. Follow-up of patients with diabetes and previously healed plantar ulcers. *Phys Ther.* 1991;71(suppl):596. Abstract.

45. Janisse DJ. Pedorthic care of the diabetic foot. In: Levin ME, O'Neal LW, Bowker JH. *The Diabetic Foot.* 5th ed. St. Louis, MO: CV Mosby; 1993;549-576.

46. Mueller MJ, Sinacore DR, Hoogstrate S, Daly L. Effect of hip and ankle walking strategies on peak plantar pressures: implications for neuropathic ulceration. *Arch Phys Med Rehabil.* 1994. In review.

47. Pecoraro RE, Ahroni JH, Boyko EJ, Stensel VL. Chronology and determinants of tissue repair in diabetic lower-extremity ulcers. *Diabetes.* 1991;40:1305-1313.

48. McKittrick LS, McKittrick JB, Risley TS. Transmetatarsal amputation for infection or gangrene in patients with diabetes mellitus. *Ann Surg.* 1949;130:826-842.

49. Miller N, Dardik H, Wolodigerr F, et al. Transmetatarsal amputation: the role of adjunctive revascularization. *J Vasc Surg.* 1991;13:705-711.

50. Fylling CP, Knighton DR. Amputation in the diabetic population: incidence, causes, cost treatment and prevention. *J Enterostom Ther.* 1989;16:247-255.

51. Gilmore JE, Allen JA, Hayes JR. Autonomic function in neuropathic diabetic patients with foot ulceration. *Diabetes Care.* 1993;16:61-67.

52. Ewing DJ, Campbell IW, Clarke BF. The natural history of diabetic autonomic neuropathy. *Q J Med.* 1980;49:95-108.

53. Reiber GE. Epidemiology of the diabetic foot. In: Levin ME, O'Neal LW, Bowker JH. *The Diabetic Foot.* 5th ed. St. Louis, MO: CV Mosby; 1993:1-15.

Chapter 11

Low-Energy Laser in Wound Management

Prem P. Gogia, PhD, PT

Laser is an acronym for Light Amplification by Stimulated Emission of Radiation. Low-energy lasers for management of open wounds have been commonly used in Eastern Europe and Russia for nearly three decades and are popular in many other European countries. However, low-energy lasers for wound healing have only been used in the United States for over a decade. Several scientific studies report the efficacy of low-energy laser for wound healing. Low-energy laser biostimulation of tissues in open wounds decreases edema, reduces inflammation, increases phagocytosis and collagen synthesis, and enhances epithelialization. In spite of this, low-energy laser is viewed with skepticism in the United States, and is still considered as an investigational device by the FDA. The purposes of this chapter are to provide the history of laser, to describe the general principles related to low-energy laser, and to provide a review of the scientific literature.

HISTORY OF LASER

Until recent years, the use of laser in the medical field revolved around its destructive property. These lasers are generally termed as high-power lasers. High-power lasers are used for photocoagulation and vaporization of tissue. Low-energy lasers, on the contrary, are used for tissue repair, reduction of inflammation and pain, and wound healing.

The theory of laser light was first suggested in 1957 by Gordon Gould, a physics graduate student at Columbia University. It was not until 1960 that an American scientist, Theodore Maiman, built the first laser, a ruby laser. The ruby laser produced an intense, millisecond beam of pure, visible red light which was used for its thermal effect, such as tissue ablation or fusion. These applications led to the development of another category of lasers—low-energy lasers. These have a number of different names such as cold, soft, low-level, low-power, and low-output lasers. A low-energy laser is essentially nonthermal and produces a temperature elevation in tissue of less than 0.1° to 0.5° C.[1] Stimulation with low-energy laser is generally referred as biostimulation.

GENERAL PRINCIPLES

The effectiveness of low-energy laser is based on a theory called the "bioluminescence theory."[2] According to this theory, the human body functions at a certain energy level under normal healthy conditions.

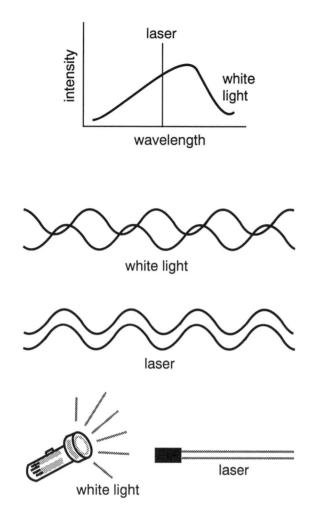

Figure 11-1. Properties of laser.

Once an injury or disease occurs, the energy level in this area decreases. Laser biostimulation of the area returns the energy level to its optimum. Many clinicians express concern regarding the effectiveness of the low-energy laser biostimulation in wound healing since the amount of stimulation it produces appears to be so small. However, low-energy laser functions according to the Arndt-Schulz Law, which states that "less is more."[3] In other words, weak stimuli excite physiologic activity, moderately strong stimuli favor physiologic effect, strong stimuli retard physiologic effect, and very strong stimuli arrest physiologic effect. Therefore, high power densities of laser irradiation have a destructive effect on tissue whereas low power densities of laser irradiation have a biostimulating effect on tissue.

Kleinkort and Foley[4] cited another possible theory for the mechanism of action of low-energy laser biostimulation. This theory was originally proposed by Moreno. The theory pustulated that low-energy laser can stimulate energy stores via adenosine triphosphate (ATP) formation and activation of enzyme activity leading to restoration of normal physiologic processes at the cell-organism levels.

PROPERTIES OF LASER

The wave of energy from a laser has three unique physical properties that distinguish it from ordinary light: monochromaticity, coherence, and divergence (Figure 11-1). Chromaticity refers to the specificity in a single, defined wavelength of stimulation produced by laser. It gives added purity to a laser which is not found in most sources of light, and provides a non-random, summative, photochemical effect. Coherence refers to the high degree of order and fixed phase relationship. There is synchronization of laser light waves for simultaneous biologic energy effects which increases the photochemical reaction. Divergence refers to the small foci and extreme parallelism of the laser light. It provides exact placement and directivity in the tissue. Due to the above physical properties, the penetration of a laser beam in tissue is much greater than with a conventional light source.

ENERGY DENSITY

The quantity of laser energy delivered to a unit surface is calculated in joules per square centimeter (J/cm^2). Clinicians must be careful in selecting energy density for treating wounds with laser. Research indicates that energy densities of 0.05 to 4.0 J/cm^2 are capable of biostimulative effects on tissues. Acute conditions require 0.05 to 0.5 J/cm^2 whereas chronic conditions require 0.5 to 4.0 J/cm^2. Research also indicates that 4.0 to 8.0 J/cm^2 causes bioinhibition effect and therefore should be avoided.

APPLICATION TECHNIQUE

Treatment guidelines are based on the amount of energy density delivered to a square centimeter of tissue surface. For open wounds with viable tissue, the "grid" technique is used. The base of the wound is visually divided into square centimeter grids. Use of any opaque substance to grid the wound area should be avoided as this may screen out the laser energy. The laser probe is held perpendicular to the center of each square at a distance of 0.5 to 1 cm from the wound surface and is swept in the entire centimeter square in a circular motion (Figure 11-2). Each square centimeter of involved tissue is stimulated equally for effective coverage of the entire tissue surface. For open wounds covered with eschar, the "surround the dragon" technique is used. The wound is stimulated around the periphery of the wound holding laser probe 0.5 to 1 cm above the surface. For cavernous wounds, one needs to fill the sinus track with normal saline. The laser probe tip should be covered with Saran that has been gas autoclaved or with OpSite dressing. The tip is placed in the cavity and the wound is treated.

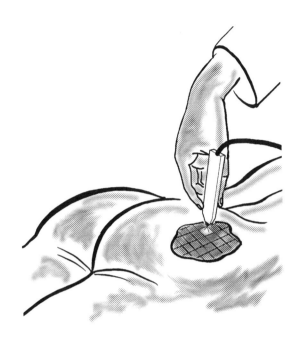

Figure 11-2. Grid technique of laser application.

FDA REGULATIONS

FDA classifies the low-energy lasers as a "nonsignificant risk investigational device." An Investigational Device Exemption (IDE) must be obtained from a committee called an Institutional Review Board (IRB) within a hospital or institution. If a clinician does not have access to an IRB, he or she may work under the IDE of the manufacturer. The IDE is intended to ensure that only qualified clinicians use the device, and they use it for investigative purposes only, not for profit. The FDA also requires that the investigator/clinician must inform patients that the device is classified as investigational without proven benefits and to obtain patients' consent. The FDA also requires that good records of the use of the device be maintained. Further, the clinician/instigator evaluates and reports unanticipated adverse effects related to the use of the device.

CONTRAINDICATIONS AND PRECAUTIONS

Contraindications and precautions of low-energy laser treatment are primarily based on the theoretical model. Biostimulation by low-energy laser during pregnancy may cause spontaneous abor-

tion when certain points in the body are stimulated. The use of low-energy laser stimulation on tumorous tissue has not been established and therefore should not be used in such cases. Laser is also contraindicated to fontanelles of growing children. Further, care must be taken to ensure that patients do not stare directly into the beam as this may cause permanent damage to the retina of the eye due to its unusual brilliance. Use of laser is also contraindicated in patients with photosensitive skin and in those patients who are taking photosensitive medications. Also, overstimulation by laser should be avoided. Exposing tissue to laser energy densities above 4 J/cm^2 should be avoided during any one treatment. Nausea and dizziness has been reported in only 2% of the patient population treated with low-energy laser. If these symptoms persist for more than 5 to 10 minutes after treatment, no further treatments are recommended.

TYPES OF LOW-ENERGY LASERS

There are a number of low-energy lasers used clinically (Table 11-1). However, the two com-

Table 11-1. Common Types of Low-Energy Lasers

Laser System	Wavelength
Argon (Ar)	488-514 nm
Carbon dioxide (CO_2)	10,600 nm
Dye	Variable
Gallium-arsenide (GaAs) or Infrared (IR)	904 nm
Gallium-aluminum-arsenide (GaAlAs)	830 nm
Helium-neon (HeNe)	632.8 nm
Neodymium:Yttrium-aluminum-garnet (Nd:YAG)	1,064 nm
Ruby	694 nm

monly used and most studied systems are the helium-neon (HeNe) and the gallium-arsenide (GaAs), or infrared (IR), lasers. HeNe is a continuous wave, low-energy laser with an average power output of 1 mW whereas IR is a pulsed, low-energy laser with an average power output of 3 mW. The primary factor which affects the actual depth to which a laser beam penetrates the tissue is the waveform of the beam. The secondary factor which affects the depth of penetration is the power output of the laser. A HeNe laser with a wavelength of 632.8 nm has a depth of penetration of 5 to 10 mm while a GaAs or IR laser with a wavelength of 904 nm has a depth of penetration up to 10 cm. The FDA classifies HeNe laser as a Class II laser and GaAs or IR laser as a Class IIIb laser.

LITERATURE REVIEW

For the purpose of simplicity and clarity, this literature review will be divided into three categories: cellular research, animal studies, and human trials.

CELLULAR RESEARCH

The effects of low-energy laser on biological systems is best understood at the cellular level. The interactions of laser at the cellular level provide the underlying rationale for clinical use.[5] Further, Basford[5] believed that the most convincing evidence for low-energy laser biostimulation is found at the cellular level. Most of the early research was done in vitro with cultured cells and tissues. The majority of these studies assessed the effects of low-energy lasers on fibroblast cells and collagen tissue. Lam and associates[6] studied the effect of both HeNe and IR lasers on collagen synthesis in human skin fibroblast cultures. They reported an approximately four-fold increase in collagen production by use of both the lasers. Similarly, Abergal and associates[7] assayed procollagen mRNA from pig skin wounds stimulated with HeNe laser. They found increased procollagen synthesis following laser biostimulation. Further research by these investigators also showed increased procollagen in human skin fibroblast cultures stimulated with low-energy laser.[8] Based on these results, Abergel and associates[7,8] postulated that the mechanism for the acceleration of wound healing with low-energy laser biostimulation involved acceleration of the mRNA transcription rate of the collagen gene or other enzymatic changes following biostimulation. Similar to the above studies, Williams[9] also found significantly higher type I and type III procollagen mRNA in wounds treated with low-energy laser at days 17 and 28, while only type III procollagen mRNA was significantly higher at day 10.

The mechanism by which these effects are produced is not clear. It is postulated that biostimulation could cause a biochemical change in the properties of the co-enzyme nicotinamide adenine dehydrogenase (NADH) which could cause a concomitant increase in cellular activity.[10] Hallman and associates[11] also treated cultured human fibroblasts in a controlled, randomized manner to assess the effect of HeNe laser. They, however, did not find a significant stimulative or inhibitive effect on replication of fibroblasts. Since several other studies reported positive results of low-energy lasers in vitro on cells and cultures, Hallman and associates[11] believed that while metabolic processes may be altered by low-energy laser biostimulation, cell proliferation may not be affected. On the other hand, Hardy and associates[12] stimulated cultured mouse fibroblast cells with pulsed ruby laser, and reported a five-fold increase in the number of cells. Kubasova and associates[13] biostimulated fibroblast cultures taken from human embryo with HeNe laser. The fibroblast cells, when stimulated four times at 24-hour intervals, showed increased binding ability to the lectin. However, when the cells were stimulated once, they did not cause any significant functional or micromorphological changes in the plasma membranes.

Increased fibroblast proliferation, as well as increased collagen synthesis, requires extra energy. Therefore, Passarella and associates[14] studied the effect of low-energy laser on ATP. They isolated mitochondria from rats and biostimulated them with HeNe laser. The investigators reported an increase in membrane potential, proton gradient, and ATP synthesis. ATP synthesis alone was reported to increase by 70% with laser biostimulation.

The effect of low-energy laser biostimulation on the immune system was studied by several investigators.[15,16] Kupin and associates[15] reported increased activity of lymphocytes in patients with a suppressed immune system when the lymphocytes were stimulated with either argon or HeNe laser. Further research of cultured human lymphocytes biostimulated with HeNe laser reported an increase in the ability of lymphocytes to bind bacteria, an increase in the frequency of binding, an increase in lymphocyte binding sites, and finally, an increase in the affinity of bacteria for lymphocytes.[16] Therefore, it was concluded that laser biostimulation increases the immune system's ability to kill invading microorganisms by increasing lymphocytes' activity and their abilities to bind pathogens. Thus, laser biostimulation may play a significant role in enhancing the healing process in chronic, infected, nonhealing wounds.

Kerotinocyte cells also play an important role in the formation of normal, functioning epidermis. Effects of low-energy stimulation on the proliferation and motility of keratinocytes has been studied in cell cultures.[17,18] Haas and associates[17] reported a three-fold increase in the rate of keratinocyte migration in cells biostimulated with HeNe laser compared to nonstimulated cells. However, laser biostimulation did not increase keratinocyte proliferation, nor did it cause an alteration in keratinocyte differentiation.[18]

ANIMAL STUDIES

Results of low-energy laser biostimulation at the cellular level are overwhelming and encouraging. This advanced research with animal studies is designed to assess the effects of low-energy laser biostimulation on both wound healing (closure) and tensile strength. Several investigators reported an increased rate of healing in animal wounds treated with low-energy laser.[19-28] Mester and associates[19] surgically created full-thickness skin wounds on the backs of mice and biostimulated the wounds twice a week for 2 weeks with ruby laser. They reported enhanced healing of the stimulated wounds. Similar results were reported in another study by Mester and associates[20] on burns in mice. The wounds healed faster when biostimulated with ruby laser than the control group. An in vivo study by Mester and Jaszsagi-Nagy[21] showed an increase in the production of collagen by 30% to 50% when the wounds were biostimulated with pulsed ruby laser.

Kana and associates[22] biostimulated full-thickness skin wounds daily in rats with ruby and HeNe laser. They reported not only faster healing of wounds but also increased collagen in wounds treated with HeNe laser compared to wounds treated with ruby laser or control wounds. The maximum effect was observed at an energy density of 4 J/cm^2. Kovacs and associates[23] also reported higher tensile strength in full-thickness skin wounds in rats when biostimulated with HeNe laser twice daily for 3 minutes for 8 and 12 days.

Complete healing of full-thickness skin wounds has also been reported in rabbits stimulated with various doses of HeNe laser.[24] These investigators also reported a higher rate of fibroblast proliferation and faster collagen synthesis in laser stimulated animals versus controls. Similarly, Lyons and associates[25] reported significant improvement in tensile strength at 1 and 2 weeks in mice wounds biostimulated with HeNe laser. They also found a significant increase in total collagen content at 2 months in laser treated wounds compared to control wounds.

Surinchak and associates[26] stimulated experimentally induced skin wounds in rabbits with HeNe laser for 30 minutes every 3 days or for 3 minutes twice daily. Although the incisions exposed to the latter treatment regime showed significantly higher tensile strengths, similar increases in tensile strength were not found in the former treatment regime. Neither dose of laser stimulation enhanced the healing process of the total skin defects.

Similar results were reported by Braverman and associates.[27] They found increased tensile strength in skin wounds of rabbits biostimulated daily with HeNe and pulsed IR lasers for a period of 21 days. However, nonstimulated wounds on the contralateral side in the same animal also showed an increase in tensile strength compared with nonstimulated control animals. The investigators suggested that some growth or tissue factor was released into the general circulation from the biostimulated side that positively influenced the development of tensile strength on the untreated side. In the same study, the investigators found no significant differences in the rate of healing and collagen synthesis in the biostimulated wounds when compared to the control wounds. Haina and associates[28] reported increased granulation tissue in rats and enhanced epidermal regeneration in guinea pigs when wounds were biostimulated with HeNe laser.

As described in Chapter 1, prostaglandin plays an important role in the early phase of inflammation. Changes in E and F types of prostaglandins contents in vivo rat skin wounds stimulated with HeNe laser were studied. At 4 days post-injury, both E and F type of prostaglandins accumulated significantly more in laser stimulated wounds, however, after 8 days of stimulation F prostaglandins were found to be higher while E prostaglandins were found to be lower compared to the control group. The reported results suggest that HeNe laser biostimulation accelerates the inflammatory phase of wound healing.[29]

On the other hand, few in vivo studies have reported no significant effect of low-energy laser on wound healing. In a randomized, controlled study, Basford and associates[30] divided six pigs into three groups of two each and created nine surgical wounds on each side of the spine. One group received cold-quartz ultraviolet irradiation, a second group received HeNe laser biostimulation, while in the third control group the wounds were covered with a semipermeable film. In their study, wounds in the control group healed faster than the other two groups. Although not statistically significant, wounds in the control group tended to be the strongest. Similar results were observed by Hunter and associates[31] who biostimulated partial-thickness wounds in pigs with HeNe laser and found no significant difference in healing when compared to a control group. Jongsma and associates[32] also found no acceleration of wound closure when biostimulated with low-energy argon laser at either 1 or 4 J/cm^2. Furthermore, McCaughan and associates[33] also observed no increased healing in pig wounds when treated with low-energy argon laser.

The effects of low-energy laser biostimulation has also been studied on skin grafts and flaps. Biostimulation by HeNe laser in animal models has been reported to increase vascularization and improve graft survival.[34] Similarly, biostimulation of experimentally designed flaps with a known potential for failure resulted in increased flap survival in animals who either received pre- or postoperative biostimulation with GaAlAs laser.[35] Increased blood supply to flaps with biostimulation was reported to be the cause of flap survival in biostimulated animals.

HUMAN TRIALS

There is a scarcity of clinical studies related to the biostimulating effects of low-energy lasers on human wound healing. Published clinical reports in this area have been either poorly controlled or uncontrolled. Further, clinical research used different doses and frequencies which severely limits an attempt to compare results from different studies.

Mester and associates[36] stimulated 1120 nonhealing human wounds with HeNe and argon lasers.

They found that 875 wounds healed completely in 12 to 16 weeks, an additional 160 wounds improved, and 85 wounds did not heal. Increased collagen synthesis, diminished cellular substance, significant vascularization, and an increase in tensile strength was observed. Kovacs and associates[37] reported a rapid regeneration of epithelium with marked reduction in healing time in cervix erosions treated with HeNe laser. Further, Kahn[38] also reported good clinical results in two patients with open wounds treated with HeNe laser. Kahn suggested that a low pulse rate of 40 pps may be more beneficial in treating chronic wounds. Similar results were reported by Gogia and associates[39] in treating two patients with chronic, nonhealing wounds with pulsed IR laser.

There have also been controlled clinical trials which have failed to demonstrate a beneficial effect of low-energy biostimulation on wound healing.[40,41] Santoianni and associates[40] reported no significant differences in chronic venous leg ulcers treated with HeNe laser. They biostimulated 16 patients using 1 J/cm^2, another 17 patients with 4 J/cm^2, while 28 patients served as control. The wounds were treated 6 days a week for at least 1 month. Similarly, Gogia and Marquez[41] reported no significant differences between treated and untreated patients with chronic leg ulcers. The results of the later study should be interpreted with great caution since both the experimental and the control groups consisted of six patients each.

CONCLUSION

Although low-energy laser research at the cellular level has been the most convincing evidence, clinical use of low-energy laser for wound management still remains a controversial area. Even though animal studies have also shown accelerated healing and improved wound strength following laser biostimulation, it is unclear how well this response generalizes to humans. These favorable results have been reported mostly in small, loose-skinned animals such as rats and rabbits. The skin of these animals differs greatly from that of humans. Pig skin has less elasticity than rats and rabbits. Further, both pigs and humans rely more on contraction than epithelialization for wound healing. Thus, a pig skin model would be more clinically applicable to humans. Unfortunately, studies on pig skins have also not reported any favorable results of HeNe irradiation on the rate of wound healing. The clinical reports, consisting of case studies, have been encouraging. However, more controlled experimental studies fail to show any significant benefit. Research concerning control groups is lacking.

The failure of some studies to find significant effects may be due to irradiation parameters. Laser wavelength, waveform, power output, energy density, and treatment schedule are critical. Clearly, there is a desperate need to establish the laser parameters to produce optimal benefit. Further, guidelines need to be established for treatment frequency. The concept of laser biostimulation has remained controversial. Obviously, further controlled clinical studies on a large number of patients are needed to confirm the clinical efficacy of low-energy lasers on wound healing in humans.

REFERENCES

1. Basford JR. Low-energy laser therapy: controversies and new research findings. *Lasers Surg Med.* 1989;9:1-5.
2. Demers LM. Overview of laser biostimulation and its application in PT. *Phys Ther Forum.* 1986;5(38):1-6.
3. *Dorland's Illustrated Medical Dictionary.* 26th ed. Philadelphia, PA: WB Saunders Co; 1985.
4. Kleinkort JA, Foley RA. Laser acupuncture: its use in physical therapy. *Am J Acupuncture.* 1984;12:51-56.
5. Basford JR. Laser therapy: scientific basis and clinical role. *Orthopedics.* 1993;16:541-547.
6. Lam TS, Abergel RP, Castel JC, et al. Laser stimulation of collagen synthesis in human skin fibroblast cultures. *Lasers Life Sci.* 1986;1:61-77.
7. Abergel RP, Lyons RF, Castel JC, et al. Biostimulation of wound healing by lasers: experimental approaches in animal and in fibroblast cultures. *J Dermatol Surg Oncol.* 1987;13:127-133.
8. Abergal RP, Lam TS, Meeker CA, Dwyer RM, Uitto J. Low-energy lasers stimulate collagen production in human skin fibroblast cultures. *Clin Res.* 1984;32:16A. Abstract.
9. Williams IF. Cellular and biochemical composition of healing tendon. In: Jenkins DHR. *Ligament Injuries and Their Treatment.* London: Chapman and Hall Ltd; 1985:43-57.

10. Pasarella S, Dechecchi MS, Quagliariello E, et al. Optical and biochemical properties of NADH irradiated by high peak power Q-switched ruby laser or by low power CW He-Ne laser. *Bioelectrochem Bioenerg.* 1981;8:315-319.

11. Hallman HO, Basford JR, O'Brien JF, et al. Does low-energy helium-neon laser irradiation alter "in vitro" replication of human fibroblast. *Lasers Surg Med.* 1988;8:125-129.

12. Hardy LB, Hardy FS, Fine S, Sokal J. Effect of ruby laser radiation on mouse fibroblast culture. *Fed Proc.* 1967;26:668. Abstract.

13. Kubasova T, Kovacs L, Somosy Z, Kokai A. Biological effect of He-Ne laser: investigations on functional and micromorphological alterations of cell membranes, in vitro. *Lasers Surg Med.* 1984;4:381-388.

14. Passarella S, Casamassima E, Molinari S, et al. Increase of proton electrochemical potential and ATP synthesis in rat liver mitochondria irradiated in vitro by helium-neon laser. *FEBS Lett.* 1984;175:95-99.

15. Kupin IV, Bykov VS, Ivanov AV, Larichev VY. Potentiating effects of laser radiation on some immunological traits. *Neoplasma.* 1982;29:403-406.

16. Passarella S, Casamassima E, Quagliariello E, Caretto G, Jirillo E. Quantitative analysis of lymphocyte-Salmonella interaction and the effects of lymphocyte irradiation by He-Ne laser. *Biochem Biophys Res Commmun.* 1985;130:546-552.

17. Haas AF, Isseroff RR, Wheeland RG, Rood PA, Graves PJ. Low-energy helium-neon laser irradiation increases the motility of cultured human keratinocytes. *J Invest Dermatol.* 1990;94:822-826.

18. Rood PA, Haas AF, Graves PJ, Wheeland RG, Isseroff RR. Low-energy helium-neon laser irradiation does not alter human keratinocytes differentiation. *J Invest Dermatol.* 1992;99:445-458.

19. Mester E, Ludany G, Sellyei M, Szende B, Tota J. The stimulating effects of low power laser rays on biological systems. *Laser Rev (Lond).* 1968;1:3.

20. Mester E, Spiry T, Szende B, et al. Effect of laser rays on wound healing. *Am J Surg.* 1971;122:532-535.

21. Mester E, Jaszagi-Nagy E. The effect of laser radiation on wound healing and collagen synthesis. *Stud Biophys.* 1973;35:227-230.

22. Kana JS, Hutschenreiter G, Haina D. Effect of low-power density laser radiation on healing of open skin wounds in rats. *Arch Surg.* 1981;116:293-296.

23. Kovacs IB, Mester E, Gorog P. Stimulation of wound healing with laser beam in rat. *Experientia.* 1974;30:1275-1276.

24. Averbakh MM, Sorokin ML, Dobkin VG, et al. The influence of helium-neon laser on the healing of aseptic experimental wounds. In: Enwemeka CS. Laser biostimulation of healing wounds: specific effects and mechanism of action. *J Ortho Sports Phys Ther.* 1988;9:333-338.

25. Lyons RF, Abergel RP, White RA, et al. Biostimulation of wound healing in vivo by a helium-neon laser. *Ann Plast Surg.* 1987;18:47-50.

26. Surinchak JS, Alago ML, Bellamy RF, et al. Effects of low-level energy lasers on the healing of full-thickness skin defects. *Lasers Surg Med.* 1983;2:267-274.

27. Braverman B, McCarthy RJ, Ivankovich AD, et al. Effect of helium-neon and infrared laser irradiation on wound healing in rabbits. *Lasers Surg Med.* 1989;9:50-58.

28. Haina D, Brunner R, Landthaler M, et al. Animal experiments in light-induced wound healing. *Laser Basic Biomed Res.* 1982;22:1-3.

29. Cseh G, Kovacs-Szabo I, Gorog P, et al. Effect of laser irradiation on the prostaglandin content of skin wounds. *Acta Physiol Hung.* 1978;52:206.

30. Basford JR, Hallman HO, Sheffield CG, et al. Comparison of cold-quartz ultraviolet, low-energy laser and occlusion in wound healing in a swine model. *Arch Phys Med Rehabil.* 1986;67:151-154.

31. Hunter J, Leonard L, Wilson R, et al. Effects of low energy laser on wound healing in a porcine model. *Lasers Surg Med.* 1984;3:285-290.

32. Jongsma FHM, Boggard AEJM, van Gemert MJC, Henning JPH. Is closure of open skin wounds in rats accelerated by argon laser exposure? *Lasers Surg Med.* 1983;3:75-80.

33. McCaughan JS, Bethel BH, Johnston T, Janssen W. Effect of low-dose argon irradiation on rate of wound closure. *Lasers Surg Med.* 1985;5:607-614.

34. Namenyi J, Mester E, Foldes I, Tisza S. Effect of laser irradiation and immunosuppressive treatment on survival of mouse skin allotransplant. *Acta Chir Acad Sci Hung.* 1975;16:327-335.

35. Kami T, Yoshimura Y, Nakajima T, et al. Effects of low-power diode lasers on flap survival. *Ann Plast Surg.* 1985;14:278-283.

36. Mester E, Mester AF, Mester A. The biomedical effects of laser application. *Lasers Surg Med.* 1985;5:31-39.

37. Kovacs L, Varga L, Palyi I, et al. Experimental investigation of photostimulation effect of low energy He-Ne laser radiation. *Laser Basic Biomed Res.* 1982;22:14-16.

38. Kahn J. Case reports: open wound management with the HeNe (6328 AU) cold laser. *J Ortho Sports Phys Ther.* 1984;6:203-204.

39. Gogia PP, Hurt BS, Zirn TT. Wound management with whirlpool and infrared cold laser treatment: a clinical report. *Phys Ther.* 1988;68:1239-1242.

40. Santoianni P, Monfrecola G, Martellotta D, et al. Inadequate effect of helium-neon laser on venous leg ulcers. *Photodermatology.* 1984;1:245-249.

41. Gogia PP, Marquez RR. Effects of helium-neon laser on wound healing. *Ostomy Wound Manage.* 1992;38:33-41.

Chapter 12

Electrical Stimulation for Wound Management

Marybeth Brown, PhD, PT

There is now a substantial body of evidence to support the use of electrical stimulation for wound healing. Guidelines (e.g., current intensity, polarity) for the use of stimulation have not yet been determined for all conditions but there is enough information in print to guide the clinician to a reasonable treatment plan. The purposes of this chapter are to present the healing properties of electrical stimulation, to review pertinent literature, to discuss treatment considerations, and to outline precautions and contraindications of electrical stimulation.

Results will be presented from animal and human studies. Unquestionably, the human results are the most significant from the standpoint of treatment efficacy, but only from animal studies can one learn what electrical stimulation (ES) does and does not do. It is hoped that information presented in this chapter will inspire practitioners to seriously consider ES as an appropriate and, at times, necessary modality for the enhancement of wound healing. The systematic utilization of ES for wounds should result in better patient care.

BACKGROUND

One of the points that will be made throughout this chapter is that there are two distinct aspects of wound healing: closure of the epithelium (i.e., the wound is no longer open) and healing of the dermis. Recovery of the dermis ultimately determines the strength of the wound. Closure is enormously important because an open wound is an avenue of infection. Without concomitant recovery of the dermis, however, there is an increased likelihood that the epidermis will reopen because wound strength is poor. Thus, ideal treatment will enhance healing events both at the epidermis and dermis.

Stimulation has been shown to influence epidermal cell proliferation and migration (i.e., closure) and dermal fibroblastic activity (collagen secretion).[1-5] While these two events are intimately related to recovery, there are other elements of the healing process that also appear to be positively influenced by ES treatment. There is evidence to indicate that ES decreases edema,[6] improves blood flow to the area being treated,[7] inhibits bacterial growth,[8] and enhances phagocytosis by attracting macrophages and neutrophils.[9] Thus, the influence of stimulation goes beyond events occurring at the skin cell level. Overviews concerning the therapeutic effects of stimulation on edema, circulation, and other cells and tissues have been presented by Snyder-Mackler,[10] Cummings,[11] and Kloth and Feedar.[12]

LITERATURE REVIEW

ANIMAL STUDIES

In one of the earliest reports, Assimacopoulos[3] applied 100 µA of direct current to full-thickness skin defects on rabbits. Negative (cathodal) current was applied continuously until wound closure was complete. Subsequently, skin pieces were examined histologically. Findings indicated that skin closure (epithelialization) occurred more quickly in treated rabbits and that the dermis appeared to have denser connective tissue when viewed microscopically. This observation was supported by higher tensile strength measures in treated rabbits compared to controls. Only two control and two experimental animals were followed in this study, however.

Alvarez and associates[13] surgically induced wounds, 0.3 mm deep, on the back of guinea pigs (normal guinea pig skin thickness is approximately 1.7 mm). The wounds were either treated with 50 to 300 µA of positive (anodal) direct current or were left untreated. The epidermis was separated from the dermis and evaluated. Wounds on the treated pigs showed a faster rate of epithelialization. The dermis showed a significant increase in collagen synthetic activity when compared with the untreated pigs. This study also appeared to indicate that electrical stimulation might influence both wound closure and wound strength. Using the same partial-thickness model as Alvarez and associates, Mertz and associates[14] also showed an increased rate of epithelialization in pigs treated with ES.

Wu and associates,[15] however, studied the effect of direct current on the tensile strength of full-thickness incisions in rabbits and found no differences between treated and untreated animals. These investigators made two parallel incisions on 33 rabbits and sutured each lesion with stainless steel or platinum wire. A 40 mV current was passed through each incision. The polarity of the current was positive for one incision and negative for another. After 7 days of treatment, tensile strength measures of the two wounds were comparable. These results should be interpreted with caution

however, as neither stainless steel nor platinum are particularly conductive. Results also could have been confounded by the possibility that the wounds were too close to each other and both wounds were receiving negative and positive polarity stimulation. Studies (unpublished) from our laboratory found that the effects of stimulation go considerably beyond the boundaries of the electrodes. Preliminary findings suggest that stimulation can affect events 2 to 3 cm away. Finally, comparisons with control animals were not included in the results. Perhaps the results for both treated groups were better than would have been found in a control group.

Several groups of investigators have examined tensile strength measures in treated and untreated animals but have not found differences between the two groups. Bach and associates[16] did not find treated wounds (1 week of treatment) to be mechanically stronger. They did note that there was an increase in collagen content in the dermis of treated wounds. Research from our laboratory did not find significantly enhanced wound strength either when stimulation treatment was given for only 7 or 8 days. However, findings indicated a different orientation of collagen fibers in treated animals suggesting stimulation effects at the dermal level.[17,18] Wound strength after 1 week of healing is very poor (10% of normal). These findings suggest that perhaps the length of treatment time in the Bach and associates[16] and Brown and associates[17,18] studies was too short for the effects of stimulation on wound strength to be realized. This hypothesis has been supported by a more recent study.

Recently Brown, Gogia, Menton, and Sinacore (unpublished) completed a study at Washington University that indicated tensile strength could be enhanced with ES. Guinea pigs were treated for 40 minutes once daily for 2 weeks. Full-thickness skin incisions of nine treated and five untreated animals were examined to failure. Statistically, the differences between control and treated animals were not quite significant. However, wounds that had been treated for 2 weeks with ES were 45% stronger than wounds that had not received treatment (552 versus 1011 gm) which can be interpreted as clinically meaningful. Following 2 weeks of treatment, an additional nine animals were allowed to recover naturally for 2 more weeks. Thus, animals in this group were a month post injury and had received ES treatment during the first 2 post-injury weeks. Wound tensile strength continued to increase during the non-treatment period in control and treated animals, but guinea pigs that had received stimulation had stronger wounds than controls. Tensile strength values averaged 2704 gm in controls versus 3419 gm in treated (p=.06). Thus, it appeared that the advantages of stimulation treatment were still apparent after its discontinuation. Whether treated wounds would still be stronger than untreated wounds in 6 months is unknown. Of additional interest in future studies is whether the ultimate tensile strength of ES treated wounds is greater than wounds that receive no attention. Wound strength in healthy skin has been reported to recover only to 70% of normal. Possibly, patients who are older men and women with diseases such as diabetes or lupus have a poorer recovery in wound strength than young, healthy adults. Perhaps ES can produce a better final outcome. Research addressing this question is needed.

Very few investigators have examined animals that were not normal. One exception is the study conducted by Smith and associates[19] who investigated the effects of ES on wound healing in diabetic mice. Mice were made diabetic within 5 days by two injections of alloxan monohydrate. Six days after injections, mice were anesthetized, and a 3 cm incision was made on the back of each mouse. Subsequently, mice were treated for 10 days with either 1 or 20 volts, 10 or 20 mA. Although authors stated that tensile strength values were higher for treated diabetic mice, there was no supporting statistical evidence given in the article.

Even though there is little to support the use of ES for an unhealthy population of animals, there is substantial evidence to support the use of ES for wound healing in unhealthy humans.

HUMAN STUDIES

Human clinical studies have appeared in the literature for decades. Most of the earlier investigations, however, were uncontrolled and much of the evidence for enhanced wound healing was anecdotal. For example, Wolcott and associates[20] treated 67 patients with ischemic ulcers with 200 to 1000 μA of low intensity direct current. The healing rate was highly variable (0% to 97%) but the overall effect of treatment appeared to be a 13.4% improvement per week. Gault and Gatens[21] also applied electrical stimulation (200 to 800 μA) to 76 patients with 106 ischemic skin ulcers. Some of the ulcers were infected and some were not. Patients were with and without sensation and circulatory compromise. A few patients with bilateral ulcers (n=6) received treatment on only one side. Results strongly suggested that ulcers that received treatment healed more rapidly than those that did not receive treatment. Even though proper controls were not used in either study, results were tantalizing and they set the stage for appropriately conducted clinical trials.

Although low intensity direct current appeared to be successful in wound healing trials, it did not become widely used in clinical settings. One reason for this failure could be the lack of treatment guidelines. Another reason may be that low intensity direct current is uncomfortable, which can affect patient acceptance and compliance. High intensity stimulators with pulsed current have been developed within the last decade. These stimulators deliver current without irritation or burning and have a higher current density, which should (theoretically) lead to better healing than low intensity direct current. Results of studies using pulsed high voltage current are very favorable. Some of the more recent studies are presented below.

Kloth and Feedar[22] randomly assigned 9 of 16 patients with Stage IV ulcers to a treatment group; the remaining 7 patients served as controls. High voltage, pulsed current was applied once a day for 45 minutes, 5 days a week. Treated ulcers healed completely in 7.3 weeks whereas untreated ulcers increased in size. Three of the untreated patients whose ulcers were not improving were later reassigned to the treatment group and healing ensued. This study clearly demonstrated that high voltage stimulation accelerates the rate of healing.

In another double-blind study, Feedar and associates[23] randomly assigned 47 patients with 50 wounds to either a treatment group or a control group. Patients had Stages II, III, and IV chronic dermal ulcers. These patients in the treatment group received negative (cathodal) pulsed ES 30 minutes twice daily. The polarity of the ES was changed every 3 days until the wound progressed to a Stage II classification. After 4 weeks of treatment, wounds in the treatment group (n=26) were 44% of their original size, while wounds in the control group (n=24) were 67% of their original size. The healing rate per week for the treatment group was 14%, but only 8.25% for the control group.

Mulder[24] also reported a more rapid rate of healing for patients treated with high voltage pulsed current. The study was designed and conducted as a double-blind, randomized, clinical trial. However, patients were given three intensities of stimulation at two different frequencies. Whether one form of stimulation was more efficacious than another was not addressed. Wounds in the stimulation groups showed an average 56% decrease in size whereas untreated wounds showed only a 33% decrease.

Griffin and associates[25] examined the effects of high voltage pulsed current on the healing of pressure ulcers in patients with spinal cord injury. After 20 days of stimulation for an hour daily, treated patients showed significantly increased healing compared to those in a placebo group. Wound measures were taken at 5, 10, 15, and 20 days.

Unger and associates conducted a series of clinical studies of the efficacy of high voltage pulsed current. In one study, 13 nursing home patients with 29 pressure ulcers were treated with ES. After 8 weeks of treatment, 82% of the ulcers healed completely.[26] In another controlled, double-blind study, 17 patients were randomly assigned to either a treatment group or a placebo group. In the treatment group, eight of nine patients were healed (89%) while in the placebo group, only three of eight patients were healed (37.5%). The average healing time with ES was 51.2 days and 460.2 mm² compared to 118.5 mm² for wounds in the placebo group.[27] Similar results were reported in another study by Unger and associates.[28] Two hundred of 233 wounds (89.7%) healed in an average 54.25 days with high voltage pulsed current. These wounds did not respond to traditional treatment for an average of 71.40 days. These studies further suggest that high voltage pulsed current can significantly increase the rate of wound closure.

COMMENTS

Results from animal and human studies support ES as a means for promoting a faster rate of healing (epithelialization). Additionally, evidence seems to indicate that wound (dermal) strength can also be enhanced with the appropriate use of stimulation. It is important to note that the treatment protocol, intensity, voltage, pulse rate, polarity, and electrode placement vary considerably from one study to another.

Criticisms often are voiced about studies that use normal animals or humans as subjects. In this instance, perhaps a point is being missed. Historically, the emphasis of wound healing studies has been on treating sick patients with recalcitrant, chronic ulcers. Obviously the healing of indolent ulcers is enormously important; the reasons are self-evident. The studies presented above suggest that clinicians could expand the scope of ES treatment to enhance wound closure in surgical patients or accident victims. Possibly ES might promote enhanced wound strength in acute care patients, thus reducing the likelihood of complications at a surgery or injury site. Studies of the effects of ES in acute care (clinical trials) are needed.

TREATMENT CONSIDERATIONS

POLARITY

Although not conclusive, there is a body of evidence that suggests that polarity is an important treatment issue, both in acute and chronic wounds. According to Vanable and associates,[29] enhancing naturally occurring bioelectric currents by applying stimulation in the proper direction of polarity does appear to enhance the healing process, whereas regeneration can be inhibited by orienting the current in the reverse direction. A series of studies conducted in our laboratory support this concept.

In the first study, rabbits were treated for 4 or 7 days with negative polarity pulsed, high voltage galvanic stimulation.[18] Full-thickness incisions of $3^1/_2$ cm were made, under anesthesia, on the back of each animal. Stimulation was applied twice daily for 2 hours each. Animals in the 4-day treated group appeared to have better healing, and a trend toward higher tensile strength values than untreated rabbits based on histological observations. After 7 days of stimulation, control rabbits had significantly higher tensile strength values than treated animals. Microscopically, 7-day treated wounds gave the impression that healing had been arrested. These conflicting results led to a second study in which rabbits were again treated for 4 or 7 days but this time positive polarity was used throughout.[17]

Wound closure for 4-day treated rabbits was significantly less than that of 4-day control animals. After 7 days, however, treated and untreated rabbits had comparable wound closure values. Tensile strength was comparable for treated and untreated animals at both time periods. Histologic examination of wounds suggested that a more rapid rate of epithelialization occurred in treated animals between days 4 and 7. Results from this study suggest that the positive polarity had an adverse effect initially, but seemed to promote a more rapid rate of healing thereafter.

In a third follow-up study examining the polarity issue, rabbits were treated for 3 days using negative polarity, high voltage pulsed stimulation.[4] After the third treatment day polarity was changed to positive and rabbits were treated with positive polarity stimulation for another 4 days. Wound closure for stimulated rabbits was 100%. This was significantly better than that of control rabbits (87%).

Histologic examination of the wounds suggested a faster rate of epithelialization in treated rabbits at both time periods. Results may indicate that wound potentials are an important determinant of polarity in acute wounds. Burr and associates[30] measured wound potentials in guinea pigs and found that, for the first 3 or 4 days of healing, wound potentials were always positive, but after the fourth day wound potentials were negative. Potentials remained negative until complete healing occurred. Thus, choosing polarity on the basis of probable wound potentials seems to be appropriate in the early phases of uncomplicated healing.

For chronic wounds, alternating polarity throughout the course of treatment appears to be important in some studies and not important in others.[2,20,22,23,31-33] Kloth and Feedar[22] reported that 4 of the 12 Stage IV skin ulcers they treated with anodal current stopped responding to treatment after an unspecified amount of time. Wound healing appeared to plateau, but when polarity was changed the healing process was once again augmented. These four patients reached a second healing plateau during the course of treatment and polarity was alternated daily thereafter. The remainder of the patients (n=8) were treated with anodal stimulation throughout the course of the study.

In another study, Feedar and associates[23] used negative polarity for the first 3 days with Stage III and IV ulcers. The polarity was then changed every 3 days until the ulcers healed to Stage II. Polarity was changed daily for stimulation of Stage II ulcers in their study.

Griffin and associates[25] used only negative polarity stimulation for 20 days on their spinal cord patients with pressure ulcers. All of the patients in this study responded favorably to treatment although the rate of healing was variable. Consistent decreases in wound surface area were observed and there was no evidence of a plateau in the rate of decrease in ulcer size. Perhaps the need to alter polarity becomes apparent with longer treatment times. Kloth and Feedar[22] treated their patients for an average of 7.3 weeks as opposed to the 20 days of treatment given by Griffin and associates.[25]

Unger and associates[27] alternated polarity for their group of patients. They began treatment using negative polarity but switched to positive polarity after the sixth day until wounds were healed. The

Table 12-1. **Polarity Effects on Wound Healing**

Negative Polarity	Positive Polarity
Epidermal proliferation, migration	Attracts macrophages to area
Increases blood flow	Epithelial growth
Fibroblast proliferation	Stimulates formation of new capillaries
Enhanced collagen synthesis in fibroblasts	Bacteriocidal effect
Attract neutrophils to area	
Lyses necrotic tissue	
Edema reduction	
Stimulates granulation tissue growth	
Capillary growth	
Bacteriocidal effect	

average time to heal was 51.2 days for treated patients and 77 days for sham treated individuals. Rate of healing was 2.4 times greater for treated ulcers.

Taken together these studies seem to indicate that for chronic wounds, polarity should be changed for some patients and left unchanged for others. Perhaps measurement of wound potentials would provide the information needed to guide clinicians in their choice of polarity.

Wound closure is affected by infection, edema, and other factors which, taken together, also should influence choice of polarity, particularly in the initial stages of treatment. A summary of polarity effects is presented in Table 12-1.

CURRENT PARAMETERS

In the earlier days of ES treatment, current was applied for many hours during the day and sometimes for entire 24-hour periods. Low intensity direct current was utilized in the studies by Assimacopoulos,[3] Wu and associates,[15] and Gault and Gatens[21] to name a few. Current density for low intensity direct current is less than the current densities available with high intensity pulsed stimulation. Theoretically, the treatment time required for successful intervention should be less with high voltage stimulation. Indeed, the results presented by Kloth and Feedar support this notion.[22] They stimulated ulcers for 45 minutes 5 days a week and achieved a comparable rate of healing as Gault and Gatens[21], for example, who treated patients for 2 hours of every 6 (8 hours of stimulation per day), 7 days a week. Relatively short treatment times (1 hour daily) were used by Griffin and associates[25] who also reported successful results. The findings of Griffin and associates[25] further support shorter treatment times for protocols using high voltage pulsed stimulation. Stimulation treatment procedures, which are reasonable to perform during daily treatment sessions in the clinic, are far more likely to be used routinely and be reimbursable.

The selection of a stimulation current is a bit like voodoo at the moment. In short, there are no standard parameters. Treatment parameters differ considerably in the studies that have achieved successful healing. Even though successful, it is unknown if treatment could have been more successful had current been weaker or stronger or applied for longer or shorter periods of time. Feedar and associates[23] believed that Stage II ulcers require low pulse frequency compared to Stage III and IV ulcers because of the risk of over charge with high frequency on Stage II ulcers.

Reich and Tarjan[35] recently attempted to clarify the ambiguities associated with dose selection. They converted known information concerning electrode size (if available) and current intensity to enable comparison of some of the studies currently in print. Using average spatial current density (amount of current per unit area) and equivalent duty cycle, they tried to get a sense of what was an appropriate treatment dose. They indicate that there is a trend suggesting that an absolute charge density of 0.1 to 2.0 mA/cm^2 may be effective. Reich and Tarjan[35] make it clear that their evidence is far from conclusive, but these treatment parameters warrant further investigation. The essentials of their findings are presented in Table 12-2.

ELECTRODE PLACEMENT

One aspect of high voltage stimulation that needs to be mentioned is that the active and dispersive electrodes are of different sizes. Typically, the active electrode, which is placed directly over the wound, is one fourth the size of the dispersive electrode. Thus, to use this form of stimulation, electrodes need to be cut to the appropriate sizes.

Placement of a dispersive or non-active electrode in reference to the active electrode is another area which has been the subject of controversy and must be addressed. Becker[34] theorized the concept of "current of injury," and found that the human body is normally polarized positively along the central spinal axis and negatively peripherally. The polarity gradient set up by the voltage potentials differential is the electromotive force driving the bioelectric circuits in the body and the current of injury. Based on the work of Becker, some researchers recommend the placement of the positive electrode proximally close to the origin of the spinal nerve root, and the negative electrode distally. In other words, while treating wounds with negative polarity, the dispersive or the positive electrode should be placed cephalically close to the spinal cord in relation to the negative electrode whenever possible, whereas while treating wounds with positive polarity, the dispersive or the negative electrode should be placed caudally farther away from the spinal cord in relation to the positive electrode whenever possible.

Kloth and Feedar[22] reported successful results by placing electrodes according to the current of injury concept. However, Griffin and associates[25] did not treat their patients using the current of injury concept but found wound closure values that were comparable to those of Kloth and Feedar.[22] Griffin and associates[25] questioned the utility of placing electrodes according to the current of injury.

PRECAUTIONS AND CONTRAINDICATIONS

ES is contraindicated in wounds associated with osteomyelitis. Stimulation of wounds with osteomyelitis may result in closure of the wound while the active infection may still be present in the bone. ES is also contraindicated in patients with cancer because of the possibility of stimulating neoplastic cells.

Table 12-2. Current Density and Published Results

Current Density (mA/cm²)	Results	Reference
.004	109% increase in collagen	13
.246	40% increase in tensile strength	19
.011	36% increase in tensile strength	17
.011	30% increase in healing rate	4
.168	56% increase in healing rate	22
.005	54% average change in wound surface area	25

Patients with demand-type cardiac pacemakers should not be treated with ES because of the possibility of interference with cardiac rhythm which may cause cardiac arrhythmia. Similarly, patients with a history of cardiac dysrhythmia should be carefully monitored during the treatment with ES. Further, application of electrode over carotid sinuses should also be avoided to prevent any sudden changes in blood pressure.

Use of ES during pregnancy is contraindicated since its safety during pregnancy has not been established. Further, while using ES, caution must be used in treating wounds which have been treated with topical agents containing metal ions such as povidone-iodine and mercurochrome. The wounds should be irrigated properly before treating with ES.

CONCLUSION

There is a growing body of literature to support the use of electrical stimulation for wound healing. Stimulation appears to speed the closure of wounds, even those that have resisted conventional care previously. Stimulation also seems to positively affect wound tensile strength, perhaps by stimulating fibroblastic activity (collagen secretion).[35-41]

There is reason to believe that high voltage pulsed stimulation is more effective than low voltage direct current. Changing polarity seems to be indicated in the early phases of wound treatment and alternating polarity may be required for chronic wounds as well. Finally, there is a charge density range that appears to be effective. It is hoped that, in another decade, decisions regarding treatment parameters can be made by clinicians with conviction, backed with the necessary evidence to support selection.

REFERENCES

1. Cruz NI, Bayron FE, Suarez AJ. Accelerated healing of full thickness burns by the use of high-voltage pulsed galvanic stimulation in the pig. *Ann Plast Surg.* 1989;23:49-54.
2. Lundeberg T, Kjartansson J, Samuelsson U. Effect of electrical nerve stimulation of healing of ischaemic skin flaps. *Lancet.* 1988;2:712-714.
3. Assimacopoulos D. Wound healing promotion by use of negative electric current. *Am J Surg.* 1968;34:423-431.
4. Brown M, McDonnell MK, Menton DN. Polarity effects on wound healing using electrical stimulation in rabbits. *Arch Phys Med Rehabil.* 1989;70:624-627.
5. Chu C-S, McManus AT, Okerberg CV, Mason AD, Pruitt BA. Weak direct current accelerates split-thickness graft healing on tangentially excised second-degree burns. *J Burn Care Rehabil.* 1991;12:285-293.
6. Mohr T, Akers TM, Landry RL. Effect of high voltage stimulation on edema reduction in the rat hind limb. *Phys Ther.* 1987;67:1703-1708.
7. Lindstrom B, Korsan-Bengtsen K, Jonsson O, Petruson B, Pettersson S, Wikstrand J. Electrically induced short-lasting tetanus of the calf muscles for prevention of deep vein thrombosis. *Br J Surg.* 1982;69:203-206.
8. Rowley BA. Electrical current effects on E. coli growth rates. *Proc Soc Exp Biol Med.* 1972;139:929-934.
9. Orida N, Feldman JD. Directional protrusive pseudopodial activity and motility in macrophages induced by extracellular electric fields. *Cell Motil.* 1982;2:243-255.
10. Snyder-Mackler L. Electrical stimulation for tissue repair. In: Snyder-Mackler L, Robinson AJ. *Clinical Electrophysiology.* Baltimore, MD: Williams and Wilkins. 1989:231-244.
11. Cummings JP. Additional therapeutic uses of electricity. In: Gersh MR. *Electrotherapy in Rehabilitation.* Philadelphia, PA: FA Davis Co; 1992:328-342.
12. Kloth LC, Feedar JA. Electrical stimulation in tissue repair. In: Kloth LC, McCulloch JM, Feedar JA. *Wound Healing: Alternatives in Management.* Philadelphia, PA: FA Davis Co; 1989:221-256.
13. Alvarez OM, Mertz PM, Smerbeck RV, Eaglstein WH. Healing of superficial skin wounds is stimulated by external electrical current. *J Invest Dermatol.* 1983;81:144-148.
14. Mertz PM, Davis SC, Eaglstein WH. Pulsed electrical stimulation increases the rate of epithelialization in partial thickness wounds. *Proceedings of the Biomedical Research and Growth Society.* Cleveland, OH; 1989. Abstract.
15. Wu KT, Go N, Dennis C, Enquist I, Sawyer PN. Effects of electric currents and interfacial potentials on wound healing. *J Surg Res.* 1967;7:122-128.
16. Bach S, Bilgrav K, Tawfiq T, et al. *Effect of electrical stimulation on healing of incisional wounds in skin.* Proc of the 2nd International Symposium on Tissue Repair. Tarpon Springs, FL: 1987. Abstract.
17. Brown M, McDonnell MK, Menton DN. Electrical stimulation effects on cutaneous wound healing in rabbits: a follow-up study. *Phys Ther.* 1988;68:955-960.
18. Brown M, Gogia PP. Effects of high voltage stimulation on cutaneous wound healing in rabbits. *Phys Ther.* 1987;67:662-667.
19. Smith J, Romansky N, Vomero J, Davis RH. The effect of electrical stimulation on wound healing in diabetic mice. *J Am Podiatry Assoc.* 1984;74:71-75.
20. Wolcott LE, Wheeler PC, Hardwicke HM, Rowley BA. Accelerated healing of skin ulcers by electrotherapy. *South Med J.* 1969;62:795-801.
21. Gault WR, Gatens PF. Use of low intensity direct current in management of ischemic skin ulcers. *Phys Ther.* 1976;56:265-269.
22. Kloth LC, Feedar JA. Acceleration of wound healing with high voltage, monophasic, pulsed current. *Phys Ther.* 1988;68:503-508.
23. Feedar J, Kloth L. Chronic dermal ulcer healing enhanced with monophasic pulsed electrical stimulation. *Phys Ther.* 1991;70:639-649.
24. Mulder GD. Treatment of open-skin wounds with electrical stimulation. *Arch Phys Med Rehabil.* 1991;72:375-377.
25. Griffin JW, Tooms RE, Mendius RA, Clifft JK, Vander Swaag R, El-Zeky F. Efficacy of high voltage pulsed current for healing of pressure ulcers in patients with spinal cord injury. *Phys Ther.* 1991;71:433-442.
26. Unger PG. Wound healing using high voltage galvanic stimulation. *Stimulus.* 1985;10:8-10.
27. Unger P, Eddy J, Raimastry S. A controlled study of the effect of high voltage pulse current (HVPC) on wound healing. *Phys Ther.* 1991;71(suppl):S119. Abstract.
28. Unger PG. A randomized clinical trial of the effect of HVPC on wound healing. *Phys Ther.* 1991;71(suppl):S118. Abstract.
29. Vanable JW, Harson LL, McGinnis ME. The role of endogenous electrical fields in limb regeration. *Prog Clin Biol Res.* 1983;110:587-596.
30. Burr HS, Harvey SC, Taffel M. Bio-electric correlates of wound healing. *Yale J Biol Med.* 1939;11:103-107.
31. Carley PJ, Wainapel SF. Electrotherapy for acceleration of wound healing: low intensity direct current. *Arch Phys Med Rehabil.* 1985;66:443-446.
32. Akers TK, Gabrielson AL. The effect of high voltage galvanic stimulation on the rate of healing of decubitus ulcers. *Biomed Sci Instrum.* 1984;20:99-100.

33. Dayton PD, Palladino SJ. Electrical stimulation of cutaneous ulcerations. *J Am Podiatr Med Assoc.* 1989;79:318-321.

34. Becker RO. The Body Electric. New York, NY: William Morrow & Co, Inc; 1985.

35. Reich JD, Tarjan PP. Electrical stimulation of skin. *Int J Dermatol.* 1990;29:395-400.

36. Gentzkow GD, Miller KH. Electrical stimulation for dermal wound healing. *Clin Podiatr Med Surg.* 1991;8:827-841.

37. Biedebach MC. Accelerated healing of skin ulcers by electrical stimulation and the intracellular mechanisms involved. *Acupun Electrother Res Int J.* 1989;14:43-60.

38. Ross CR, Segal D. High voltage galvanic stimulation: an aid to post-operative healing. *Current Podiatry.* 1981;30:19-25.

39. Becker RO. Electromagnetism and life. In: Marino AA. *Modern Bioelectricity.* New York, NY: Marcel Dekker; 1988:1-15.

40. Binder SA. Applications of low and high-voltage electrotherapeutic currents. In: Wolf SL. *Electrotherapy, Clinics in Physical Therapy.* New York, NY: Churchill Livingstone; 1981:1-24.

41. Carley LC, Lepley D. Effect of continuous direct electric current on healing wounds. *Surg Forum.* 1962;13:33-35.

Chapter 13

Oxygen Therapy for Wound Management

Prem P. Gogia, PhD, PT

Tissue oxygen studies indicate that most occurrences of nonhealing in wounds are due to tissue hypoxia. Tissue hypoxia causes increased edema, ischemia, and infection. It affects all phases of normal wound healing including phagocytosis, angiogenesis, wound contraction, epithelialization, and collagen synthesis. On the other hand, increased oxygen tension ameliorates the healing process. Increased oxygen tension improves phagocytic capabilities of leukocytes to destroy bacteria and other foreign materials. It enhances epithelialization and wound contraction, and it also causes increased collagen synthesis as well as improved cross-linking of the collagen fibers, thus improving wound tensile strength. Clinically, increased oxygen tension can be achieved by using oxygen therapy.

Currently, there are two forms of oxygen therapy: hyperbaric oxygen therapy and topical oxygen therapy. In hyperbaric oxygen therapy, patients inhale oxygen at barometric pressure greater than sea level. In topical hyperbaric oxygen therapy, oxygen is administered topically at intermittent pressures in an extremity or a sacral chamber. The purposes of this chapter are to describe the effects of tissue hypoxia and increased oxygen tension on wound healing, to review wound healing literature pertinent to hyperbaric oxygen therapy and topical oxygen therapy for most common types of ulcers, and to review their indications, contraindications, and side effects.

TISSUE HYPOXIA

Tissue hypoxia is a fundamental problem that results in chronic nonhealing wounds. Adequate supply of oxygen is vital for a rapid and effective wound healing and hypoxia can inhibit or disrupt the normal healing sequence in almost all phases. Anaerobic metabolism is possible in hypoxic tissue but aerobic metabolism and energy production is severely diminished in hypoxic wound environment. The amount of ADP and ATP decreases in hypoxic wounds as does the body's immune system's ability to fight against infection. It also impairs the leukocytes' capabilities of killing common aerobic organisms found in wound infections and creates an ideal environment in which anaerobic organisms flourish.[1]

Fibroblast cells are highly susceptible to damage in a hypoxic environment and the rate of fibroblast proliferation decreases. Thus, collagen synthesis is significantly impaired with hypoxia, resulting in decreased wound strength.[2] Proliferation of epithelial cells is significantly diminished and wound contraction is also altered in a hypoxic wound environment. If long-term hypoxia is present in the wound during the course of healing, the healing process gradually comes to a halt.[3]

ROLE OF OXYGEN

The clinical importance of oxygen has been well established in all phases of wound healing. Oxygen is important for cell growth and cell division. Increased oxygen tension in the wound causes an increased RNA/DNA ratio indicating an enhanced differentiation of wound cells.[4] Oxygen is an essential component for elimination of pathogens, stimulation of phagocytosis as well as degradation of dead tissue structures, and synthesis of new tissue structures.[3] Hunt and Pai[5] and Niinikoski and Kulonen[6] investigated the effects of oxygen on several aspects of wound healing and demonstrated that the healing can be enhanced by raising the oxygen tension in the wound. This is partly due to improved energy supply provided by oxidative rather than glycolytic metabolism. Both laboratory and clinical studies indicate that oxygen is a precondition for various phases of normal wound healing such as phagocytosis and wound infection, epithelialization, angiogenesis, and collagen synthesis.

PHAGOCYTOSIS AND WOUND INFECTION

Oxygen deficiency is the most common contributor to inadequate wound repair and defense mechanism against infection. The probability of wound infection is significantly decreased when oxygen tension is increased. LaVan and Hunt[7] recommend use of supplemental oxygen in all patients who are at high risk of infection, who are undergoing a surgical procedure, or who are in the acute recovery phase following injury. Phagocytosis of bacteria by leukocytes is important to intracellular killing.[8] This process stimulates a ten- to thirty-fold

increase in leukocyte oxygen consumption.[9] Infection results when sufficient bacteria are present to overwhelm the phagocytic response or to diminish its already poor oxygen supply to the point that intracellular killing cannot prevent infection.[10] Once leukocytes have internalized bacteria they must destroy them. This mechanism is also oxygen dependent.

Increased oxygen tension ameliorates the ability of leukocytes to destroy invading microorganisms. Raising the PO_2 from 45 to 150 mmHg has been shown to increase leukocyte killing effectiveness by 40% in in vitro studies.[11,12] In the presence of oxygen, leukocytes marginate, migrate, and digest bacteria by the process of phagocytosis. Phagocytosis activates a membrane-bound enzyme that reduces extracellular molecular oxygen to superoxide which it inserts into phagosomes. Within phagosomes, an enzyme system converts superoxide to a number of high energy, bactericidal oxygen radicals without which bacterial killing is less than optimal. Oxygen is also required by neutrophils for creation of free oxygen radicals that kill bacteria.[8] Infection is reported to become less invasive or even failed to develop in hyperoxygenated guinea pigs when bacteria were injected into the skin.[9] Hunt and associates[10] reported that the susceptibility of wounds to infection could be diminished by increasing wound oxygen supply thereby changing the phagocytic defense system.

EPITHELIALIZATION

It is commonly observed that wounds heal poorly at high altitude where the oxygen tension is low,[5] while they heal quickly under the sea level where oxygen tension is high.[13] Epithelial cell migration is highly energy dependent. Their replication rate is also oxygen dependent. Silver[14] suggested that direct access of pure oxygen to the surface of open wounds would promote both epidermal cell migration and proliferation. Cultured epithelium has also been reported to preserve its viability under strictly anaerobic conditions for at least a week, but oxygen availability was an essential component for cell growth and cell division.[15] Regeneration of epithelial cells is increased by five- to ten-fold in an oxygen enriched environment in open wounds.[5] The closure rate of open, full-thickness skin wounds is reportedly enhanced in rats exposed to increased oxygen.[5] Fischer[16] reported improved epithelialization and contraction of chronic pressure ulcers when pure oxygen was administered topically, and under pressure. Increased epithelialization, wound contraction, collagen synthesis, and maturation has been reported with topical application of humidified oxygen on experimental third-degree burns in unrestrained guinea pigs.[17]

COLLAGEN SYNTHESIS

Fibroblast cells are aerobic cells and require oxygen for both division and collagen synthesis. They do not migrate properly when the tissue oxygen tension is less than 10 mmHg.[18] Fibroblast cells can survive but cannot synthesize collagen without oxygen.[5] Fibroblasts in vitro are reported to produce an intracellular polypeptide collagen precursor, but fail to release it in hypoxia. However, collagen is produced when oxygen is made available once again. Hydroxylation of lysine and proline molecules are required for export of protein and its incorporation into fibers. Tsurufuji and Ogata[19] suggested that synthesis and maturation of collagen depend on aerobic cellular activities. Kao and associates[2] found a significant increase in collagen synthesis when the atmospheric oxygen was increased from 21% to 95%. Similar results were also obtained by Lampiaho and Kulonen.[20] It is suggested that the atmospheric derived oxygen is necessary to form both intermolecular and intramolecular cross-linking in the collagen tissue.[21] Udenfriend[22] showed that intermolecular cross-linking and the final assembly of the molecule of the protein cannot proceed without oxygen. Cross-linking and maturation of collagen filaments in chick embryo skin slices were reported to increase linearly when the oxygen concentration of incubation gas was elevated from 20% to 95%.[23]

Hunt and Pai[5] also reported correlation between inspired oxygen and collagen synthesis over the range of 14% to 40%. Breathing a 45% oxygen mixture promoted healing of full-thickness skin wounds in rats while reduced oxygen tension resulted in a slower healing rate. Experimentally incised wounds in rats breathing a high concentration of oxygen had increased tensile strength.[24] Niinikoski[25] reported that a critical wound oxygen tension under which accumulation of collagen is definitely impaired is approximately 20 mmHg. In animals, the rate of collagen synthesis and the tensile strength are reported to increase approximately 50% by increasing arterial pressure of oxygen from 80 to 200 torr (approximately 0.1 to 0.26 atmospheric pressure absolute).[26] Niinikoski[27] reported an increase of 25% in tensile strength in 50% oxygen.

ANGIOGENESIS

Formation of new granulation tissue is dependent on the formation and extension of new blood vessels into the wound space. Knighton and associates[28] have shown that a high arterial oxygen pressure drives angiogenesis into hypoxic spaces. On the other hand, exposure of the central wound to high levels of oxygen arrests vessel growth. This is due to production of angiogenesis factor by macrophages when the wound environment is hypoxic. Wound oxygen tensions do not reach sufficiently high levels to terminate production of this factor until sufficient capillary ingrowth has occurred.[29,30]

OXYGEN THERAPY

Oxygen tension in hypoxic wounds can be increased by using oxygen therapy. Oxygen therapy is used to enhance oxygenation of the affected tissues in the wound. Increased tissue oxygen enhances the growth of fibroblasts, production of collagen tissue, angiogenesis, and the phagocytic capabilities of the hypoxic leukocytes.[31] A number of animal as well as clinical studies support its efficacy of enhanced healing of open wounds.

There are two forms of oxygen therapy: hyperbaric oxygen therapy and topical oxygen therapy. The hyperbaric oxygen therapy delivers oxygen via the dermal capillaries to the wound vicinity, and thereafter by diffusion through granulation tissue with inadequate blood supply.[32] The topical oxygen therapy delivers the oxygen directly to the wound bed and dissolves in tissue fluids.[32]

HYPERBARIC OXYGEN THERAPY

Hyperbaric oxygen therapy (HBO) was first used in 1964 to prevent necrosis of skin grafts and flaps and to treat traumatic and vascular ulcers.[34] Thereafter, HBO has been commonly recommended for chronic, nonhealing, open wounds. HBO is defined as the intermittent administration of 100% oxygen inhaled at barometric pressure greater than sea level. It is believed that wounds with markedly compromised blood flow and oxygen supply respond favorably to HBO. The HBO increases capillary PO_2 tension and promotes perfusion of oxygen, thereby increasing the amount of oxygen available for the repairing cells. Enhanced healing of rat and pig skin wounds has been reported by intermittent treatment in hyperbaric oxygen. Both clinical and experimental studies demonstrate that HBO enhances wound healing, improves flap survival, and also limits necrosis in free composite graft.[33,35] Rates of epithelialization in normal and ischemic wounds have been reported to be enhanced when HBO is administered at 1 to 2 atmospheric pressure absolute (ATA). LaVan and Hunt[7] recommend the use of HBO if an infected space in the wound cannot be sufficiently vascularized with debridement and flap reconstruction. However, a few studies have also shown either no effect or only marginal effect on wound healing from HBO.[36-38] Although infrequent, the adverse effects of HBO on wound healing have also been reported.[39] It is recommended that tissue oxygen tension be carefully monitored when wounds are treated with HBO. HBO can stop progression of infection in open wounds. Cohn[31] believes that HBO is an adjunct treatment only and must always be used with appropriate antibiotic therapy and surgical debridement. If large vessels are occluded and collateral circulation is compromised, HBO may not be beneficial in wound healing.[40]

There are two types of full body HBO chambers: monoplace chambers and multiplace chambers. Monoplace chambers (Figure 13-1) accommodate a single patient while the multiplace chambers can accommodate several patients who breathe 100% oxygen through a face mask, head hood, or endotracheal tube at ambient air pressures. Patients inhale oxygen at 2 to 2.5 ATA for 90 to 120 minutes, once or twice a day depending on the condition of the wound. Clinical applications of HBO include treatment of a variety of open wounds such as nonhealing surgical wounds, crush injury wounds, frostbite, animal bites, pressure ulcers, venous and arterial ulcers, and diabetic wounds. For the purpose of this chapter, HBO literature related to most common types of ulcers such as venous, arterial, diabetic, and pressure ulcers will be reviewed.

VENOUS ULCERS

Slack[41] used HBO to treat 15 patients with varicose ulcers of the legs. The patients were treated at 2.5 ATA once a day in a monoplace chamber. He reported improvement in healing of the ulcers. Many ulcers remained healed for more than 6 months. Duration of treatment and healing time was not documented. Slack recommended use of HBO for varicose ulcers when conventional treatment fails. Bass[42] treated 19 patients with chronic venous stasis ulcers. The patients received HBO at 2 ATA for 2 hours daily. Complete healing of the ulcers was obtained in 17 of 19 patients with a mean of 60.7 hours of treatment. Usually, HBO is not recommended for uncomplicated venous ulcers since these ulcers usually heal well by ligation and stripping of the veins. However, HBO may be beneficial in venous ulcers prior to skin graft.

ARTERIAL ULCERS

Kidokoro and associates[43] used HBO at 2 to 2.5 ATA in 22 patients with pain and leg ulcers due to arterial insufficiency. Fifteen of their patients obtained relief of pain at rest while ulcers healed in 12 patients. Hart and Strauss[44] used HBO at 2 ATA to treat 16 patients with arterial insufficiency ulcers. These patients failed to respond to conventional treatments. They reported complete healing of ulcers in 75% of their patients. Similarly, Perrins and Barr[45] treated 50 patients with HBO at 1.5 to 3.0 ATA and reported complete healing of arterial insufficiency ulcers in 52% of their patients. Yagi[46] treated 95 patients with infected ischemic ulcers using HBO and reported healing in 62 of 95 patients (65%). The HBO may play little or no role in advanced arterial insufficiency and inadequate microvascular circulation.

DIABETIC ULCERS

In diabetic ulcers, HBO promotes healing by supplementing host defenses and by exerting a bacteriostatic effect on anaerobic organisms.[47] Hart and Strauss[44] used HBO at 2 ATA to treat 11 patients with diabetic ulcers of the lower extremities. They reported observing a fair response in all patients, but only two of their patients achieved complete healing. On the contrary, Weisz and associates[48] treated 14 patients with chronic, nonhealing diabetic ulcers with HBO at 2.5 ATA and reported complete healing in 11 patients and partial healing in one patient. Doctor and associates[49] reported better control of infection and decreased number of amputations in patients with chronic diabetic ulcers. Perrins and Barr[45] also reported healing in 67% of their patients with diabetic ulcers who received HBO. Further, amputation was avoided in 18% of the cases. Similarly, Baroni and associates[50] performed a prospective controlled clinical study in patients with diabetic foot infections and partial foot gangrene. They reported complete healing in 16 of the 18 patients who received daily HBO at 2.5 to 2.8 ATA for 90 minutes. Two patients had amputation while, in the control group, 4 of the 10 patients underwent amputation and only 1 patient improved. Similar results were observed among older patients with diabetic ulcers and large vessel disease.[51] It is believed that HBO may not be of benefit in the most extreme diabetic wounds, however, its benefit in the marginally perfused diabetic ulcers may be significant.

PRESSURE ULCERS

Rosenthal and Schurman[52] used HBO to treat 18 patients with pressure ulcers. The patients had 38 pressure ulcers. Complete healing of the ulcers was reported in 58% of the cases while an additional 13% were reduced by at least half their original size. Similarly, Eltorai[53] used HBO to treat 27 patients with pressure ulcers covered by inadequately vascularized skin flaps. He reported complete intake of 74% of the flaps. Eltorai recommended use of HBO when a skin flap is in danger of ischemia during surgery for pressure ulcers. Generally, the HBO is not recommended for uncomplicated pressure ulcers since proper dressing changes and skin flaps are usually successful in treating these ulcers.[1]

CONTRAINDICATIONS AND SIDE EFFECTS

HBO is contraindicated during uncontrolled fever and untreated pneumothorax. It is also contraindicated in upper respiratory infection, chronic sinusitis, and emphysema with carbon dioxide retention. Further, it is not recommended to use for patients with a history of asymptomatic pulmonary lesions and congenital spherocytosis. Although HBO is not contraindicated during pregnancy, clinicians might avoid treating a pregnant woman for a chronic, nonhealing wound.

There are several side effects of HBO. Oxygen seizures are reported in patients with prior history of seizure disorders, febrile patients, and patients who have been on steroids for a long time. Pulmonary toxicity is common due to prolonged treatments at high pressures of oxygen which produces lung tissue damage, irritation of the large airways, and a decrease in vital capacity. HBO is also reported to cause changes in visual acuity by enhancing growth of cataracts resulting in permanent visual changes. Pressure trauma to soft tissue-lined cavities such as the sinus and middle ear may occur with the application of HBO.

TOPICAL OXYGEN THERAPY

Topical oxygen therapy (THO) was first used

in 1932 as an "oxygen boot" to treat gangrene of the feet. Since that time, THO has been clinically used on the extremities as well as on pressure ulcers. THO is defined as the application of 100% surface equivalency of oxygen applied by pressure in a closed container sealed to a body part while the patient is maintained in a one atmospheric environment. THO directly forces oxygen into the wound base and directly diffuses the granulated tissue. With THO, increased oxygen tension in the open wound can be achieved without the risk of systemic oxygen toxicity. THO penetrates superficial tissues of the open wound and does not cause systemic absorption of oxygen. Further, much lower pressures of oxygen are needed to stimulate the superficial tissues, thereby reducing the risk of toxicity. Fischer[54] believed that THO is a simple, safe, and inexpensive means of increasing rate of wound healing and preparing wounds for surgical intervention. Complete healing of lower extremity ulcers of various etiologies has been reported,[55] however, endothelial cell toxicity has been reported in leg ulcers[56] treated with THO.

THO causes increased oxygen tension, promotes microcirculation, and also suppresses growth of bacteria in the wound. THO also eliminates or significantly reduces tissue edema, thereby reducing the chances of chronic inflammatory conditions. THO is reported to be more successful in patients with a good vascular supply.[55] THO is also more effective when the ulcers are free of nonviable tissue. Therefore, all necrotic tissue should be debrided prior to administration of THO. All topical ointments should be removed prior to the use of THO to improve the possibility of oxygen perfusion. However, LaVan and Hunt[7] believe that oxygen, when administered topically, has poor penetration through the skin, and that compromised blood flow secondary to external pressure makes it a less than optimal treatment. They believe that topical oxygen may be beneficial in minimizing superficial bacterial infections when blood supply and oxygen penetration are of less concern.

There are several different types of chambers used for THO therapy. One type is a disposable, one-piece polyethylene bag used for extremity ul-

cers. The disposable bag is placed over the involved extremity and the pressure is usually monitored by sphygmomanometer connected to bag. Another type of chamber is a nondisposable, two-piece plexiglas chamber used for extremity ulcers (Figure 13-2). This type of chamber is built to fit around the involved extremity and seals around it. The oxygen is delivered to the chamber through rubber tubing and the regulated pressure is monitored through a control box. Yet another type of chamber is a nondisposable, single piece rubber cushion used for ulcers located on the sacrum. This type of chamber is built to fit around the sacrum and to secure in place with a body strap. The oxygen is delivered to the chamber through rubber tubing and the regulated pressure is monitored through a control box.

The recommended treatment varies from twice a day for 90 minutes each, to once a day for 120 minutes. Oxygen compression ranges from 10 to 50 mmHg while decompression is to 0 mmHg. Oxygen is cycled every 20 to 30 seconds and flow rates range from 1 to 4 L/min. Clinical applications of THO include treatment of a variety of open wounds such as: nonhealing crush injury wounds, frostbite, animal bites, pressure ulcers, venous and arterial ulcers, and diabetic wounds. For the purpose of this chapter, THO literature related to most common types of ulcers such as arterial, venous, diabetic, and pressure ulcers will be reviewed.

VENOUS ULCERS

THO has been most successful in treating venous ulcers.[55] Fischer[16] used THO at 22 mmHg and oxygen flow rate of 2 to 8 L/min to treat 16 patients with venous stasis ulcers of 5 months to 24 years duration. The average healing time was 15 days. All ulcers had been unsuccessfully treated by other conservative treatments before being treated with THO. In another similar study, Fischer[54] treated three cases of venous stasis ulcers of 6 months to 35 years of duration with THO at 22 mmHg and oxygen flow rate of 4 L/min. These ulcers also had failed to respond to other local treatments. Fischer observed a prompt arrest of inflammation, a decrease in edema, and an increase in granulation

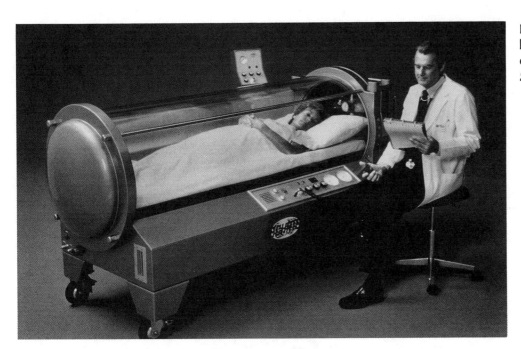

Figure 13-1. Monoplace hyperbaric oxygen therapy (HBO) chamber. *Photo courtesy of Sechrist Industries, Inc.*

tissue in these wounds. The wound closure took 2 to 7 weeks. Kravitz[57] treated 20 patients with chronic venous stasis ulcers of 6 months to 9 years duration. Ten patients received whirlpool treatment, while the remaining 10 patients received THO daily for 12 weeks. She concluded that the THO was a more beneficial approach than the conventional whirlpool treatment both for re-epithelialization and edema reduction. Jackson and associates[58] presented their experience with THO and pinch grafting. Patients with stasis ulcers of 4 months to 10 years duration were treated daily for 3 days to 2 weeks with THO. Patients then received pinch grafts.

Follow-up examinations made 8 to 28 months later revealed complete healing of three grafts without complications, loss of one pinch graft because of infection but healed with THO. The use of THO for the initial treatment of these wounds seemed to increase granulation tissue and decrease necrotic tissue. No side effects were observed and the patients receiving THO were observed to have shorter hospitalization compared to similar patients not treated with THO. In treating venous ulcers, Heng[59] recommended 18 to 20 mmHg above atmospheric pressure. Higher pressure is considered detrimental since in venous ulcers, the venous pressure is so high that the pressure driving blood from the arteriolar end of the capillary to the venous end may be less than 1 mmHg.

ARTERIAL ULCERS

THO is reported to be most effective in ulcers with adequate blood supply. A higher rate of failure is found in ulcers with poor blood supply.[55] Heng and associates[60] treated chronic arterial ulcers with THO. In the experimental group, 18 of 27 ulcers healed within 6 to 21 days while 7 other ulcers reduced 50% to 90% of their original size after 3 weeks of treatment. In the control group, none of 10 ulcers healed. In another study, Heng[61] reported the effects of THO on leg ulcers, including ischemic ulcers. Ulcers developed abundant granulation tissue which filled up the wound from the base towards the epidermal surface. Heng[62] also treated a patient with polyarteritis and a deep ulcer of the heel. The ulcer healed completely without the need of a skin graft. Olejniczak and Zielinski[63] also reported 33% healing of ischemic ulcers treated with THO at 5 to 12 mmHg (depending upon patients' tolerance) for 20 minutes twice daily.

DIABETIC ULCERS

Ignacio and associates[64] used THO at 16 to 20 mmHg to treat 17 patients with diabetic ulcers. The

Figure 13-2. Topical hyperbaric oxygen therapy (THO) chamber.

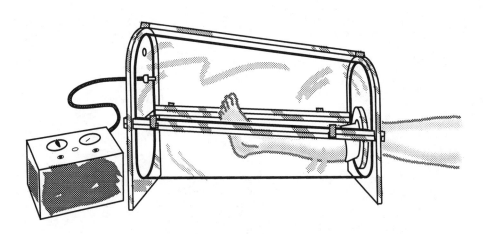

patients were treated for 45 minutes twice a day, 6 days a week. They observed excellent healing in their diabetic patients. Similarly, Singer and associates[65] treated 65 patients who had diabetic ulcers with THO at 2 ATA. Fifteen patients were treated with THO while the remaining 50 patients were treated with conservative treatments not described. The wounds treated with THO healed significantly faster and with significant granulation tissue compared with the other group. The time spent in bed was also significantly shorter for patients treated with THO. On the contrary, Leslie and associates[66] observed no benefit of THO in an experimental group of 12 patients with diabetic foot ulcers who were treated for 90 minutes twice a day at pressures that cycled between 0 and 30 mmHg every 20 seconds. The control group consisted of 15 patients.

PRESSURE ULCERS

Torelli[67] used THO to treat nursing home patients with pressure ulcers. They reported successful healing of ulcers when treated with THO in conjunction with standard medical care. Similarly, Fischer[17] treated 26 patients with pressure ulcers on the hips and sacral areas using THO and reported improvement in almost all patients within 6 hours of treatment. Increased granulation tissue and epithelialization was observed in lesions less than 6 cm in diameter. In lesions greater than 6 cm, THO sup-

pressed bacterial growth and stimulated granulation tissue. Fischer[54] also reported well-vascularized tissue in 16 patients with pressure ulcers on the ankle, heels, and medial aspect of knee when treated with THO. The duration of ulcers ranged from 2 months to $4^1/_2$ years. The ulcers did not respond to conventional treatment. With THO, total healing was achieved in all cases in a period of 2 weeks to 2 months. Similar results were reported by Gorecki[68] in a patient with bedsores infected of 9 months duration, located at the sacrum and right hip. In this case report, Gorecki used THO at a pressure of 15 mmHg for 15 minutes three to four times daily with oxygen flowing at 12 to 15 L/min. Both areas healed completely after about 4 weeks of treatment.

CONTRAINDICATIONS AND PRECAUTIONS

THO is contraindicated in the presence of acute thrombophlebitis because of the possibility of thrombus dislodge due to pressure variations. THO is also contraindicated in patients with large vessel occlusions. In patients with pseudomonas bacteria in the wound, the wound should be covered with a gauze soaked in acetic acid during THO administration. The acetic acid increases pH level in the wound and suppresses the growth of pseudomonas bacteria. Further, application of acetic acid dressings for 3 to 4 hours is recommended, following application of THO, when pseudomonas bacteria are present. Finally, while using THO, precautions must be taken with patients having altered mental status and for those who are unable to remain relatively immobile, since each treatment session lasts for 90 to 120 minutes.

CONCLUSION

Tissue hypoxia is the most common cause of chronic, nonhealing wounds. It causes increased edema, ischemia, and infection. Increased oxygen tension ameliorates the healing of wounds and results in enhanced epithelialization, improved contraction, and increased collagen synthesis and tensile strength. Hyperbaric oxygen therapy and topical oxygen therapy are used to increase oxygen tension in wounds. Hyperbaric oxygen therapy, although quite successful in treating open wounds, is expensive, requires specialized equipment, and has substantial risks of systemic oxygen toxicity to the central nervous system and the lungs. On the other hand, topical oxygen therapy is a low cost modality, equipment is readily available, and lacks systemic oxygen toxicity. However, the results presented in the literature pertinent to oxygen therapy should be interpreted with great caution. Many studies lack controls and the methods have not been described in detail. Further controlled, experimental studies are needed to establish the efficacy of these treatment modalities.

REFERENCES

1. *Hyperbaric Oxygen Therapy: A Committee Report.* Be thesda, MD: Undersea and Hyperbaric Medical Society; 1989.
2. Kao KY, Hitt WE, Dawson RL, McGavack TH. Connective tissue. VIII. Factors affecting collagen synthesis by sponge biopsy connective tissue. *Proc Soc Exper Biol.* 1963;113:762-766.
3. Kuhne HH, Ullmann U, Kuhne FW. New aspects on the pathophysiology of wound infection and wound healing: the problem of lowered oxygen pressure in the tissue. *Infection.* 1985;13:52-56.
4. Niinikoski J. Oxygen and wound healing. *Clin Plast Surg.* 1977;4:361-374.
5. Hunt TK, Pai MP. The effect of varying ambient oxygen tensions on wound metabolism and collagen synthesis. *Surg Gynec Obstet.* 1972;135:561-567.
6. Niinikoski J, Kulonen E. Reparation at increased oxygen supply. *Experientia (Basel).* 1970;26:247-248.
7. LaVan FB, Hunt TK. Oxygen and wound healing. *Clin Plast Surg.* 1990;17:463-472.
8. Hohn DC, Hunt TK. Oxidative metabolism and microbicidal activity of rabbit phagocytes: cells from wounds and from peripheral blood. *Surg Forum.* 1975;26:85-87.
9. Knighton DR, Holliday B, Hunt TK. Oxygen as an antibiotic: a comparison of the effects of inspired oxygen concentration and antibiotic administration on in vivo bacterial clearance. *Arch Surg.* 1986;121:191-195.
10. Hunt TK, Linsey M, Grislis G, Sonne M, Jawetz E. The effect of differing ambient oxygen tensions on wound infection. *Ann Surg.* 1975;181:35-39.
11. Hohn MD, MacKay RD, Holliday B, Hunt TK. The effect of oxygen tension on the microbicidal function of leukocytes in wounds and in vitro. *Surg Forum.* 1976;27:18-20.
12. Mader JT, Brown GL, Guckian JC, Wells CH, Reinarz JA. A mechanism for the amelioration by hyperbaric oxygen of experimental staphylococcal osteomyelitis in rabbits. *J Infect Dis.* 1980;142:915-922.
13. Gilbert DL. Perspective on the history of oxygen and life. In: Gilbert DL. *Oxygen and Living Processes. Interdisciplinary Approach.* New York, NY: Springer Verlag; 1981:1-43.
14. Silver IA. Wound healing and cellular microenvironment. Final technical report. *US Army R and D Command Contract DAJA.* 1971;37:70-2328.
15. Medawar PB. The behaviour of mammalian skin epithelium under strictly anaerobic conditions. *Quart J Microsc Sci.* 1947;88:27-37.
16. Fischer BH. Topical hyperbaric oxygen treatment of pressure sores and skin ulcers. *Lancet.* 1969;2:405-409.
17. Kaufman T, Alexander JW, Nathan P, MacMillan BG. Microclimate wound chamber: topical treatment of experimental deep burns with humidified oxygen. *Surg Forum.* 1982;33:607-609.
18. Jain KK. Hyperbaric oxygen therapy in wound healing. In: Jain KK. *Textbook of Hyperbaric Medicine.* Lewiston, NY: Hogrefe & Huber Publishers; 1990:193-202.
19. Tsurufuji S, Ogata Y. Biosynthesis of collagen in skin minces in relation to the mechanism of the formation of insoluble collagen. *Biochem Biophys Acta (Amst).* 1965;104:193-199.
20. Lampiaho K, Kulonen E. Metabolic phases during the development of granulation tissue. *Biochem J.* 1967;105:333-341.
21. Tanzer ML. Crosslinking of collagen. *Science.* 1973;180:561-566.
22. Udenfriend S. Formation of hydroxyproline in collagen. *Science.* 1966;152:1335-1340.
23. Chvapil M, Hurych J, Ehrlichova E. The influence of various oxygen tensions upon proline and hydroxylation and the metabolism of collagenous and non-collagenous proteins in skin slices. *Z Physiol Chem.* 1968;349:211-217.

24. Stephens EO, Hunt TK. Effect of changes in inspired oxygen and carbon dioxide tensions on wound tensile strength: an experimental study. *Ann Surg.* 1971;173:515-519.

25. Niinikoski J. *The effect of blood and oxygen supply on the biochemistry of repair.* Symposium on Wound Healing and Wound Infection. San Fransisco, CA; 1975.

26. Hunt TK. Disorders of wound healing. *World J Surg.* 1980;4:271-277.

27. Niinikoski J. Effect of oxygen supply on wound healing and formation of experimental granulation tissue. *Acta Physiol Scand.* 1969;337(suppl):1-72.

28. Knighton DR, Silver IA, Hunt TK. Regulation of wound-healing angiogenesis: effect of oxygen gradients and inspired oxygen concentration. *Surgery.* 1981;90:262-270.

29. Hunt TK, Conolly WB, Aronson SB. Anaerobic metabolism and wound healing: an hypothesis for the initiation and cessation of collagen synthesis in wounds. *Am J Surg.* 1978;135:328-332.

30. Jensen JA, Hunt TK, Scheuenstuhl H, et al. Effect of lactate, pyruvate and pH on secretion of angiogenesis and mitogenesis factors by macrophages. *Lab Invest.* 1986;54:574-578.

31. Cohn GH. Hyperbaric oxygen therapy: promoting healing in difficult cases. *Postgrad Med.* 1986;79:89-92.

32. Heng MCY. Topical hyperbaric therapy for problem skin wounds. *J Dermatol Surg Oncol.* 1993;19:784-793.

33. McFarlane RM, Wermuth RE. The use of hyperbaric oxygen to prevent necrosis in experimental pedicle flaps and composite skin grafts. *Plast Reconstr Surg.* 1964;37:422-430.

34. Slack W. Hyperbaric oxygen in the treatment of trauma, ischemic disease of limbs and vericose ulcers. In: Brown IW, Cox B. *Proceedings of the Third International Conference on Hyperbaric Medicine.* National Academy of Sciences, National Research Council. Washington, DC: 1966:621-624.

35. Niinikoski J. Viability of ischemic skin flaps in hyperbaric oxygen. In: Trapp WG, Banister EW, Davison AJ, et al. *Fifth International Hyperbaric Congress Proceedings.* Vol 1. Canada: Simon Fraser University Press; 1974:244-252.

36. Kernahan DA, Zingg W, Kay CW. Effect of hyperbaric oxygen on the survival of experiment skin flaps. *Plast Reconstr Surg.* 1965;36:19-25.

37. Kulonen E, Niinikoski J. Effect of hyperbaric oxygenation on wound healing and experimental granuloma. *Acta Physiol Scand.* 1968;73:383-384.

38. Lundgren C, Sandberg N. Influence of hyperbaric oxygen on the tensile strength of healing wounds in rats. In: Ledingham IM. *Hyperbaric Oxygenation: Proceedings of the Second International Cogress.* London: ES Livingstone Ltd; 1965:393-396.

39. Irvin T, Smith G. Treatment of bacterial infections with hyperbaric oxygen. *Surgery.* 1968;63:363-376.

40. Strauss MB. Role of hyperbaric oxygen therapy in acute ischemia and crush injuries: an orthopaedic perspective. *Hyperbaric Oxygen Review.* 1981;2:87-106.

41. Slack WK. A hyperbaric unit for your hospital? *Hospital Practice.* 1966;1(3):42-47.

42. Bass SH. The treatment of varicose leg ulcers by hyperbaric oxygen. *Postgrad Med J.* 1970;46:407-408.

43. Kidokoro M, Sakakibara K, Takao T, et al. Experimental and clinical studies upon hyperbaric oxygen therapy for peripheral vascular disorders. In: Wanda J, Iwa T. *Proceedings of the Fourth International Congress on Hyperbaric Medicine.* Baltimore, MD: Williams and Wilkins; 1969:462-488.

44. Hart GB, Strauss MB. Responses of ischemic ulcerative conditions to OHP. In: Smith G. *Proceedings of the Sixth International Congress on Hyperbaric Medicine.* Aberdeen, WA: Aberdeen University Press; 1977:312-314.

45. Perrins JD, Barr PO. Hyperbaric oxygenagation and wound healing. In: Schmutz J. *Proceedings of the First Swiss Symposium on Hyperbaric Medicine.* Foundation for Hyperbaric Medicine. Basel; 1986:119-132.

46. Yagi H. On the hyperbaric oxygen therapy for severe infected granulation wounds (ulcers) of upper and lower extremities. *Jpn J Hyperbaric Med.* 1987;22:27-40.

47. Magnant CM, Milzman DP, Dhindsa H. Hyperbaric medicine for outpatient wound care. *Emegency Med Clin N Am.* 1992;10:847-860.

48. Weisz G, Ramon Y, Melamed Y. Treatment of the diabetic foot by hyperbaric oxygen. *Harefuah.* 1993;124:678-681.

49. Doctor N, Pandya S, Supe A. Hyperbaric oxygen therapy in diabetic foot. *J Postgrad Med.* 1992;38:112-114.

50. Baroni G, Porro T, Faglia E, et al. Hyperbaric oxygen in diabetic gangrene treatment. *Diabetes Care.* 1987;10:81-86.

51. Kucan J, Robson M. Diabetic foot infections: fate of the contralateral foot. *Plast Reconstr Surg.* 1986;77:439-441.

52. Rosenthal AM, Schurman A. Hyperbaric treatment of pressure sores. *Arch Phys Med Rehabil.* 1971;52:413-415.

53. Eltorai I. Hyperbaric oxygen in the management of pressure sores in patients with injuries to the spinal cord. *J Dermatol Surg Oncol.* 1981;7:37-40.

54. Fischer BH. Treatment of ulcers on the legs with hyperbaric oxygen. *J Dermatol Surg.* 1975;1:55-58.

55. Diamond E, Forst MB, Hyman SA, Rand SA. The effect of hyperbaric oxygen on lower extremity ulcerations. *J Am Pod Assoc.* 1982;72:180-185.

56. Heng MCY, Kloss SG. Endothelial cell toxicity in leg ulcers treated with topical hyperbaric oxygen. *Am J Dermatol.* 1986;8:403-410.

57. Kravitz S. *Comparison of whirlpool and hyperbaric oxygen in the healing of venous stasis ulcers.* New York University; 1984. Thesis.

58. Jackson B. *Topical hyperbaric oxygen therapy.* Presented at the Scientific Study area at the 1987 AAD Meeting. Veterans Administration Hospital and University of Tennessee, Memphis, TN. Unpublished material; 1987.

59. Heng MCY. Venous leg ulcers: the post-phlebitic syndrome. *Int J Dermatol.* 1978;26:14-21.

60. Heng MCY, Pilgrim JP, Beck FWJ. A simplified hyperbaric oxygen technique for leg ulcers. *Arch Dermatol.* 1984;120:640-645.

61. Heng MC. Local hyperbaric oxygen administration for leg ulcers. *Br J Dermatol.* 1983;109:232-234. Editorial.

62. Heng MCY. Hyperbaric oxygen therapy for a foot ulcer in a patient with polyarteritis nodosa. *Aust J Dermatol.* 1983;24:105-108.

63. Olejniczak S, Zielinski A. Low hyperbaric therapy in the management of leg ulcers. *Mich Med.* 1975;74:707-712.

64. Ignacio DR, et al. *Treatment of extensive limb ulcers with the use of topical hyperbaric oxygen therapy.* Greater Southeast Community Hospital, Washington DC; 1983.

65. Singer P. *Concerning the initial results from the treatment of diabetic gangrene with a chamber for local high pressure oxygen treatment.* Berlin: Berlitz Translation Service, Berlitz School of Language of America, Central Institute for Cardiac and Circulatory Research, 1978.

66. Leslie CA, Sapico FL, Ginunas VJ, Adkins RH. Randomized controlled trial of topical hyperbaric oxygen for treatment of diabetic foot ulcers. *Diabetes Care.* 1988;11:111-115.

67. Torelli M. Topical oxygen for decubitus ulcers. *Am J Nurs.* 1973;73:494-496.

68. Gorecki Z. Oxygen under pressure applied directly to bedsores: case report. *J Am Ger Soc.* 1964;12:1147-1148.

Chapter 14

Ultrasound for Wound Management

Mary Dyson, PhD, CBiol, MIBiol

Ultrasound, a mechanical vibration transmitted at a frequency above the range of human hearing, can be used both therapeutically to stimulate the rate of wound healing and diagnostically to monitor the rate of healing. The purpose of this chapter is to present both of these applications of ultrasound as they relate to wound management.

THERAPEUTIC ULTRASOUND

When used correctly, ultrasound therapy can be a highly effective means of increasing the rate of healing of acute wounds and of stimulating the healing of some types of chronic wounds, such as venous stasis ulcers and pressure ulcers, provided that the health of the patient is not too greatly impaired and that suitable environmental conditions are maintained. There is now considerable evidence that ultrasound therapy can act as a stimulus to cells involved in the process of wound healing, particularly those of the inflammatory and early proliferative phases of healing. The main features of ultrasound therapy will be briefly described, followed by its effects on the cellular events which follow soft tissue injury and which result in repair.

DIAGNOSTIC ULTRASOUND

Until recently, many of the reports of the clinical effectiveness of ultrasound therapy and other forms of therapy in the treatment of wounds were based on subjective assessment of the progress of healing. There was clearly a need for a clinical method that is noninvasive, painless, and objective as well as reliable and repeatable to assess wound healing. Recent advances in high resolution diagnostic ultrasound and image analysis have led to the development of portable scanners which provide the information required in a readily interpretable form. It is envisaged that the use of this equipment, which will be briefly described in this chapter, will allow clinicians involved in the treatment of wounds the ability to monitor the effectiveness of their treatments and modify them as required.

PROPERTIES OF ULTRASOUND

Like sound, ultrasound is a mechanical disturbance in which molecules of the medium into which it is transmitted vibrate in a cyclical fashion. Both sound and ultrasound are transmitted as waves consisting of regions where the molecules are alternately pulsed together and separated. In the case of sound the frequency of this cyclical vibration is low enough to be detected by the human ear, whereas in the case of ultrasound the frequency is above this limit of 20 kiloHertz, that is, 20,000 cycles per second. In liquids and soft tissues the waves are longitudinal, i.e., the molecules are displaced parallel to the direction in which the wave travels. At the interphase between soft tissue and hard tissue, such as bone, mode conversion occurs with the result that some of the ultrasound is transmitted as transverse or shear waves in which the molecules are displaced at right angles to the direction in which the wave is propagated. This is clinically important because mode conversion produces an increase in temperature at the interface in the case of soft tissue and at the periosteum in the case of bone.[1] If the incident intensity is too high, it can cause tissue damage and associated pain. It is therefore recommended that the intensities used be kept to low levels which have been found to be therapeutically effective,[2] typically 0.1 to 0.2 W/cm^2 when averaged in space and time. Other clinically significant features of ultrasound are its frequency (to which wavelength is inversely proportional) and amplitude.

Frequency is the number of times per second that a molecule is displaced by the ultrasound and returns to its original position. Most therapeutic ultrasound equipment produces ultrasound at frequencies of 0.5 to 3.0 MHz, but equipment operating at lower KHz frequencies is also available and has been used to cleanse the skin, debride necrotic tissue,[3] reduce pain, and relieve muscular spasm.[4] High frequency ultrasound is more readily absorbed and less penetrative than lower frequencies, therefore, 3.0 MHz is a suitable frequency for treating superficial tissues such as those of injured skin, whereas lower frequencies are more appropriate for deeper tissues such as tendon, muscle, and the joint capsule. When ultrasound reaches the interface between materials with different acoustic properties (e.g., tissue fluid and collagen) some of the ultrasound is transmitted and some reflected. Transduc-

ers used to produce ultrasound can also be used to receive the reflected signals which can then be digitized and converted into images of the tissues exposed to the ultrasound. Provided that sufficiently high frequencies (20 MHz) are used, ultrasound can be used diagnostically to image injured and healing tissues noninvasively. High resolution ultrasound, having higher frequencies than those used therapeutically, has been used to detect the depth of burns and, by using fractal analysis of B-scans, to monitor repair objectively.[5,6] Frequency (f), wavelength (l), and resolution are related in such a manner that the higher the frequency, the shorter the wavelength and the greater the resolution. Wavelength is thus inversely proportional to frequency but also directly proportional to the velocity (c) of ultrasound. In soft tissue c is approximately the same as in water (about 1500 m/s). So if, for example, f = 1 MHz (a typical therapeutic frequency), then l = 1.5 mm. With the higher frequencies used to image superficial tissues the wavelengths are much shorter and the resolution therefore much greater.

Amplitude is the maximum molecular displacement produced when ultrasound is transmitted. Amplitude increases with intensity, the latter usually being measured in W/cm^2. The intensity and amplitude have to be sufficiently great to produce permeability changes in cell membranes for biologically and clinically significant effects to occur. The levels of all these parameters are important in determining what effects ultrasound has on the tissues it is absorbed by.

Ultrasound can be transmitted through, reflected, refracted, or absorbed by different components of tissues. Only when ultrasound is absorbed, and at a sufficient level, can it produce any therapeutic effect. However, if too much ultrasound is absorbed, the effects can be damaging.[2] Partial or total reflection occurs when the ultrasound wave reaches an interface between two media of differing acoustic impedance. A change in the direction of wave propagation also occurs at these interfaces due to refraction. The amount of reflection and refraction is directly proportional to the difference in acoustic impedance of the two media forming the interface.

Since water and soft tissue have closely similar acoustic impedances, little reflection or refraction occur at the interfaces between them, whereas much more occurs between air and soft tissue or between soft tissue and bone, whose acoustic impedances are dissimilar. Unless the operator is aware of the position, type, and shape of these interfaces, the energy reaching the target tissues cannot be predicted. The medium used to transmit ultrasound from the treatment head to the patient should have a similar acoustic impedance to that of soft tissue to avoid excessive reflection and refraction.[7] For similar reasons, it should also be free of air bubbles. Some aqueous gel-based wound dressings, which can also be used to dress the wound after ultrasound treatment,[8] are suitable. With reflection, the interaction of the incident and reflected traveling waves can result in production of a stationary or standing wave; here the peaks of the two traveling waves coincide and summate at fixed positions. Damaging amplitudes can be produced from standing waves from an incident wave of an innocuous amplitude; the observed effects of stationary waves on tissue include the interruption of the flow of blood cells and damage to the endothelium lining the blood vessels.[9] There is also an increased risk of transient cavitation and associated free radical release with damaging consequences.[10] These responses can be avoided by moving the applicator throughout treatment so that the position of the peaks relative to the tissue is constantly changing. As the ultrasound travels through the tissues it is absorbed by them, its kinetic energy decreasing exponentially as it is transduced into heat. The half-value depth of penetration, that is the distance from the treatment head at which the energy remaining at the beam is half that emitted, varies with the absorption coefficient of the medium and the ultrasound frequency. Tissues with a high protein content and with little fat and water, such as muscle, tendon, and ligaments, absorb more ultrasound and are therefore heated by it more readily than are tissues with less protein and more water and fat such as areolar and adipose tissue.[11] Furthermore, low frequencies are absorbed less readily than high frequencies. Therefore, by selecting a lower frequency it is possible to deliver ultrasound to deeply located lesions such as joint capsules without excessively heating the more superficial adipose and areolar tissues.

PHYSICAL EFFECTS OF ULTRASOUND THERAPY

Therapeutic intensities of ultrasound can affect the activity of cells and tissues in a manner which stimulates wound healing, whereas higher intensities can be damaging.[12] An understanding of the physical mechanisms by which the therapeutic and damaging effects are produced can increase the ability of the clinician to use ultrasound effectively and safely. The physical mechanisms by which ultrasound produces its effects are usually classified as being predominantly either thermal or nonthermal.

THERMAL MECHANISMS

The temperature of the tissues exposed to ultrasound increases when the ultrasound is absorbed by them. The extent of this local heating is controlled by a number of factors, including the frequency and intensity of the ultrasound, the acoustic properties of the tissues in the path of the ultrasound, and the effectiveness of the circulation in dissipating the heat generated. If the local temperature reaches between 40° and 45° C, significant clinical effects such as hyperemia and decreased pain occur; however, temperatures greater than 45° C are damaging and must be avoided. Since some structures (e.g., periosteum) absorb ultrasound more readily than others, care must be taken when ultrasound is used over them.

NONTHERMAL MECHANISMS

Nonthermal mechanisms include stable and transient cavitation, acoustic streaming, and standing wave formation. They can accompany ultrasonically induced, clinically significant heating and may contribute to it, but they can also occur at lower intensities than those needed to produce heating, that is, less than 0.5 W/cm^2 spatially and temporally averaged in adequately perfused tissue. While there is evidence that stable cavitation and acoustic streaming can produce therapeutic changes in cells and tissues, transient cavitation and standing wave formation are damaging and should be avoided.

Cavitation

Cavitation is the formation of minute cavities (a few microns in diameter) by ultrasound. Low intensity, low amplitude ultrasound causes these cavities to vibrate in response to the variations in the pressure which occurs during each ultrasonic cycle. This is termed stable cavitation and can produce reversible changes in the permeability of the plasma membranes of cells located next to the cavities, acting as a signal to which the cells can respond.[13] High amplitude ultrasound can, however, cause the cavities to implode violently, which is termed transient cavitation, and this produces irreversible mechanical and chemical damage, the latter due to free radical formation affecting cells and some tissues adversely. Stable cavitation occurs readily in suspensions of cells in vitro when exposed to ultrasound therapy and may also occur in living tissues,[14] although the latter has been challenged by Watmough and associates.[15] Transient cavitation has not been detected in living tissues exposed to ultrasound therapy but has been produced in blood plasma exposed to therapeutic levels of ultrasound under conditions which produce standing waves.[10]

Acoustic Streaming

Acoustic streaming is the unidirectional flow of fluid induced by radiation forces. High velocity gradients are produced at boundaries between fluid and the cells and cavities it contains. High viscous forces associated with these gradients can modify membrane structure, temporarily changing the membrane permeability to second messengers such as calcium ions. This can stimulate cell activity with therapeutically valuable results.[2,16] There is evidence of increased uptake of calcium ions by fibroblasts exposed to therapeutic levels of ultrasound which could be due to the action on the plasma membrane of shear forces produced by acoustic streaming in the presence of stable cavitation.[13] Acoustic streaming can also occur in the absence of cavitation as a result of radiation torque.[17] Temporary increase in intracellular calcium ions could act as a signal for changes in the cell activity leading to a cascade of events as a result of which wound healing is accelerated. For example, in fibroblasts, protein synthesis is stimulated by ultrasound therapy,[18] in platelets the release of serotonin (and presumably stimulators of wound healing such as platelets derived growth factor) is induced,[19] in mast cells the release of histamine (and possibly angiogenic heparin) is stimulated,[20] and in macrophages growth factor release is increased.[21] The observed acceleration of wound healing following exposure to ultrasound therapy could be due to the collective effects of these cellular events.

Standing Wave Formation

Standing waves may be formed when ultrasound is reflected at the interface between two acoustically different media such as soft tissue and bone or soft tissue and air. When a standing wave is produced the pressure antinodes (peaks) of the incident and reflected waves are superimposed, stationary, and separated by half a wavelength. Midway between adjacent pressure antinodes are nodes where the pressure is zero. In gas-containing suspensions of cells, bubbles or cavities collect at the pressure antinodes whereas cells are forced toward the nodes.[22] Acoustic streaming is enhanced around the gas bubbles, and if excessive, it can irreversibly damage the plasma membranes of immobile cells such as the endothelial cells lining blood vessels.[9] Blood cell stasis can also be induced, the cells forming bands half a wavelength apart, centered on the pressure nodes. Tissue damage can be avoided by moving the ultrasound applicator continuously during ultrasound treatment so that the positions of the nodes and antinodes are continually altered.

In summary, both thermal and nonthermal ultrasonically induced effects can produce changes in cells and tissues that could be of clinical benefit and lead to the acceleration of wound healing. However, excessive healing is dangerous, and should be avoided by reducing the intensity. Similarly, although some of the nonthermal effects of ultrasound such as acoustic streaming and stable cavitation are beneficial, others such as transient cavitation and standing waves are dangerous and should be avoided.

EFFECTS OF ULTRASOUND THERAPY ON THE CELLULAR EVENTS FOLLOWING INJURY

Injury is generally followed by repair, although this can be delayed to such an extent that wounds can become chronic. As described in Chapter 1, repair normally consists of a cascade of interrelated cellular events which are divided into inflammatory, proliferative, and remodeling phases. Ultrasound therapy can affect each of these phases, resulting in the acceleration of healing.

INFLAMMATORY PHASE

Treatment with ultrasound is most effective as a therapeutic agent if applied shortly after injury, that is, in the inflammatory phase of the repair. It has been shown in excised wounds that treatment with therapeutic levels of ultrasound is followed by a shortening of the inflammatory phase with the result that the proliferative, fibroplastic phase begins earlier, thus accelerating healing.[16]

There is evidence that exposure to therapeutic levels of ultrasound can increase the release of growth factors by degranulation and other materials stimulating healing from cells involved in the early part of the inflammatory process, namely mast cells,[20] platelets,[23] and macrophages.[24] This may be why treatment with ultrasound is particularly effective if applied shortly after injury.

Fyfe and Chahl[20] demonstrated that a single treatment with ultrasound delivered at a spatial average and pulse average output intensity of 0.5 W/cm², typical of that used clinically to produce nonthermal therapeutic changes, could stimulate mast cell degranulation in injured tissues. This is considerably lower than the level needed to induce

mast cell degranulation in uninjured intact tissue,[25] indicating that mast cells previously exposed to the conditions found in injured tissue have an increased sensitivity to ultrasound. Mast cells usually degranulate in response to environmentally induced changes in their plasma membranes which lead to an increase in intracellular calcium ions.[26] Although it is not known if this is the mode of action of ultrasound on mast cells, increased uptake of calcium ions following exposure to therapeutic levels of ultrasound has been found in fibroblasts.[13] It is therefore possible that ultrasound can produce similar changes in other types of cells including mast cells.

Chemotactic agents released from mast cells and platelets attract blood-borne neutrophils and monocytes to the wound site. On arrival at the wound site the monocytes develop into activated macrophages. In addition to clearing the wound site of bacteria and debris by phagocytosis, neutrophils and activated macrophages also release other chemotactic agents and growth factors which stimulate fibroblasts and endothelial cells to produce granulation tissue at the wound site. Young and Dyson[24] have shown that the exposure of macrophage-like U937 cells to therapeutic levels of ultrasound can increase the release of mitogenic growth factors which stimulate fibroblast proliferation, an essential part of the healing process.

Therapeutic ultrasound is an accelerator of the inflammation process; it is not an anti-inflammatory. Although like anti-inflammatory drugs it reduces edema and pain, ultrasound achieves this by shortening the duration of the inflammation phase[21] so that the proliferative phase begins earlier. This may be caused by an ultrasonically induced increase in the release of mitogenic and angiogenic growth factors from mast cells, platelets, and macrophages.

PROLIFERATIVE PHASE

As well as reducing the duration of the inflammation phase, thus causing the proliferative phase of wound healing to begin earlier, there is also evidence that exposure to ultrasound therapy during the proliferative phase can reduce its duration with the result that the remodeling phase begins earlier.

An increase in secretion of mitogenic growth factors from platelets[23] and macrophages[24] increases fibroblast proliferation. The synthesis and secretion of collagen by fibroblasts is also stimulated when they are exposed to therapeutic levels of ultrasound.[27] It has been shown that the exposure of fibroblasts to ultrasound is followed by a temporary increase in calcium ion content as a result of changes in plasma membrane permeability.[28] There is evidence that these changes may be due to shear stresses associated with acoustic streaming and possibly with stable cavitation.[13] Intensities of ultrasound that are too low to produce physiologically significant increases in temperature can stimulate some aspects of fibroblast activity, e.g. collagen synthesis, at the wound site[18]; similar intensities have been shown to produce stable cavitation-like events within living tissue,[14] suggesting, but not proving, that stable cavitation may be the physical mechanisms involved in producing these effects.

An important part of the proliferative phase of healing is wound contraction. Dyson and Smalley[29] demonstrated that this could be accelerated by ultrasound in vivo. Hart,[23] using fibroblast populated collagen lattices as an in vitro model of wound contraction, showed that this acceleration could be induced via substances, presumably including growth factors released by ultrasound from platelets.

There is evidence that the stimulation of wound healing by ultrasound is due to an acceleration of the inflammatory phase, so that the proliferative phase is entered earlier. Differential cell counts made of tissue samples at different times after injury have shown that macrophages, fibroblasts, and endotheliocytes,[21] cells characteristic of the proliferative phase of repair, arrive at the wound site more rapidly in wounds treated with low level (0.1 W/cm^2 spatial and temporal average intensity) ultrasound therapy than in sham-irradiated control wounds. They also leave more rapidly as the proliferative phase is succeeded by the remodelling phase.

REMODELING PHASE

The mechanical properties of the scar tissue that develops at the wound site can be increased dramatically if the wounds are treated with therapeutic ultrasound during inflammation and proliferation. Webster[18] found that treatment of full-thickness excised skin wounds with low levels of ultrasound (0.1 W/cm^2 spatial and temporal average intensity) for 5 minutes three times a week during the first 2 weeks after injury led to the production of scar tissue which was significantly stronger and more elastic than that of control, sham-irradiated wounds. The increase in tensile strength was associated with an increase in collagen synthesis while the increase in elasticity was associated with changes in collagen fiber pattern.[30] Similar improvements have been reported in injured tendons with low-level ultrasound.[31]

APPLICATION TECHNIQUES

One of three techniques can be selected for transmission of ultrasound for wound healing.

INDIRECT TECHNIQUE

Periwound area, i.e., the intact skin around the periphery of the wound, can be treated with ultrasound using an acoustic coupling cream or a water-based gel/lotion. These coupling agents have the advantage of lubricating the skin so that the applicator can be moved over it easily and also cause little attenuation of the ultrasound. Prior to the application of ultrasound therapy, the skin should be cleaned thoroughly to remove any topical substances. Clinicians need to be careful to avoid moving the ultrasound head over the wound bed. After the completion of treatment, the skin as well as the wound should be cleaned thoroughly to remove the coupling agent.

DIRECT TECHNIQUE

The wound area can be directly treated with ultrasound using an aqueous gel-based sterile dressing. Prior to the application of ultrasound therapy, the wound bed as well as the surrounding skin should be cleaned thoroughly to remove any topical substances. The dressing should be applied directly over the wound bed and then covered with a thin layer of a coupling agent as described above. The same dressing, if appropriate, can also be used to dress the wound after the ultrasound treatment.

UNDERWATER TECHNIQUE

This technique can be used to treat wounds over irregular surfaces and bony prominences if they can be immersed. The container used to submerge the wound area and the ultrasound applicator should be lined with an ultrasound absorbing material such as rubber matting to minimize reflection at the interface between the water-filled container and the surrounding skin. Using this technique, the wound bed can be treated directly with ultrasound.

CONTRAINDICATIONS AND PRECAUTIONS FOR WOUND MANAGEMENT

Although ultrasound therapy has an impressive record of safety and efficiency when used in a correct manner, it is potentially dangerous when used inappropriately. Ultrasound therapy is contraindicated with malignancies and precancerous lesions, the gonads and the structures associated with them, and the cranium. It is also contraindicated over bony prominences, over epiphyseal plates, over the pregnant uterus, over the eye, and over the cardiac area. Ultrasound therapy should not be used to treat acute infections because of the fear of spread of infection. Further, it is also contraindicated to irradiate ultrasound over tissues previously treated by deep x-ray or other radiation. It is also contraindicated in vascular abnormalities including deep vein thrombosis, emboli, severe arterial occlusion, and severe atherosclerosis. Hemophiliacs who are not covered by factor replacement should not be treated with ultrasound therapy.

The following precautions should be observed when using ultrasound therapy in the therapeutic range:

- Only adequately trained clinicians should administer ultrasound therapy.
- Lower intensities should be used which are con-

sistent with producing the desired therapeutic effects.
- The applicator should be constantly moved throughout the treatment to avoid the effects of standing waves.
- Anesthetic areas should never be treated with ultrasound.
- If the patient feels any additional pain during treatment, irradiation should be ceased immediately.
- If in any doubt, ultrasound therapy should not be administered.

CONCLUSION

It would appear that the treatment of wounds with therapeutic levels of ultrasound can accelerate healing and improve the mechanical properties of the scar that develops at the wound site during the remodeling phase of healing. The inflammatory phase is accelerated so that subsequent phases occur more rapidly. There is evidence to support the hypothesis that this acceleration could be caused by ultrasound modifying the permeability of the plasma membrane of growth factor secreting cells such as platelets and macrophages. The subsequent release of these factors could lead to a more rapid recruitment of fibroblasts and endothelial cells to the wound site so that the proliferative and remodeling phases occur more rapidly. Nonthermal mechanisms such as acoustic streaming and stable cavitation are considered to be more responsible for producing the changes in membrane permeability observed. Ultrasound therapy is an effective, economic way of accelerating the repair of both acute and chronic wounds provided that it is used by suitably trained clinicians who understand its biological and clinical effects and are aware of the mechanism by which these effects are produced.

REFERENCES

1. Williams AR. Production and transmission of ultrasound. *Physiotherapy.* 1987;73:113.

2. Dyson M. The role of ultrasound in wound healing. In: Kloth LC, McCulloch JM, Feedar JA. *Wound Healing: Alternatives in Wound Management.* Philadelphia, PA: FA Davis; 1990:259-258.

3. Bradnock B. Long-wave ultrasound in soft-tissue injury. *Int J Sports Med.* 1994;6:6-7.

4. Weichenthal M, Mohr T. 30kIIz ultrasound treatment of chronic leg ulcers. *Proc 4th Ann Meeting Europ Tissue Rep Soc.* Abstract 26.

5. Whiston RJ, Yound SR, Lynch JA, Harding KG, Dyson M. Application of high frequency ultrasound to the objective assessment of healing wounds. *Proc 2nd Conference on Advances in Wound Management.* London: Macmillan Press; 1992:26-29.

6. Young SR, Lynch JA, Liepins PJ, Dyson M. Ultrasound imaging: a non-invasive method of wound assessment. *Proc 2nd Conference on Advances in Wound Management.* London: Macmillan Press; 1992:29-31.

7. Docker M, Foulkes DJ, Patrick MK. Ultrasound couplants for physiotherapy. *Physiotherapy.* 1982;13:124-125.

8. Brueton RH, Campbell B. The use of Geliperm as a sterile coupling agent for therapeutic ultrasound. *Physiotherapy.* 1987;73:653-654.

9. Dyson M, Pond J, Woodward B, Broadbent J. The production of blood cell stasis and endothelial cell damage in the blood vessels of chick embryos treated with ultrasound in a stationary wave field. *Ultrasound Med Biol.* 1974;1:133-148.

10. Crum LA, Daniels S, Dyson M, ter Haar GR, Walton AJ. Acoustic cavitation and medical ultrasound. *Proc Inst Acoust.* 1986;8:137-146.

11. Hoogland R. *Ultrasound Therapy.* Holland: Delft. Enraf-Nonius. 1987.

12. Dyson M. The effect of ultrasound on the biology of soft tissue repair. In: McLatchie GR, Lennox CME. *The Soft Tissues-Trauma and Sport Injuries.* Oxford: Butterworth-Heinemann Ltd; 1993:200-212.

13. Mortimer AJ, Dyson M. The effect of therapeutic ultrasound on calcium uptake in fibroblasts. *Ultrasound Med Biol.* 1988;14:499-506.

14. ter Haar GR, Daniels S. Evidence for ultrasonically induced cavitation in vivo. *Phys Med Biol.* 1981;26:1145-1149.

15. Watmough DJ, Davies HMN, Quan KM, Wytch R, Williams AR. Imaging microbubbles and tissues using a linear focused scanner operating at 20 MHz; possible implications for the detection of cavitation thresholds. *Ultrasonics.* 1991;29:312-318.

16. Dyson M. Mechanisms involved in therapeutic ultrasound. *Physiotherapy.* 1987;73:116-120.

17. Nyborg WL. Acoustic streaming. In: *Physical Acoustics.* Vol 2, part B. New York: Academic Press; 1985:265.

18. Webster D. The effect of ultrasound on wound healing. University of London, 1980. Thesis.

19. Williams AR. Release of serotonin from human platelets by acoustic streaming. *J Acoust Soc Amer.* 1974;56:1640-1643.

20. Fyfe MC, Chahl LA. Mast cell degranulation: a possible mechanism of action of therapeutic ultrasound. *Ultrasound Med Biol.* 1982;8(suppl):62.

21. Young SR. The effect of therapeutic ultrasound on the biological mechanisms involved in dermal repair. University of London, 1988. Thesis.

22. NCRP Scientific Committee 66. *Biological effects of ultrasound: mechanisms and clinical implications.* NCRP Report No. 74 1983, Bethesda, MD: National Council on Radiation Protection and Measurements.

23. Hart J. The effect of therapeutic ultrasound on dermanl wound repair with emphasis on fibroblast activity. University of London, 1993. Thesis.

24. Young SR, Dyson M. Macrophage responsiveness to therapeutic ultrasound. *Ultrasound Med Biol.* 1990;16:809-816.

25. Dyson M, Luke DA. Induction of mast cell degranulation in skin by ultrasound. *Inst Elec Electron Eng, Trans Ultra Ferroelec Freq Cont.* 1986;URRC-33(2):194-201.

26. Yurt RW. Role of mast cells in trauma. In: Dineen B, Hildick-Smith G. *The Surgical Wound.* Philadelphia, PA: Lea and Febiger; 1981:125.

27. Harvey W, Dyson M, Pond J, Grahame R. The in vitro stimulation of protein synthesis in human fibroblasts by therapeutic levels of ultrasound. In: *Proc 2nd Europ Cong Ultrason Med, Excerpta Medica Congress Series No. 363.* Amsterdam: Excerpta Medica; 1975:10-21.

28. Mummery CL. The effect of ultrasound on fibroblasts in vitro. University of London, 1978. Thesis.

29. Dyson M, Smalley D. Effects of ultrasound on wound contraction. In: Millner R, Corbet U. *Ultrasound Interactions in Biology and Medicine.* New York: Plenum Press; 1983:151-158.

30. Dyson M. The effect of ultrasound on the rate of wound healing and the quality of scar tissue. In: Mortimer AJ, Lee N, Winnipeg, Canadian Physiotherapy Association. *Proc Internat Symp Therap Ultrasound.* 1981:110-123.

31. Enwemaka C. The effects of therapeutic ultrasound on tendon healing. A biomechanical study. *Am J Phys Med Rehabil.* 1989;68:283-287.

Chapter 15

Review of Surgical Procedures for Wound Management

David J. Wainwright, MD, FRCS(C), FACS

The open wound presents both the patient and the medical personnel with a multiplicity of problems which persist until closure is finally achieved. Pain from exposed nerve endings is a constant concern for the patient and is augmented by the dressing changes and other wound manipulations necessary to facilitate healing. The open wound restricts the patient's ability to participate in normal daily activities and results in functional limitations secondary to pain, edema, and restrictive scar tissue, or the immobilization necessary for treatment. The required, regular wound care further limits the patient and is a continual inconvenience. Patients are susceptible to infection, both locally and systemically, secondary to the loss of the barrier function. Metabolic, nutritional, and electrolyte derangements may be experienced with large open wounds such as those encountered with large burn injuries. Regular wound care and dressings also result in significant health care costs.

In previous chapters, the range of nonoperative treatments has been described. Occasionally, the most suitable treatment for a particular wound is surgical intervention. This generally involves a combination of cleansing and debridement combined with definitive closure. This chapter describes various options for surgical wound closure, an overview of the indications for each, the specific technique that is involved, and the special postoperative care and precautions that are necessary. The factors that influence the decision of the most appropriate management for a particular wound are reviewed. Finally, the specific surgical management of the more commonly encountered wounds is described.

WOUND PREPARATION

DEFINITIONS

Debridement

This indicates removal of non-viable tissue, adherent wound exudate, or occasionally, unwanted viable tissue, i.e., hypertrophic granulation tissue. The actual technique of debridement can vary considerably and includes the action of wet-to-dry dressings, hydrotherapy or jet lavage, enzymatic or surgical scraping, or excision of tissue. Its primary purpose is to cleanse the wound of unwanted debris or non-viable tissue and produce a healthy wound base which would be conducive to wound healing.

Excision

The term excision implies the formal, surgical removal of necrotic or unwanted tissue using a variety of instruments including dermatomes, scalpels, etc.

Tangential Excision

Tangential excision is a technique commonly used for burn injuries and first described by Janzekovic.[1] In this method, the surgeon uses a special knife or dermatome to remove thin, sequential slices of the necrotic tissue until a bleeding, viable tissue base is present. The goal is to preserve the maximum amount of viable tissue possible to minimize subsequent deformity and functional loss and is perfectly applicable to the burn wound which often has a variable depth of necrosis. In the classic description of this technique, the excision is accompanied by simultaneous skin grafting.

Eschar

This is another term for the necrotic skin and subcutaneous tissue found after injury.

TECHNIQUE

Regardless of the form of wound closure anticipated, the wound must be prepared to optimize conditions for wound healing. Wound preparation consists of removal of necrotic tissue and cleansing the surface of bacterial contamination and wound exudate. Simple dressing changes, with or without hydrotherapy, may be sufficient to prepare the wound for delayed primary closure or skin grafting. More highly contaminated wounds or those with a significant amount of adherent eschar may require more invasive modalities such as jet lavage and surgical excision, often necessitating general anesthesia.

Although formal hydrotherapy, in combination with dressing changes, is sufficient to cleanse open wounds of superficial, loosely adherent, nonviable material, occasionally a more aggressive technique is necessary for those with more significant contamination. Jet lavage allows the clinician to clean the wound with a saline solution spray applied under pressure to mechanically debride the wound, thereby removing adherent material that would be unaffected by conventional techniques. Often an antimicrobial solution will be used as the lavage solution. This technique has the advantages of cleansing the wound in a shorter period of time compared with standard dressing changes and hydrotherapy, and minimizes the removal of viable tissue that accompanies the more aggressive excisional procedures.

Surgical debridement may be performed at the time of definitive closure or as a separate procedure if the contamination and tissue necrosis is extensive enough to warrant multiple cleansings. Formal excision of eschar is performed to obtain a wound bed that is completely covered with viable tissue and can actively participate in the wound healing process. A unique excision technique called tangential excision is used for removal of necrotic tissue in burn injuries. Regardless of the form of debridement employed, meticulous hemostasis is mandatory to prevent complications such as hematoma and infection following definitive wound closure.

WOUND CLOSURE

GENERAL CONSIDERATIONS

Regardless of the technique of closure planned, there are several points that need to be addressed to ensure a favorable environment for wound healing.

General Medical Condition

The patient's physiologic state must be such that satisfactory wound healing will occur. There are a number of general medical conditions that may affect wound healing which have been covered in Chapter 1. Certain laboratory parameters will provide the clinician with a general idea of the patient's condition and the wound's ability to heal. Serum hemoglobin and the arterial blood gases provide some indication of oxygen delivery. Nutritional status can be evaluated by the level of serum proteins and especially those representative of current status (i.e., the acute phase proteins such as transferrin, pre-albumin). A number of conditions may result in the production of substances toxic to wound healing such as sepsis, renal failure, hyperbilirubinemia, etc. When operative management is considered, more demanding requirements are necessary since the metabolic needs of the wound will be increased with surgical intervention and a general anesthetic.

Wound Bed

The wound must be clean, uncontaminated, and for the most part, have a healthy, viable granulating base before it can be expected to close satisfactorily. It is well recognized that high bacterial counts will adversely affect wound healing. Bacterial counts over 100,000 per gram of tissue have been shown to be incompatible with successful skin graft take.[2] If there is a concern, biopsies can be performed prior to wound closure with quantitative analysis of bacterial numbers. The granulation tissue may or may not be removed prior to definitive wound closure.

INDICATIONS FOR SURGICAL WOUND CLOSURE

As in most fields of medicine, there is no single solution for the problem of the open wound. There are a number of considerations that must be assessed prior to choosing the most appropriate method of accomplishing wound closure. Each wound and each patient must be analyzed on an individual basis and the advantages and disadvantages of the different treatment modalities must be weighed. The first decision must be whether the wound can be expected to close satisfactorily with daily local wound care alone or whether surgical intervention is required. The following factors will influence the decision whether or not to proceed with surgical repair.

Wound Factors

Size

The size of the wound is directly proportional to the time necessary to accomplish closure and is the most important factor to be considered. The location of the wound will also determine what size open wound will be tolerated. For example, an open wound 1 cm or more, located on the face or hand, would be best closed in an expedient manner to improve function and/or appearance. On the other hand, larger wounds on the trunk or lower extremities could be appropriately managed with dressing changes and time. However, there is a limit to the wound size that can be adequately treated with dressing changes only. Generally, a wound of 7 cm or more in diameter will close much more rapidly with suturing, if possible, or a simple skin graft. This reduces the period of pain and the requirement for dressing changes and allows the patient to resume his normal lifestyle in a shorter period of time.

Location

Location is important for several reasons. The surgeon will be more aggressive in the management of open wounds that are located in areas that are important aesthetically or functionally, such as the face or the hand. Smaller wounds should be closed earlier and perhaps with a more sophisticated technique such as a flap to maximize the aesthetic or functional result and prevent the significant scarring that occurs with delayed closure. On the other hand, areas such as the hand and face have very little loose tissue adjacent to the open wound which is necessary to permit undermining, advancement, and direct closure. Larger open wounds on the trunk and occasionally, the proximal extremities, can be closed simply by direct closure by wide undermining of the adjacent uninjured skin, thus permitting approximation of the wound edges and eliminating the need for more involved techniques such as skin grafts or flaps.

Pain

All patients will experience some degree of pain during the treatment of an open wound. If this pain is severe and/or is anticipated to persist for a long time because of the size of the wound, the patient and physician may decide that surgical closure would be the more preferable course of treatment. Some patients are either very stoic or would prefer to experience even significant pain if it means the possibility of avoiding surgery. On the other hand, certain patients have a very low pain tolerance and might benefit from surgical closure for wounds that routinely would be managed nonoperatively. Another consideration is the amount of aggressive debridement that is necessary. Some degree of necrotic tissue removal is possible in combination with hydrotherapy and/or dressing changes, but if the amount of tissue to be debrided is large or it is particularly adherent, this may be much too painful to be carried out without a general anesthetic.

Time Course

Wounds close by a combination of epithelial migration and wound contraction, and a general idea of just how long a wound will take to close can be estimated based on its size. However, some wounds do not follow the rules and remain open well beyond the date that was predicted for closure. In these instances the wound closure may be facilitated by a simple procedure, generally a skin graft. As indicated in the section on size, wounds that are large, and are expected to take a long time to heal, are best managed surgically.

Exposed Structures

Most tissues will support skin grafting or at the very least produce granulation tissue. However, there are a number of tissues which will not do so and when these tissue types or structures are exposed, the wound is unlikely to close spontaneously. In these instances, there is not sufficient vascularity to produce granulation tissue in a timely fashion or to support and revascularize an overlying skin graft. In addition, the migration of granulation tissue from well-vascularized, adjacent tissues is impaired, which further delays and prevents wound closure. The treatment of choice then becomes coverage by tissue with its own blood supply, i.e., flap closure. A local flap can be used if sufficient, dependable tissue is available adjacent to the wound, otherwise it must

be obtained from an alternate source, either a distant or free flap. Those tissues where skin grafting is not possible include bone without periosteum, cartilage without perichondrium, tendon without peritenon, and nerve without perineurium.

Sensation

Occasionally it is important for sensation to be restored to provide a good functional result or to prevent future problems with breakdown as a result of the lack of sensation. Although full-thickness skin grafts provide better sensation than their split-thickness counterparts, the best sensation is provided when a flap is designed to incorporate a sensory nerve within it. This will provide the normal donor site sensation to the recipient site. An example is a neurovascular island flap from the ring finger to the index finger to restore precise sensation to this functionally important area in cases where there has been substantial tissue loss at the fingertip. Certain free flaps which include a known sensory nerve (i.e., tensor fascia lata—lateral cutaneous nerve of the thigh) are ideal for heel and sole of the foot reconstruction since sensation is so critical for normal ambulation.

Padding

As with sensation, there are certain areas where adequate padding is critical to restore function and to prevent further deterioration in the future. Specific examples include restoration of normal fingertip bulk or heel padding, and provision of additional soft tissue over bony prominences when treating decubitus ulcers, i.e., sacrum, ischial tuberosity, and greater trochanter of the femur. The only technique that will accomplish this goal is flap closure. Sometimes a simple skin flap which includes the subcutaneous fat is sufficient, but muscle or myocutaneous flaps are commonly used because of their increased padding, greater blood supply, and more dependable skin vascularity.

Vascularity

Periodically it is useful to augment the blood supply to the open wound site. This is particularly important in infected or potentially infected wounds since it improves the delivery of circulating inflammatory cells and antibiotics. The healing of bone grafts or fractures at the base of an open wound may be facilitated if coverage is achieved with well-vascularized tissue. The method of choice in these instances is a muscle or myocutaneous flap since there is a significantly increased blood supply with this technique. This is also important for wounds that occur in tissues that have received a significant amount of radiation. In these instances, the recruitment of additional blood supply that is provided with flap coverage may assist with ultimate wound closure and healing.

Patient Factors

Patient Compliance

The patient must be willing and capable of performing regular dressing changes if spontaneous closure is planned. This may not be possible with some patients, therefore, surgical closure may be necessary to achieve healing. On the other hand, some surgical techniques also necessitate patient participation and may not be practical if the patient is unwilling or incapable of cooperating.

Patient Preferences

Patients differ widely on their concern over surgical intervention. Their desires must be considered and this information included in formulating a plan of treatment. Some patients prefer to avoid surgery unless absolutely necessary and willingly perform prolonged dressing changes. Others may elect to have the wound closed as soon as possible so they may resume their prior lifestyle. Patient preferences, therefore, may provide additional useful information for decision making in those patients where the treatment choice is not clear.

Failure of Nonoperative Treatment

Despite optimal, nonoperative management, some wounds are resistant to closure by these techniques. If problems arise in treatment, the wound may not close and a change to surgical management may be indicated.

METHODS OF SURGICAL WOUND CLOSURE

Definitions

Forms of Healing

Forms of closure, i.e., primary intention, secondary intention, and delayed primary closure, have been discussed in Chapter 1.

Graft

A graft is a portion of tissue which has been completely removed from the body, and therefore its blood supply, and is transferred to another site. Its survival entirely depends upon revascularization from the recipient site. As a result, there are significant restrictions in the size or thickness of grafts as there may be cell death if revascularization or nutrition is not restored within an acceptable length of time.

Flap

A flap is a portion of tissue which is transferred with its own blood supply. The tissue to be transferred is elevated from the body but remains attached by a pedicle or stalk which contains the flap's blood supply. This includes free flaps whose vascular supply is restored through the anastomosis of vessels. Flaps do not have the size and thickness restrictions of grafts and can be composed of multiple tissue types, i.e., a combination of bone, muscle, and skin.

Treatment must be individualized and a number of factors play a role in the decision making process. If surgery is selected, the goal is to perform the simplest procedure with the greatest chance of success and the most appropriate technique for that particular wound and patient. In plastic surgery, the concept of the "reconstructive ladder" with gradually increasing levels of complexity to the techniques is used (Table 15-1).

Spontaneous Healing

This topic has been covered in Chapters 1, 5, and 8 describing wound care and dressing techniques.

Table 15-1. **Reconstructive Ladder**

Spontaneous (secondary) healing
Direct closure (primary or delayed)

Skin graft
    Split thickness
    Full thickness

Local flap
    Random/axial cutaneous
    Fasciocutaneous
    Muscle plus split-thickness skin graft
    Myocutaneous

Distant flap
    Adjacent area
    Tube transfer
    Free flap

Specialized flap
    Sensory
    Osseocutaneous
    Compound
    Composite

Direct Closure

Indications

Lacerations; surgical wounds; small, clean, open; and wounds in anatomically permissible sites.

Technique

This is the simplest form of surgical wound closure and is the technique used for most acute, uncomplicated lacerations. Prior to closure, the wound must be irrigated to remove contamination and debrided of all necrotic and marginally viable tissue. Even when some tissue loss has occurred, undermining of the wound edges will often permit direct closure under an acceptable amount of tension. Occasionally, if a wound is deemed too contaminated to close primarily, the wound can still be closed directly on a delayed basis once the wound is sufficiently clean and free from contamination and necrotic debris. Although the wound margins have often retracted from the action of the elastic fibers in the skin, generous undermining of the wound edges

can considerably relax the tissues and permit closure.

Suturing is the most commonly used method for accomplishing closure. In all but very superficial wounds, deep sutures in the subcutaneous tissues are used to decrease the tension on the skin closure itself and to minimize dead space. Surgical staples are occasionally used and taping alone is rarely used for definitive skin approximation. The size of the suture material will depend on the anatomic location and the amount of tension on the repair.

Precautions

Most directly closed wounds can be cleansed from the onset to prevent blood and serous drainage from accumulating. Although dressings are often applied, patients are permitted to bathe after several days as long as they avoid stress along the incision. Physical and occupational therapy can be initiated early if care is exercised to avoid excessive tension across the site of closure. Generally, full range of motion exercises are resumed by 1 to 2 weeks, especially in functionally important locations such as the hands.

Skin Grafts

Indications

Skin grafts are used for the closure of open wounds that are not expected to close spontaneously within a reasonable length of time and where sufficient vascularity exists to revascularize the skin graft. Besides direct closure, they are the simplest form of wound closure. Skin grafts are not an appropriate form of closure if the wound has special needs such as padding, aesthetic considerations, or the tissue bed lacks sufficient vascularity.

Technique

Split-thickness skin grafts (Figure 15-1) are composed of the epidermis and a variable depth of dermis. They are harvested with an instrument called a dermatome. The dermatome has an adjustable setting, which permits the surgeon to remove grafts of variable thickness. Standard thicknesses range from .0008

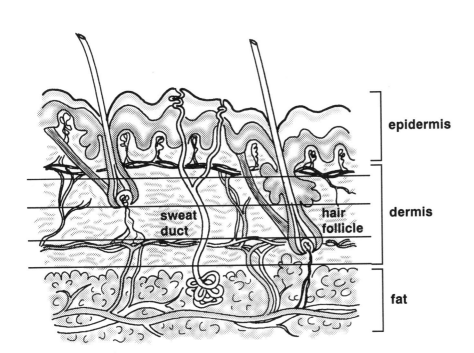

Figure 15-1. Cross-section of the skin showing epidermis and dermis.

epidermis

dermis

sweat duct

hair follicle

fat

to .0015 inches. Split-thickness skin graft sites close by epithelial migration from the transacted epidermal appendages onto the raw dermal surface.

Split-thickness skin grafts are used as either sheet or meshed grafts. Meshing is performed using a special instrument, or mesher, which produces multiple linear slits along the graft (Figure 15-2). Several meshing ratios are available which determine the degree of expansion possible. Meshing of split-thickness skin grafts provides a number of advantages. Once the skin graft is meshed, it can be stretched or expanded and therefore cover a larger area. This is particularly important in burn injuries where the amount of available donor skin may be limited. Another purpose of meshing is to provide drainage. If fluid, whether it be serum or blood, accumulates beneath the skin graft, revascularization will be impaired or prevented. By meshing, the fluid is allowed to escape through the interstices of the meshed graft into the dressing, therefore ensuring good approximation of the skin to the wound bed. Meshed grafts have also been shown to tolerate slightly higher bacterial concentrations than non-meshed or sheet grafts. Mesh grafting also limits the

amount of donor skin required. The main disadvantage to mesh grafting is the cosmetic appearance of the "pebblestone" pattern.

Full-thickness skin grafts, on the other hand, involve the harvesting of the epidermis and the entire thickness of the dermis (see Figure 15-1). As a result, there are no epithelial remnants available at the base of the wound to participate in wound closure. Small, full-thickness skin graft donor sites are closed primarily with suturing, while larger areas may be closed with application of a thin, split-thickness skin graft. The characteristics of the two types of skin grafts are depicted in Table 15-2. In general, split-thickness skin grafts take more readily, have less demanding recipient site characteristics, and contract to a greater extent. Full-thickness skin grafts, on the other hand, demand a more meticulous technique but contract less and provide a more satisfactory cosmetic and functional result.

Recent investigations in wound care have widened the options that may soon be available to the surgeon. Cultured epithelial autografts (CEA) are sheets of epithelium that are grown in culture from

Local Flaps	**Distant Flaps**

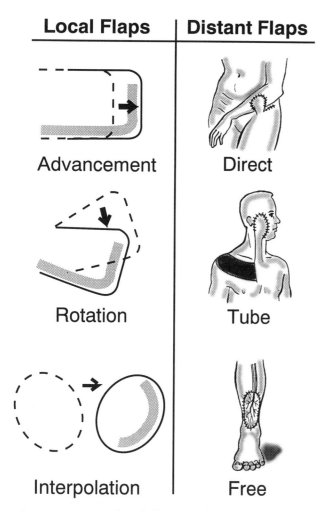

Advancement	Direct
Rotation	Tube
Interpolation	Free

Figure 15-2. Local and distant split-thickness skin flaps.

small skin biopsies excised from the patient. This would permit closure of the wound with the patient's own epithelium without extensive donor site harvesting. This would be especially important when donor skin is minimal such as in extensive burn injuries. Although the concept is quite attractive, this has not proven to be a technique appropriate for the routine closure of wounds needing a skin graft. The CEA take is often less than that of standard skin grafts and the resultant skin cover has the tendency to be fragile and break down easily with minimal trauma. For this reason, occupational and physical therapy must often be delayed much beyond the time practiced with standard skin graft techniques. This technique is also considerably more expensive than standard skin grafting.

Another advance which may prove beneficial is the use of synthetic or processed materials to augment the dermis. It is well recognized that the thicker the skin graft, the less contracture and the more aesthetically desirable the result. Several investigators have attempted to synthesize a dermal equivalent with mixed success. Our institution has been using a processed acellular cadaveric dermal matrix to augment the resulting dermis in full-thickness burn injuries. Initial results have been encouraging with take comparable to standard skin grafts. In addition there has been significant fibroblast infiltration with no evidence of rejection. Unlike scar tissue, the complex dermal collagen ultrastructure and elastin is preserved in the dermal matrix. This material has the potential of minimizing undesirable scarring and contracture. Reconstructive efforts could be significantly improved by providing tissue of a thickness equal to full-thickness skin grafts in quantities previously unattainable without producing significant donor site problems.

Precautions

Postoperative care revolves around prevention of infection and immobilization of the graft to permit revascularization. The grafts are left undisturbed for 3 to 4 days to prevent disruption of the delicate vascular connections developing during this time. Following this, daily dressings may be initiated but care must be taken not to disturb the graft. The grafts are fragile for the first 7 to 14 days and shearing forces between the graft and its underlying bed must be prevented as this can lead to disruption of the neovascularization and graft loss. Once the graft has taken, it can be left exposed but will require lubricating lotions to replace the natural lubricants lost in the grafting process.

Once the vascular supply is restored, mobilization can be initiated. Following the initial period of immobilization, gentle range of motion exercises are initiated with splinting of that site during periods of rest and/or at night. If the graft crosses a joint, that site should be immobilized with a splint for at least 3 to 5 days. Splinting is discontinued at 7 to 10 days to permit full mobilization. This protec-

Table 15-2. Characteristics of Split-Thickness and Full-Thickness Skin Grafts

	STSG	FTSG
Take	Earlier; easier; less demanding	Longer to develop blood supply; more demanding conditions
Color	Hypo/hyperpigmentation common	Closer color match

Contraction
  Primary
  Secondary
	
	Minimal
	Moderate
		
		Moderate
		Minimal

Sensation	Returns earlier; less complete	Delayed; closer to normal
Hair Growth	None	Potential exists
Durability	More fragile; easily injured	Better quality
Donor Site	Re-epithelialization spontaneously	Direct closure or split-thickness skin graft if large

tion is particularly important when grafts are applied to the lower extremity. The standing position will result in increased pressure within the venous system and can lead to graft edema, blister formation with either blood or serum, and disruption of the graft's adherence to the underlying bed. Patients should be advised to wear elasticized wraps or garments when upright and encouraged to walk and not stand. In this way they will use the natural pumping action of the leg musculature to prevent venous pooling and elevated pressures.

Occasionally sheet grafts can be managed by an exposure technique soon after surgery. This allows continual inspection of the graft and "gardening." The latter involves removal of crusting and exudates, lubricating generously and expressing small hematomas and seromas by cutting the surface of the graft. Mesh grafts, particularly expanded ones, cannot be treated by an exposure method immediately after surgery since there is a high risk of desiccation.

Flaps

Indications

Flaps are required when there are special demands for wound closure. Flaps provide tissue that most closely matches the tissue that is missing; they also provide more bulk than simpler skin grafting techniques. Flaps are indicated when the following characteristics are required to optimally manage the wound.
- Better quality skin cover/durability
- Sensation
- Padding
- Coverage of exposed structure or foreign body (i.e., orthopedic plate)
- Augmented blood supply
- Cosmesis
- Functional restoration

Classification

Several methods of classifying flaps have been described. The most useful descriptions to identify the flap are either the composition or type of tissue transferred or the site from which the donor tissue is removed (Figure 15-3).

Tissue Type
- Skin and subcutaneous tissue (random/axial)
- Muscle flaps plus or minus overlying skin
- Bone flaps plus or minus overlying skin and/or muscle

Random Flap

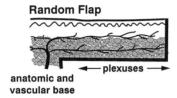

anatomic and
vascular base

Fasciocutaneous Flap

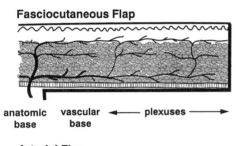

anatomic   vascular   ◄— plexuses —►
base   base

Arterial Flap

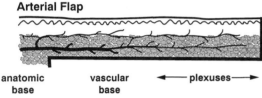

anatomic   vascular   ◄— plexuses —►
base   base

Myocutaneous Flap

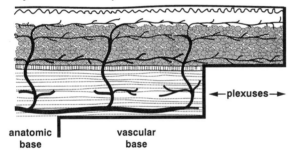

◄—plexuses—►

anatomic   vascular
base   base

Figure 15-3. Various types of skin flaps.

Donor Site Location

- Local: The tissue lies adjacent or near the defect to be closed.
- Distant: The donor tissue is transferred from a site distant to the wound to be closed but is still attached to that donor site, at least temporarily until adequate blood supply forms, i.e., cross finger flap.
- Free flap: The donor tissue was removed from a distant site and its blood supply reattached to blood vessels adjacent to the wound to be closed.

Technique

Skin Flaps   Skin flaps (Figure 15-4) contain skin and the underlying subcutaneous fat tissue. A blood supply can either be haphazard, random, or axial, indicating that a single vessel supplies the entire flap. The length and size of random flaps is limited because of the unpredictable blood supply. Axial flaps, which have a major feeding vessel along their length, have a much more dependable vascular supply, and their lengths and sizes can be proportionately larger.

Muscle Flaps   Muscle can be transferred alone or with the overlying skin. If transferred alone, the surface of the muscle is covered with a split-thickness skin graft. There are a number of advantages to muscle flaps which make them more desirable in certain clinical situations. They are:
- The blood supply to muscle flaps is usually axial with a single nutrient vessel, therefore allowing a good arc of rotation or its possible use as a free flap.
- The musculocutaneous perforating vessels will supply a more dependable vascularity to the overlying skin and therefore the skin transfer is more dependable.
- The bulk of the transferred muscle may be beneficial to provide padding over bony prominences or fill in cavities to prevent dead space, e.g., decubitus ulcers.
- The rich blood supply to muscle may improve healing of underlying structures such as bone grafts or fractures, e.g., open tibio-fibula fracture.
- The rich blood supply in the muscle may help decrease infective complications by providing improved blood supply and therefore better delivery of antibiotics and inflammatory cells, e.g., osteomyelitis.

Free Flaps   Free flaps are flaps that are moved to a new location and receive their blood supply through the microsurgical anastomosis of their nutrient vessels to vessels in the recipient bed. A number of skin, muscle, and myocutaneous flaps

Figure 15-4. Sample of skin flap.

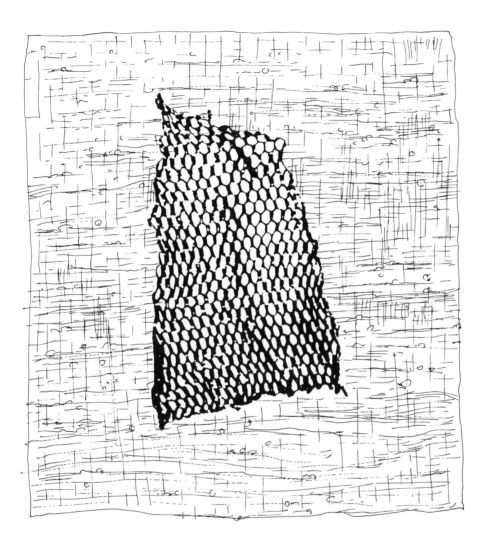

have a single, identifiable arterial supply and can potentially be used as a free flap. The artery must be of sufficient caliber and appropriately sized draining veins should be present. In addition, there must be adequate vessels available at the recipient site for the vascular anastomosis.

The major advantage of free flaps is the ability to provide good quality, well-vascularized tissue to areas where the required tissue is not available locally. In certain instances, the free flap can also provide a nerve that can be sutured to another nerve at the recipient site and provide sensation to the injured area. This is particularly important for heel reconstruction and resurfacing since the perception of pressure and touch is critical for normal ambulation.

Other Flaps   Other, more sophisticated flaps are occasionally used in special circumstances to reconstruct specific deficits and restore function. Examples include situations where bone is needed to reconstruct defects such as those seen in the mandible following ablative tumor surgery. Certain flaps may also contain vascularized nerves which can either facilitate bridging of a nerve gap or provide sensation to a critically important area, i.e., the sole of the foot. Jejunal free flaps have been used to reconstruct esophageal defects and free omental flaps to provide coverage for exposed skull in extensive degloving injuries of the scalp.

Precautions

Although flap surgery results in the transfer of a segment of viable tissue, a portion of its blood supply has been divided and therefore, the skin is not as robust. The blood supply may be somewhat tenuous, and additional tension or pressure on the flap may compromise its vascular inflow leading to tissue ischemia and necrosis. In instances where pressure cannot be avoided in the supine position, i.e., flap coverage of a sacral pressure ulcer, the patient should be managed in a special air-fluidized bed. Care must be taken by medical personnel when moving the patient to avoid tension on the closure and to minimize any shearing forces on the surface of the flap which can lead to partial-thickness injury. Although hydrotherapy is uncommonly required after surgery, it can be resumed soon after surgery as long as efforts have been made to minimize tension and pressure. The wound is generally sealed sufficiently by 2 or 3 days to permit cleansing.

Range of motion exercises, with gentle active and passive motion, can be resumed early as long as care is taken not to stress the site to the extent that tension occurs across the suture line. Sutures may be left in place for 2 to 3 weeks to help support the wound. Stretching and strengthening exercises and dynamic splinting should be avoided for 2 to 3 weeks if there is suspicion that excessive tension might be placed on the wound closure.

SPECIFIC WOUNDS

The following is a brief overview of the role of surgery in selected common wounds encountered in everyday practice.

TRAUMATIC WOUNDS

Lacerations

Most simple lacerations can be managed under local anesthesia in the emergency room or office with simple suturing techniques. This must be performed in conjunction with adequate debridement.

Abrasions

Most abrasions result in partial-thickness loss of skin and therefore should re-epithelialize spontaneously in 1 to 2 weeks. Occasionally they extend through the full thickness of the skin and will require resurfacing with skin grafts. Traumatic tattooing can occasionally result from this injury by the impregnation of the dermis or subcutaneous tissue with debris which is forced deep into the tissues by the force of the abrading injury. This debris is most easily removed at the time of the injury by vigorous scrubbing of the wound while the wound surface is still open. This scrubbing may require general anesthesia to permit complete removal. If left alone, significant discoloration will occur and more aggressive techniques such as dermabrasion will be necessary.

Avulsion/Degloving Injuries

If possible, every effort should be made to replace the avulsed or degloved tissue soon after injury. Contamination is often present and aggressive irrigation with jet lavage and debridement is required. The wound may be closed but the site should be well drained. The area may require further surgical care in the operating room in the form of irrigation and debridement to further clean the wound and to excise tissue that was marginally viable on initial exam. Skin grafting or flap coverage may be necessary for areas where skin loss occurs.

Burns

Partial-thickness burns are characterized by blistering and can be managed successfully with dressing changes alone. Third-degree or full-thickness injuries, on the other hand, will require split-thickness skin grafting once the necrotic tissue has been removed. Burn eschar is generally removed by the sequential removal of thin slices of necrotic tissue until a viable, bleeding base is produced. Mesh skin grafting is most often employed to minimize donor site requirements and to maximize graft take, although sheet grafts are used in small burns or those that occur in aesthetically (face) or functionally (hand) important areas. Generally no more than 10% to 15% of the body surface can be excised at one operative procedure due to anesthetic and blood loss considerations.

SURGICAL WOUNDS

Elective surgical sites are generally closed by simple direct closure techniques.

CHRONIC ULCERS

Peripheral Vascular Disease/Venous/ Diabetic

These wounds will be discussed together since many of the wound management techniques and approaches are similar. Basic to the treatment of these conditions is an attempt to define and manage the underlying condition that initially led to the ulcer. In general, these ulcers tend to be small and are at least initially treated with the expectation that they will close spontaneously. If this does not take place within a reasonable length of time, surgical closure may be considered. Skin grafting is generally the technique of choice since it is simple and the demands of a skin graft on the open wound bed are less when compared with flap techniques. Occasionally, flaps are necessary if important structures have been exposed.

Pressure Ulcers

Decubitus ulcers usually present with significant tissue necrosis which may extend to the underlying bony prominence. Pressure over this bone is often responsible for the wound in the first place. Small, superficial wounds can be managed with simple dressing changes and occasionally skin grafts once a viable base has developed. However, if there is bone exposure, flap coverage is the technique of choice. Following complete excision of all necrotic tissue, including the ulcer cavity itself, and removal of infected bone and any sharp prominences, local flaps are developed to close the wound. Flaps are preferable as they not only provide well-vascularized tissue to contribute to wound healing and to the

prevention of infection, but also result in additional padding over the underlying bone. Muscle or myocutaneous flaps are the technique of choice in this clinical setting for the reasons outlined previously.

Postoperatively, the patients are managed in an air-fluidized or similar bed for 2 to 3 weeks to prevent pressure on the incision and flap. It should be emphasized that flap coverage does not eliminate the need to avoid pressure on these areas with regular turning and cushioning devices. The flap does not have special qualities which will resist injury by excessive or prolonged pressure but does provide the patient with a "second chance" to prevent the development of a second pressure ulcer.

Radiation

Radiation ulcers are characterized by extremely poor vascularity and therefore are prone to remain open for prolonged periods and to be very resistant to closure. In addition, successful skin grafting is difficult to accomplish since there is insufficient vascular supply to support even a simple split-thickness skin graft. Occasionally hyperbaric oxygen treatment can be coordinated with skin grafting to improve graft take. Unfortunately, this success may only be temporary with graft loss occurring once the hyperbaric treatment is discontinued. Many times the only recourse is to use a well-vascularized flap to achieve closure. Often the adjacent tissues have also sustained some degree of damage and distant or free tissue transfers are required.

INFECTED WOUNDS

Initial management of infected wounds is to permit adequate drainage by incision and drainage and to remove all infected, necrotic tissue, by surgical means if necessary. Dressing changes, hydrotherapy, and appropriate use of topical and systemic antibiotics are then instituted until the wound closes spontaneously, or is clean enough to consider surgical closure. Skin grafting is the method of choice since the risk of reinfection or abscess formation is high if the area is closed directly or with a flap. This risk must be taken, however, if an important structure has been exposed by the original injury. Infected wounds with underlying osteomyelitis or exposed bone are best managed by muscle or myocutaneous flap coverage following adequate debridement. This improves the blood supply and the delivery of important inflammatory cells and antibiotics and therefore facilitates the eradication of the infection.

CONCLUSION

Surgical intervention may be the most suitable choice in certain wounds, particularly large and deep wounds. However, local care of wounds prior to surgical intervention is very important. This may include debridement, application of topical medications, supplemental nutrition, and dressing changes. Goals of the local preoperative care are to maintain wounds free of infection and increase the granulation tissue as much as possible. Patients should be carefully monitored to obtain a highly successful wound healing following surgical intervention.

REFERENCES

1. Janzekovic Z. A new concept in the early excision and grafting of burns. *J Trauma.* 1970;10:1103-1108.
2. Krizek TJ, Robson MC, Kho E. Bacterial growth and skin graft survival. *Surg Forum.* 1967;18:518-519.

Chapter 16

Conducting Clinical Research

Lia van Rijswijk, RN, ET, and Mary Matwhich, RN, CCRN

An editor once asked: "Does research make for better doctors?"[1] Similarly, will a clinician be a better clinician if he or she is conducting clinical studies? The editor concluded that, even after leaving academia, persons who have been involved in research will benefit for the rest of their careers, since they have acquired critical thinking capabilities and an ability to read between the lines of research reports. Anyone who has ever attempted or completed a clinical study will tell that, if nothing else, they learned a lot. The future of every group of health care professionals can only be sustained if their interventions are valuable. Specifically, health care professionals must be able to show that their interventions are safe and effective, that they increase the patient's quality of life, or that they save time and money. The term "outcome research" is relatively new, but it is here to stay. All over the world, providers are seeking ways, often based on outcomes data, to determine whether or not they are getting value for the money spent.[2] Since 1989 the US Department of Health and Human Services has had an agency (the Agency of Health Care Policy and Research, or AHCPR) that is solely concerned with enhancing the quality, appropriateness, and effectiveness of health care services as well as access to these services. With respect to wound care, there are many territories to explore since there is not only a paucity of controlled clinical studies

establishing the efficacy of many commonly used treatment modalities, but research into the effect of treatments on other variables, for instance pain, rehabilitation, quality of life, or cost, is sparse.[3] It is not within the scope of this book to provide an in-depth review of research methods, tools, and data analysis concerns. Rather, this chapter describes different types of studies and their basic requirements, and it also addresses the basic practical concerns and problems that may be encountered along the way. No matter why or to what extent one is involved in clinical studies, one should expect obstacles along the way when dealing with people. However, in the end, it is always exciting and rewarding to be able to document how the care can make a difference in the patient's life.

NEW TREATMENTS VERSUS APPROVED TREATMENTS

From a practical point of view, there are two types of studies: those involving new and unapproved drugs or devices or the unapproved use of an existing product, and studies involving established procedures or marketed products. Making this distinction is important because it affects the clinician's responsibilities as an investigator as well as the extent, if any, of manufacturer involvement

Phase	Description	Purpose
I	First use of new drug or device in humans. Usually healthy volunteers, sometimes patients or special populations.	Determine safety, action, toxicity, metabolism, absorption, elimination, dosage, route of administration.
II	Trials involving limited number of patients. Usually randomized and controlled.	Test safety, efficacy, and establish dosage for phase III studies.
III	Trials involving larger number of patients in treatment and control groups.	Gather more data on product safety, efficacy, and optimal dosage.
IV	Postmarketing studies.	Monitor safety; continuation of phase III studies to enroll more patients, comparative studies against other available products or usage of drug in secondary indications.

Table 16-1. **Study Phases of Investigational Drugs/Devices**

in the project. For example, health care professionals can take legal responsibility for the unapproved use of marketed products. However, a manufacturer is not allowed to sponsor these types of studies without first obtaining approval from the FDA.

DRUGS

The use of new, investigational drugs and some devices is carefully regulated by the FDA (Table 16-1).[4] Prior to initiating Phase I studies, the manufacturer of the drug has to file an Investigational New Drug Application (INDA) with the FDA. They cannot start studies with humans until approval has been obtained. Usually, upon completion of Phase II and III studies, FDA approval to market the product is requested. When studying the unapproved use of an approved drug, the company also has to request the FDA's permission to do so.

DEVICES

The situation, with respect to devices, varies depending on the type of device involved which, in turn, will effect what one has to do when asked to conduct a clinical study with a device. The majority of products encountered by clinicians are so-called Class I devices. These devices are not "life-supporting or life-sustaining or for a use which is of substantial importance in preventing impairment of human health, and which does not present a potential unreasonable risk of illness or injury."[5] In regard to wound management, they include a variety of products including examination gloves and most devices used to cover wounds. The manufacturing and marketing (including labeling) of most Class I devices is regulated by the FDA. However, testing as outlined in Table 16-1 is not required. Many are cleared for marketing based on "essential equivalence," i.e., they are similar to an already marketed product, the so-called premarket notification or 510(k). Some products, mainly those considered for "general hospital" use, can be marketed with filing a premarket notification with the FDA. Class III devices include life-supporting or life-sustaining equipment and implants. They are more stringently regulated, and proof of safety and efficacy must be established prior to marketing. Before testing a Class III device in humans, the FDA must approve the so-called Investigational Device Exemption (IDE). Finally, there are Class II devices. With respect to manufacturing, marketing, and labeling requirements, these products are treated as Class I devices, however, they also must meet federally defined, general performance standards. Examples include low-energy or cold lasers. Finally, since devices were first regulated in 1976, many changes have occurred.[6,7] In recent years many products have been reclassified, and if unsure of the status of a device, it is always best to call the manufacturer or the FDA.

ESTABLISHED PROCEDURES AND APPROVED USE OF PRODUCTS

If a clinician is interested in studying the effect of established procedures or the use of marketed products for an approved indication, the general principles of protecting human rights and study design apply. Approved indications can be found in the package insert of drugs as well as devices.

COMMON DEFINITIONS AND TYPES OF STUDIES

There are a number of ways to evaluate the effect of care (Figure 16-1). When conducting a retrospective study, records are reviewed and a population is studied after the event or intervention has occurred. If one defines study guidelines and enrolls patients for "future" follow-up, the study is prospective. The design of the study is usually characterized by whether or not there is a control group, i.e., treatment outcomes can be compared. As a rule, a noncontrolled study provides information about the safety of the intervention. Following a non-controlled or case study, treatment efficacy can only be assessed against the background of the clinician's own experience or the existing literature. However, if one evaluates the same parameters during and following application of different treatment modalities, one can compare the results. There are different ways of comparing treatment outcomes. The study design, i.e., the method of studying the hypothesis, could include patients who serve as their own control, or two groups of patients who are randomly assigned to different treatment modalities. For instance, the use of a mirror-image design is very common when studying skin graft donor site healing. Each patient receives both treatment modalities on their skin graft donor sites. In a crossover design, patients receive one type of treatment, and then

cross over to the other treatment modality. Both study designs allow for within-person comparisons, but crossover studies are not very suitable when a carry over effect from the treatments can be expected to occur, or when the study period is limited.[8] If patients are randomized to different methods of intervention, it is important to try and keep the number of variables that may effect outcome to a minimum. For example, when evaluating a topical agent for healing pressure ulcers, try to get all patients to use the same type of pressure-relieving device. Finally, choose data collection instruments with care. Search the literature and try to use methods that have been shown to be valid (i.e., they measure what they are supposed to), sensitive (they can discriminate between different treatment groups), reliable (different investigators using the same tool will reach the same conclusion), and practical.[9] The above is of particular concern when measuring subjective phenomena (for instance pain, quality of life, and body image) and the use of reliable and valid tools is imperative.[10]

RELIABILITY AND VALIDITY

There are two main reasons for carefully designing and conducting the study: the results must be reliable and have external validity, i.e., other investigators reach the same conclusions if they conduct the same study and the results can be applied to other populations. A well-designed study does not "stand on its own," rather, it builds upon the work of others. One of the problems of studies related to chronic wounds is that many do "stand on their own." Results cannot be compared because they are reported differently by different investigators, data collection instruments vary, adequate controls have not been included, and/or patient variables have not been taken into account.[3] Finally, a good study design, incorporating an appropriate control treatment, also balances the placebo effect, particularly if the study can be blinded. The placebo effect can be very powerful, particularly when studying subjective variables. For instance, it has been shown that the power of the placebo can be doubled by an enthusiastic clinician, compared with a skeptic.[11]

Figure 16-1. Commonly used designs in clinical studies.

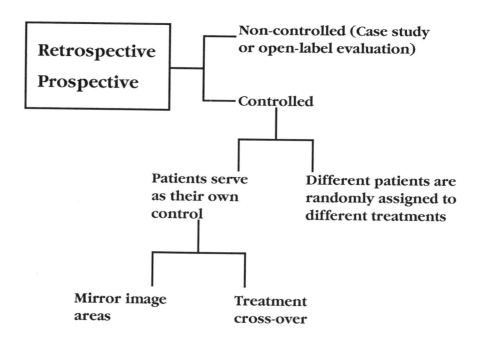

Similarly, studies have shown that, providing the control treatment consists of basic, good wound care practices, a number of chronic wounds heal without further interventions.[12]

PRACTICAL CONSIDERATIONS

Preparation is the key to successful completion of the study. If study plans are well defined, it will be easier to complete the research project. First, it is important to consider both the resources available at the institution where research is being conducted as well as the practical problems likely to be encountered. For example, will others be able to do assessments if the primary investigator is not available and will the staff be supportive of the efforts? If help is needed from the staff, to provide special care or provisions, it is imperative to educate them about the goals of the study and how this project might benefit patients.[13] Creating an environment in which everyone involved feels empowered and part of the project will benefit the study, the patient, and even the staff. This is one reason why conducting a pilot study can be very useful. During the pilot study the investigator can solicit comments from staff and evaluate the feasibility of conducting the larger scale study envisioned.

HYPOTHESIS

A clear and concise definition of the research question asked will help the investigator focus his or her efforts.[14] The investigator may be looking for multiple answers. However, it is always easier when the number of questions asked are restricted. Also, at this time, the investigator must consider how many patients are needed to enroll in the study. Ideally, the sample size should be calculated based upon the estimated difference in response to treatments. The aim is to maximize statistical power of the test for a given level of significance. In general, a power of 80% or 90% is sufficient.[15] Of course, the help of a statistician, at this time as well as upon completion of the study, is invaluable. To estimate the difference in response to treatments and to help formulate the hypothesis, the investigator must read all pertinent materials on the subject.

REVIEW OF THE LITERATURE

A thorough review of the literature will help the investigator formulate the hypothesis, design the study, and calculate the statistical power. If the investigator has access to a medical library, becoming familiar with what it has to offer in the way of services can save a lot of time. Even though not all publications on a particular subject may be relevant to the investigator, reviewing most of what is available will reveal current trends in a particular area of research. Also, there are a number of textbooks that can help the investigator in getting started.[15-18] Last, but not least, consultation with peers and experts in the field can be very helpful. There may be people in one's own facility who share an interest or have experience doing research. Also, attending a few professional meetings can be very productive (and a lot of fun!). Current research is usually presented at professional meetings and most speakers are eager to discuss their work and experiences during the lunch and coffee breaks.

HUMAN RIGHTS AND INFORMED CONSENT

No matter what type of study you plan to conduct, one major concern is the protection of human rights. Following World War II, specifically after the Nuremberg Military Tribunals, the first international code of ethics for research involving humans was developed.[19] In 1964, the World Medical Association adapted the Nuremberg Code and the Declaration of Helsinki was issued.[20] The declaration has been updated periodically, but the basic principles have remained virtually unchanged (Table 16-2). Basically, whenever a patient is randomly assigned to any type of intervention, or when a treatment is provided in order to increase medical knowledge or understanding, informed consent must be obtained. Finally, the success of the study depends, to a large extent, on the cooperation of the patient. An honest review of what will be involved and a good investigator-patient relationship will reduce the "drop-out" rate.[9]

HUMAN RIGHTS COMMITTEE/INSTITUTIONAL REVIEW BOARD

The human rights committee or institutional review board at the institution where research will be conducted will be able to help design appropriate patient consent forms. Often, basic guidelines for protocol preparation can also be obtained from the board or committee. These committees consist of a variety of disciplines, i.e., medical, nursing, administrative, legal, clerical, and laypersons. Their purpose is to review and approve all study protocols, particularly with respect to the protection of human rights. If the investigator works in a private practice and is not affiliated with a hospital, approval to conduct research must still be obtained. Some hospitals will accept "outside" protocols for review, but the investigator can also submit a protocol to an independent board. These review boards charge a fee for review and approval of the protocol. Prior to submission, the investigator should make sure that this board works in compliance with FDA regulations. When in doubt, call the Department of Health and Human Services, FDA, in Rockville, Maryland. In Europe, Ethics Committees take the place of Institutional Review Boards. As a rule, Ethics Committees permit studies whereas US Institutional Review Boards or Human Rights Committees scrutinize the study protocol as well as approve it.[21]

FUNDING

Funding for the study may or may not be a concern. If the investigator does not need special tools or equipment and is able to get help from colleagues and a statistician, funding may not be needed. Also, there may be times when the investigator does not want to receive funds, particularly from commercial sources. However, an often underestimated aspect of conducting studies is the amount of time involved. Everything, from searching the literature and preparing the paper work, to talking with the patients and following them up, is time consuming. The five most common types of funding are grants, fellowships, donations, gifts, and contracts (Table 16-3).[22]

Government Funding

Applying for a grant from the government can be an intimidating process. However, the National Institute of Health (NIH) provides brochures and guidelines free of charge (*NIH Guide for Grants and Contracts*), and some excellent

---

Table 16-2. Basic Principles of Protecting Human Rights in Biomedical Research

Medical progress is based on research which ultimately must rest in part on experimentation involving human subjects.

The research must conform to generally accepted scientific principles.

The design and performance of each experimental procedure should be clearly formulated in the protocol which should be submitted for evaluation to a committee independent of the investigator and sponsor.

The responsibility for the subject must always rest with a medically qualified person.

The importance of the objective of the study must be in proportion to the inherent risk to the subject and refusal of the patient to participate should never interfere with the health care provider-patient relationship.

Concern for the interests of the subject, including his or her integrity and privacy, must always prevail over the interests of science and society.

Investigations should be discontinued if the hazards are found to outweigh the potential benefits.

When publishing the results of the investigation, the researcher is obliged to preserve the accuracy of the results.

Each potential subject must be adequately informed of the aims, methods, anticipated benefits, potential hazards, and the discomfort the study may entail and informed consent should be obtained.

Every patient, including those of a control group, should be assured of the best proven diagnostic or therapeutic methods.

Based on the declaration of Helsinki/World Medical Association, 1964/1975/1983.

---

publications on the topic have been published.[23-25] Also, the AHCPR, an agency of the US Public Health Service, awards research grants and contracts for their programs, including cost and financing, primary care research, and subjects related to technology and quality assessment.[26] With respect to wound care, particularly pressure ulcers, the investigator may consider requesting grant information to study areas of care that were defined as requiring further research in the AHCPR *Clinical Practice Guidelines*.[27,27a] Finally, the political climate at the time of application will make a difference as well. As mentioned earlier, outcome-oriented research, previously a novelty, has become more popular. Similarly, the cost of health care has received increased attention. This means that the outcome of debates within government as to whether biomedical research drives costs higher or keeps costs down, will influence the availability of government funding for a particular project.[28]

Corporate Funding

Industry provides an increasingly significant portion of the total health research and development costs (Figure 16-2).[29,30] From a practical point of view, one of the most important reasons for seeking corporate funding is that the investigator does not have to go through a maze of paperwork to apply for a grant. However, depending on the type of study, the product involved and the philosophy of the sponsor, there may still be a significant amount of administrative work involved. Particularly if the investigator is involved in Phase I, II, or III studies of new drugs or some new devices, the responsibilities are considerable and carefully regulated by the FDA.[31] When participating in these types of studies, one must remember that the information gathered through research work will probably be included in documents submitted to the FDA to obtain approval for a new product or for a new indication of an existing product. The investigator's name and credentials will be submitted along with the results of the study. The FDA requires the investigator to maintain scrupulous records, and measures designed to disqualify investigators following "clinical investigator misconduct" (including submitting false information) when evaluating new drugs will probably be expanded to include evaluation of devices.[32]

Table 16-3. **Types of Research Funding**	
Funding Type	**Description**
Contract	A fee-for-service agreement between two parties. This is the most common form of study sponsorship by corporations.
Donations	A donation may or may not be earmarked for a particular type of research, investigator, or department.
Fellowships	Individual support during advanced training. Most commonly obtained from a not-for-profit or government source. If provided by a corporation, the field of research activities is usually specified.

GOOD CLINICAL PRACTICE GUIDELINES

When conducting studies for corporations, one must comply with the so-called Good Clinical Practice (GCP) Guidelines.[21,31] First approved by the FDA in 1978, these study guidelines apply to sponsors and investigators alike. Though they are standard in the United States, the European community has not yet fully accepted them into practice, but it is expected that they will be completely adopted in the near future. Worldwide acceptance of GCP guidelines will make investigators accountable to their peers, and more importantly, to the patients who participate in the research. The Standard Operating Procedures, a fundamental component of the GCP guidelines, regulate record-keeping procedures. Many sponsors employ clinical monitors who work between the sponsor and the investigator. They coordinate the research, standardize record-keeping procedures, and monitor compliance with the GCP guidelines. Regulators can audit the investigator or sponsor at any stage of the study. Specific information regarding the patients enrolled in studies is often reviewed by the sponsor on an ongoing basis, and reporting adverse experiences is an important responsibility of the investigator. Adverse reactions should not be viewed as negative, rather, they may provide important information about the product used. Adverse experience reporting procedures are provided by both the study sponsor and the institutional review board that approved the study. The investigator is usually required to report them immediately, or at least within 24 hours. All events should be reported; no event is insignificant, and at the time of the event, the investigator must assume that it is related to the treatment studied. Adverse Experiences can include:

- Overdose
- Malignancy
- Fatality
- Congenital defect
- A reaction that prolongs or requires hospitalization
- A significant worsening of a patient's condition

CONTRACTS AND AGREEMENTS

Prior to starting the process of obtaining funds for the research project, the investigator must consider different options and how to handle possible problems along the way. If the investigator is going to get corporate sponsorship, he or she should have a contract or letter of agreement with the sponsor. The contract should discuss confidentiality issues, reimbursement, rights to data, responsibilities of both parties, supplies needed/provided, adverse reactions, and indemnification.[33] Confidentiality may pertain to one or both parties and may or may not affect rights to publication. The sponsor will often discuss their rights to names or data for promotional materials and, if applicable, patent and copyright considerations. Reimbursement in the case of study termination is an important consideration as well. Finally, in the case of new drugs or devices, companies often indemnify (i.e., secure against hurt, loss or damage; make compensation to for incurred

Figure 16-2. Research funding provided by various sources.

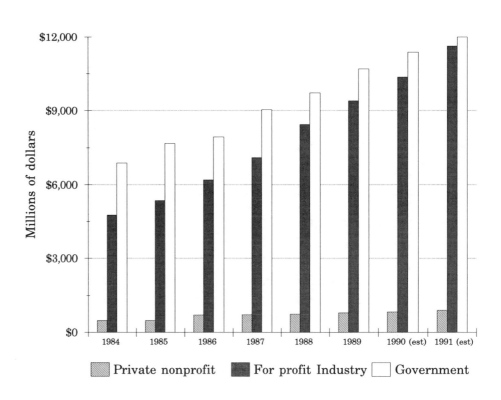

Private nonprofit   For profit Industry   Government

hurt, loss, or damage) the investigator and/or the institution against claims or legal actions initiated by patients as a direct result of the proper use of the study products.[33]

CONFLICT OF INTEREST

When signing the study agreement and later, when presenting or publishing the data, the issue of conflict of interest should be considered. For instance, a conflict of interest can arise if the investigator wants to publish information but the sponsor has requested confidentiality. Similarly, the investigator may be asked to report certain aspects of the study only. As a rule, genuine, unbiased results are desirable for all involved. It allows industry to make accurate decisions, resulting in maximum benefit to the patient and health care professionals while maintaining the researcher's integrity.[33] Financial conflicts of interest in health care and health care research have recently received an abundance of attention.[34,35] As a result,

almost all peer-reviewed journals have adopted conflict-of-interest policies, and the FDA continues to develop its regulations on continuing education and the AMA's Council on Scientific Affairs and Council on Ethical and Judicial Affairs has adopted guidelines for their members.[36-38] However, conflicts of interest are not necessarily limited to money. A conflict of interest is "a set of conditions in which professional judgment concerning a primary interest (such as a patient's welfare or the validity of research) tends to be unduly influenced by a secondary interest."[39] These secondary interests can be financial, but they can also be a tenaciously held belief in specific scientific theories or, for instance, the sexual orientation of the researcher (such as a homosexual studying homosexuality).[40,41]

A conflict of interest by itself does not indicate wrongdoing, rather, it refers to a setting in which factors that might influence one's conduct exist. According to some, the problem lies with "the conventional view that where the potential for such influence exists, there is reason for concern, and moreover, this potential implies an increased probability of misconduct."[42] The primary responsibility of health care professionals, that is, the well-being of the patient and the longevity of a career regardless of funding or interests, depends on the credibility and the quality of the work produced. Because it is difficult to ignore one's own views, controlled studies should be conducted and, if at all possible, the studies should be double-blind as well. Similarly, masking the identity of an author and his or her affiliation has been shown to help journal reviewers focus on the substance of the work, subsequently increasing objectivity.[43] There is no doubt that disclosing economic ties should be practiced at all times. In so doing, one exhibits honesty and integrity.[33] At the same time, the investigator must remember that judging someone's work by any characteristic other than the content, results in substituting prejudice for reason and could be considered unethical.[42]

WRAPPING IT UP

Before the investigator can start preparing the publication, one last and very important step must be taken. The data must be tabulated and analyzed. If the study was sponsored by a corporation, the investigator needs to write a report for the sponsor and review options to present/publish the data. Do not forget to share the findings with the individuals who have helped along the way. For instance, a presentation to the staff will not only help them understand the value of their involvement, but also make them feel connected to the institution's goals of improving future patient care.

Research is a privilege for those who have the time and resources to perform it. With this privilege comes the responsibility of integrity. The system of sharing information about research work, whether by means of presentation or publication, is based upon the inherent trust that the data presented are accurate and reliable. After all, the findings can have serious implications for patient care. Therefore, the investigator must approach the data analysis part of the study as systematically as the study. Even though everyone likes to pre-

sent exciting, positive findings, it is important to remember that negative findings are just as valuable. For example, the research findings that some type of intervention did not improve the outcome can result in significant cost savings. Data analysis procedures should be carried out according to well-established methods. It is well known that "if you torture your data long enough, they will tell you whatever you want to hear."[44] However, this practice is neither statistically sound nor clinically prudent, and can result in the dissemination of incorrect information to colleagues and patients.

Analysis of all study data and preparation of a manuscript can take as long as the study itself. In addition to publishing the results of the study, consider presenting them at a professional meeting. First, it enables the investigator to share the work sooner; after all, the publication process does take time. Second, it is very rewarding, albeit intimidating at times. If the investigator is very nervous about public speaking, consider doing a poster presentation first. During the poster presentation the investigator will be able to talk about research one-on-one and get feedback from participants which, in turn, will help the investigator when preparing the manuscript.[45] When preparing a presentation, discuss the contents with co-workers or colleagues who are not familiar with what has been done. Sometimes the investigator becomes so familiar with a subject that it may be difficult to explain it clearly.

PUBLISHING THE RESULTS

Before writing the manuscript, the investigator must decide on which journal he or she wants to submit it to. They should become familiar with its style and get a copy of the instructions for authors. Also, make sure that the subject is appropriate for the journal. If the investigator is very interested in publishing in a particular journal but is not sure if the topic is appropriate, call the editor. The process of publication can be very intimidating. However, remember that editors are always interested in receiving high quality manuscripts that meet the needs of their readers. By talking to the editors one can gauge their level of interest and very often they will tell exactly what it is they are looking for. Since the journal will obtain the copyrights to the publication immediately following submission, the manuscript is to be sent to only one journal at a time. If the manuscript is rejected, they will return the copyrights back to the investigator. Some journals plan publishing "theme" issues, and unless the investigator talks to them, he or she does not know that they would like to see the manuscript before a particular date. Even if the editor says that they are very interested, do not take short cuts on style, content, and clarity. If the instructions advise one to adhere to the AMA manual of style, purchase the manual or borrow it from the library.[46] The reviewers usually do not know that the editor would like to publish the manuscript, and they will read it as they would any other submission. The peer-review process takes time. Count on not hearing anything from the journal for at least 2 to 3 months. Editorial review board members are usually busy professionals themselves who volunteer their time to look at the work. Also, some journals have adopted the "blind" peer-review process, i.e., the reviewers do not know who submitted the manuscript. Their comments and suggestions are based solely upon the work itself. It is important to remember not to take these things personally because after all the hard work, one of the most maddening experiences is getting the manuscript back with comments, revisions, and (sometimes) downright criticism.

First, take a deep breath and remember that everyone who has ever published anything has had the same experience. Second, review everything as dispassionately as possible and you will discover that, most of the time, once the comments are incorporated, the publication will look much better indeed. After all, if something was not clear to the reviewer, it will not be clear to the reader either. If the manuscript is rejected, put it away for a couple of weeks and think about the reasons for rejection (the editors will almost always give a reason). Then, start again. Edit it and submit it for publication to another journal. If it is accepted, get ready to wait some more. The manuscript will now go "in the pipeline" and often the next thing one sees is the so-called galley proofs, mailed to the author by the printer. The author usually gets 48 hours to review them and this is the time to proofread very carefully. Remember that someone else keyed in the manuscript and mistakes are made. Now, the author's work is finished and the author can sit back and wait for the issue to arrive in the mail.

CONCLUSION

After all the hard work that went into conducting the study, analyzing the data, and writing up the results, is the clinician a better health care professional? Maybe, but the clinician certainly learned a lot, and the experience will be very useful when the next study is started. Conducting studies is not only exciting, but also a great learning experience, because for every answer obtained, 10 questions will arise. Finally, research can influence patient care now, as well as in the future, and that is, by far, the most rewarding experience of all.

REFERENCES

1. Does research make for better doctors? *Lancet.* 1993;342:1063-1064. Editorial.
2. Outcomes data: a key to Aetna payment decisions. *Devices & Diagnostics Letter.* 1993;20:1.
3. van Rijswijk L. General principles of wound management. In: Gogia PP. *Clinical Wound Management.* Thorofare, NJ: SLACK Inc; 1995:31-52.
4. Iber FL, Riley WA, Murray PJ. *Conducting Clinical Trials.* New York, NY: Plenum Publishing Corp; 1987.
5. Code of Federal Regulations. Food and Drugs. CFR 21;1987: §860.3.
6. Pub L No. 94-295, 90 Stat 539 (1976), codified at 21 USC Sections 360c-360k (1982).
7. Kessler DA, Pape SM, Sundwall DN. The federal regulation of medical devices. *New Engl J Med.* 1976;317:357-365.
8. Woods NF. Designing prescription-testing studies. In: Woods NF, Catanzaro M. *Nursing Research, Theory & Practice.* St. Louis, MO: CV Mosby; 1988;202-218.

9. van Rijswijk L. Nursing research and dermatology: where to start. *Derm Nurs.* 1990;2:158-161.

10. Frank-Stromberg M. *Instruments for Clinical Nursing Research.* Norwalk, CT: Appleton & Lange; 1988.

11. Benson H, McCallie DP. Angina pectoris and the placebo effect. *N Engl J Med.* 1979;300:1424-1429.

12. Steed DL, Moosa HM, Webster MW. The importance of randomized prospective trials in evaluating therapy for wound healing. *Wounds.* 1991;3:111-115.

13. Ouslander JG, Schnelle JF. Research in nursing homes: practical aspects. *J Am Ger Soc.* 1993;41:182-187.

14. Carpenter LM. Is the study worth doing? *Lancet.* 1993;342:221-223.

15. DeAngelis C. *An Introduction to Clinical Research.* New York, NY: Oxford University Press; 1990.

16. Bailar JC, Mosteller F. *Medical Uses of Statistics.* 2nd ed. Waltham, MA: Mass Med Society; 1992.

17. Domholdt E. *Physical Therapy Research: Principles and Applications.* Philadelphia, PA: WB Saunders; 1993.

18. Currier DP. *Elements of Research in Physical Therapy.* 3rd ed. Baltimore, MD: Williams and Wilkins; 1990.

19. Perley S, Fluss SS, Bankowski Z, Simon F. The Nuremberg code: an international overview. In: Annas GJ, Grodin MA. *The Nazi Doctors and the Nuremberg Code: Human Rights in Human Experimentation.* New York, NY: Oxford University Press; 1992:149-173.

20. CIOMS/WHO. *International Ethical Guidelines for Biomedical Research Involving Human Subjects.* Geneva: CIOMS; 1993.

21. Allen ME. *Good Clinical Practice in Europe.* Essex, UK: Rostrum Pub; 1991.

22. Larson E. Guidelines for collaborative research with industry. *Nursing Economics.* 1986;4:131-133.

23. Office of Grants Inquiries, Division of Research Grants, National Instititutes of Health. *Helpful Hints on Preparing a Research Grant Application to the National Institutes of Health.* Bethesda, MD: National Institute of Health; 1990.

24. Gordon SL. Ingredients of a successful grant application to the National Institutes of Health. *J Orthop Res.* 1989;7:138-141.

25. Cuca JM, McLoughlin WJ. Why clinical research grant applications fare poorly in review and how to recover. *Cancer Invest.* 1987;5:55-58.

26. Agency for Health Care Policy and Research. *AHCPR Purpose and Programs.* Rockville, MD: Department of Health and Human Services, Public Health Service; 1990.

27. Panel for the Prediction and Prevention of Pressure Ulcers in Adults. *Pressure Ulcers in Adults: Prediction and Prevention. Clinical Practice Guideline, No. 3.* AHCPR Publication No. 92-0047. Rockville, MD: Agency for Health Care Policy and Research, Public Health Service, US Department of Health and Human Services; 1992.

27a. Bergstrom N, Bennett MA, Carlson CE, et al. *Treatment of Pressure Ulcers. Clinical Practice Guideline, No. 15.* AHCPR Publication No. 95-0652. Rockville, MD: Agency for Health Care Policy and Research, Public Health Service, US Department of Health and Human Services, December 1994.

28. Anderson C. Research and healthcare costs. *Science.* 1993;261:416-418. News.

29. Clemmitt M. US drug industry's research support. *Nature.* 1993;361:757-760.

30. National Institute of Health. *National Institute of Health Data Book.* Bethesda, MD: Author; 1991.

31. Code of Federal Regulations, Food and Drugs. CFR 21;1992, §50,56 & 312.

32. FDA proposes rules for disqualifying investigators. *Devices & Diagnostics Letter.* 1993;20:2-3.

33. van Rijswijk L, Caldwell-Brown D. Industry and dermatology research: how well can they work together? *Derm Nurs.* 1990;2:339-342.

34. Chase M. Mixing science, stocks, raises questions of bias in the testing of drugs. *Wall Street Journal.* 1989;January 26:1.

35. Blumenthal D. Academic-industry relationships in the life sciences: extent, consequences, and management. *JAMA.* 1992;268:3344-3349.

36. Council on Scientific Affairs and Council on Ethical and Judicial Affairs. Conflict of interest in medical center/industry research relationships. *JAMA.* 1990;263:2790-2793.

37. Koshland DE Jr. Conflict of interest policy. *Science.* 1992;257:595. Editorial.

38. Relman AS. New information for authors and readers. *N Engl J Med.* 1990;323:56. Editorial.

39. Thompson DF. Understanding financial conflicts of interest. *N Engl J Med.* 1993;329:573-576.

40. Marshall E. The perils of a deeply held point of view. *Science.* 1992;257:621-622.

41. Marshall E. Sex on the brain. *Science.* 1992;257:620-621.

42. Rothman KJ. Conflict of interest: the new McCarthyism in science. *JAMA.* 1993;269:2782-2784.

43. McNutt RA, Evans AT, Fletcher RH, Fletcher SW. The effects of blinding on the quality of peer review: a randomized trial. *JAMA.* 1990;263:1371-1376.

44. Mills JL. Data torturing. *N Engl J Med.* 1993;329:1196-1199.

45. McDaniel RW, Bach CA, Poole MJ. Poster update: getting their attention. *Nurs Res.* 1993;42:302-304.

46. American Medical Association. *Manual of Style.* 8th ed. Baltimore, MD: Williams and Wilkins; 1989.

Appendix A

Support Surface Categories for Pressure Relief

Mattress Overlays (Static or Dynamic)
- Foam
- Air
- Gel
- Water
- Combination

Mattress Replacements (Static or Dynamic)
- Foam
- Air
- Combination

Specialty Beds
- Low Air Loss
- Air Fluidized

Chair Cushions (Short Term or Long Term)
- Foam
- Air
- Gel
- Combination

Wedges

Heel Elevators

Appendix B

Resources and Sources of Information

Journals

Decubitus
Dermatology Nursing
Journal of the Wound, Ostomy, and Continence Nurses Society
(formerly *Journal of ET Nursing*)
Ostomy/Wound Management
Wound Repair and Regeneration
Wounds

Organizations:

Agency for Health Care Policy and Research (AHCPR)
AHCPR Clearinghouse
P.O. Box 8547
Silver Spring, MD 20907
1-800-358-9295
301-227-8364

National Pressure Ulcer Advisory Panel (NPUAP)
SUNY at Buffalo
Beck Hall
3435 Main Street
Buffalo, NY 14214
716-881-3558

Wound, Ostomy and Continence Nurses Society (WOCN)
27241 LaPaz Road
Suite 121
Laguna Niguel, CA 92656
714-476-0268

Appendix C

Manufacturer/Product Information

Jobst Inst.
P.O. Box 653
Toledo, OH 43694

Omni Medical Specialties
Suite L
5555 Magnatron Blvd.
San Diego, CA 92111

GypsonaII Plaster Bandage
National Patent Development Corp.
Dayville, CT
Chaston Medical
Melville, NY 11746

3M Orthopedic Products
17132 Pullman
Irving, CA 92714

F-scan In-Shoe Pressure Monitoring Device
F-scan Inc
451 D Street
Boston, MA 02210

Index